Harty's Dental
DICTIONARY

Commissioning Editor: Michael Parkinson
Development Editor: Janice Urquhart
Project Manager: Elouise Ball
Design Direction: Stewart Larking
Illustrator: Antbits
Illustration Buyer: Merlyn Harvey

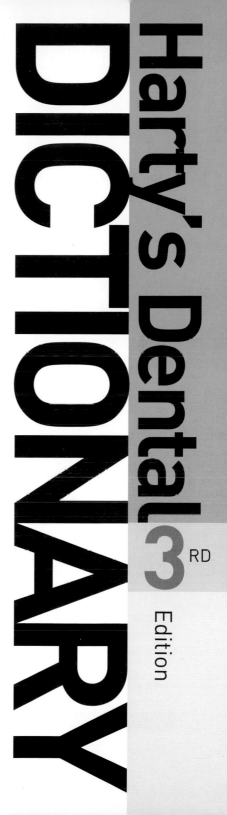

Harty's Dental DICTIONARY

3RD Edition

Edited by

Peter **Heasman**
BDS MDS PhD
FDSRCPS DRDRCS
Professor of Periodontology,
University of Newcastle upon Tyne, UK

Giles **McCracken**
BDS PhD FDSRCPS
Lecturer in Restorative Dentistry,
University of Newcastle upon Tyne, UK

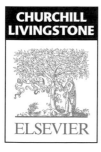

CHURCHILL
LIVINGSTONE

ELSEVIER

Edinburgh London New York Oxford
Philadelphis St Louis Sydney Toronto 2007

CHURCHILL
LIVINGSTONE
ELSEVIER

An imprint of Elsevier Limited
Previously published as *Concise Illustrated Dental Dictionary*

© IOP Publishing 1987
© Elsevier Limited 1994
© 2007, Elsevier Limited. All rights reserved.

The right of Peter Heasman and Giles McCracken to be identified as editors of this work has been asserted by them in accordance with the Copyright, Designs and Patents Act 1988.

First edition 1987
Second edition 1994
Third edition 2007

ISBN-13: 9780443102530

British Library Cataloguing in Publication Data
A catalogue record for this book is available from the British Library

Library of Congress Cataloging in Publication Data
A catalog record for this book is available from the Library of Congress

Note
Knowledge and best practice in this field are constantly changing. As new research and experience broaden our knowledge, changes in practice, treatment and drug therapy may become necessary or appropriate. Readers are advised to check the most current information provided (i) on procedures featured or (ii) by the manufacturer of each product to be administered, to verify the recommended dose or formula, the method and duration of administration, and contraindications. It is the responsibility of the practitioner, relying on their own experience and knowledge of the patient, to make diagnoses, to determine dosages and the best treatment for each individual patient, and to take all appropriate safety precautions. To the fullest extent of the law, neither the Publisher nor the Editors assume any liability for any injury and/or damage to persons or property arising out or related to any use of the material contained in this book.

The Publisher

 your source for books,
journals and multimedia
in the health sciences
www.elsevierhealth.com

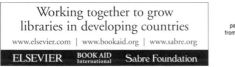

Working together to grow
libraries in developing countries
www.elsevier.com | www.bookaid.org | www.sabre.org

ELSEVIER BOOK AID International Sabre Foundation

The publisher's policy is to use paper manufactured from sustainable forests

Printed in China

Preface to the Third Edition

The second edition of this dictionary was first printed in 1994 and the continued and unqualified success of the book has subsequently necessitated 9 further reprints, almost on an annual basis. We, therefore, considered it a privilege to have been approached by Michael Parkinson of Elsevier with a view to working on the third edition of the book.

In his preface to the second edition, Fred Harty outlined the difficulty that he had encountered in deciding which terms had become outdated during the 7 years since the first edition was published. We faced the same challenge in preparing the third edition and acknowledge that a dictionary should not only present contemporary terminology and definitions but also contain entries that students may encounter in their reading of classic as well as more recent texts on dental science and clinical subjects.

Quantitatively, the size of this new edition has changed little from the previous publication with the number of new entries approximately balancing the deletions that we made. Such omissions were only considered when it was felt that the terms were so outdated that students may have been misinformed during their study of the relevant subject. Nevertheless, we also wish to reiterate the request made in previous editions that readers inform us of any errors, shortcomings and omissions that they identify in this book so that we can work towards further modifications in future editions.

We must also acknowledge that the production of this edition has been a genuine team effort with contributions from many of our academic and consultant colleagues at the University of Newcastle upon Tyne and Newcastle Dental Hospital. This was indeed the only practical way to approach our challenge as the required breadth and depth of dental specialty terminology could only be achieved through contributors from the range of dental specialities. We offer our sincerest thanks.

Finally, we are also indebted to Janice Urquhart, the Development Editor at Elsevier, for her valuable advice and input into the production the new edition.

PH
GMcC

Preface to the First Edition

This dictionary is the brain-child of Robin Ogston. Sadly he did not live to see it published and it is to be hoped that the completed volume will serve as an epitaph to a life enthusiastically devoted to the practice of dentistry.

It was originally conceived as an addendum to his tape/slide presentations and lectures aimed at the dental surgery assistant. However, this concept was expanded to meet the needs of dental surgeons, students, both undergraduate and postgraduate, and also the auxiliary dental and secretarial staff on whom the profession relies to form an efficient dental team.

Dictionaries are generally concerned with words as materials for speech. Scientific dictionaries have to go further and attempt to define the word in its scientific sense. For example, the word 'bite' in dentistry means something completely different from its meaning to a non-dentally educated person. Alas, the problems of defining dental words do not cease there, for sometimes the same word has a different meaning to dentists in different countries and, all too often, to dentists within the same country but educated in different schools.

Spelling and hyphenation were two other areas that immediately created problems, and in order to obtain a semblance of uniformity the following texts were consulted and used as prime sources. *Butterworth's Medical Dictionary* (2nd Edition 1978). Where a specific word was not included in this dictionary, *A Guide to the Preparation of Typescripts and Notes on House Style*, issued by the *British Dental Journal*, 1984, was consulted and wherever possible the preferred form and usages given in that guide were used.

The definition of terms caused considerable difficulties for, often, two or more terms have the same meaning or, alternatively, the same term has two or more definitions depending on the branch of dentistry to which it is applied. In such cases, the prime source was taken to be that given in *The British Standards Institution's-British Standard Glossary of Dental Terms-BS 4492:1983*.

Inevitably, dental terminology contains many obsolescent or deprecated terms and, although many have been included for historical reasons, the preferred term has been stressed.

Dictionaries are concerned with words, whilst encyclopaedias go further and explain the object that the word describes, since this may be necessary to allow the word to be used correctly. So in this dictionary I have sometimes expanded an entry to facilitate understanding. Also expanded entries have been used where it was thought that they would be beneficial to the student dental surgery assistant. At the other end of the scale, the postgraduate student has been catered for by including definitions of exotic and rarely encountered conditions which he or she must know about if only for examination purposes.

Appendices have been added, the object being to collect useful and frequently used information from various sources and make it readily available between the covers of one book.

The compilation of a dictionary is a certain way of finding out just how little one knows about many subjects and it is therefore inevitable that I shall be guilty of many omissions and errors. To those who will take the trouble to inform me of my shortcomings, I would like to express my thanks in advance and to assure them that I will take note of even the most minor criticism.

Contributors

Justin Durham, Clinical Fellow in Oral and Maxillofacial Sciences

Nick Girdler, Professor of Sedation Dentistry

Ross Hobson, Senior Lecturer in Orthodontics

Steve Hogg, Senior Lecturer in Oral Biology

Iain MacLeod, Consultant in Dental and Maxillofacial Radiology

Anne Maquire, Senior Clinical Lecturer in Child Dental Health

John Meechan, Senior Lecturer in Oral Surgery

Sarah Rolland, Clinical Fellow in Restorative Dentistry

Mike Reeson, Chief Instructor of Dental Technology

John Whitworth, Senior Lecturer in Restorative Dentistry

Contents

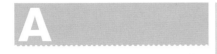

A point An orthodontic cephalometric landmark defined as the position of the deepest concavity on the anterior profile of the maxilla.

a-(an) Prefix signifying absence or without.

abacterial Free from bacteria.

abatement Reduction in the severity of pain or symptoms.

Abbé Estlander's operation Transfer of a full-thickness flap from one lip to repair a defect in the other lip, using an arterial pedicle to ensure survival of the graft.

abdomen That part of the body lying between the diaphragm of the thorax and the groin, containing, among other organs, the liver, kidneys, spleen, pancreas, stomach and intestines.

abdominal Pertaining to the abdomen.

aberrant Deviating from the normal.

aberration 1. Deviation from the normal. 2. Unequal refraction of light rays by a lens.

abnormal 1. Unusual, not normal, in growth or development. 2. In statistics, a departure from the mean of distribution.

abnormality 1. Any abnormal condition. 2. A defective or malformed organ.

abrasion 1. Grazing of the surface tissues. 2. Abnormal wearing away of a substance or structure by a mechanical process. *Dental a.* Loss by wear of tooth substance or a restoration, caused by factors other than tooth contact, e.g. incorrect tooth brushing.

abrasive Substance which wears away, scours or grinds down a surface, sometimes in preparation for polishing, e.g. diamonds, carborundum, sand, emery, garnet, pumice, cuttle. *A. disc. See*

1

disc. *A. paste.* Paste used for polishing or cleaning, e.g. prophylactic paste *A. strip.* Metal, linen or plastic strip coated with an abrasive on one or both sides and used to modify and polish the surface of a tooth or restoration. *A. wheel.* Wheel-shaped rotary instrument containing an abrasive in a rubber base and used to shape and polish metal restorations and prostheses.

abscess Localized collection of pus in a cavity, formed by the breakdown of tissues, commonly by infection with pyogenic bacteria. *Acute a.* Relatively short-lived abscess accompanied by painful local inflammation. *Apical a. See* periapical a. *Blind a.* An abscess without an external opening or draining sinus. *Chronic a.* One of slow development, mild inflammation, slow to heal and generally draining through a sinus. *Periapical a.* An acute or chronic inflammation with pus formation and tissue destruction at the apex of a tooth whose pulp has become infected. *Periodontal a.* An abscess in the periodontal tissues which occurs when there is an increase in the concentration or virulence of plaque micro-organisms. *Phoenix a.* A periodontal abscess which, after a symptom-free period, becomes symptomatic with all the characteristics of an acute periodontal abscess. *Pulp (or pulpal) a.* An acute or chronic abscess in the pulp tissue of a tooth due to an irritant such as dental caries, cavity preparation, bacterial leakage around a restoration or traumatic injury.

absorbed dose In radiology, the energy per unit mass imparted to matter by ionizing radiation. Formerly expressed in rads, the SI unit is the gray (Gy). 1 Gy = 100 rad.

absorbent Substance which attracts and takes up gases or liquids.

absorbent point *See* paper point.

absorption 1. Incorporation of a fluid, gas or other substance into the body of a material or tissue. 2. In radiology, the process whereby the energy of a beam of radiation is reduced during its passage through matter.

absorptive Able to absorb, absorbent.

abut To have a common boundary. To touch or border upon.

abutment Support to receive lateral and horizontal thrust. In dentistry, a tooth, crown or part of an implant used to provide support, stabilization, anchorage or retention for a fixed or removable prosthesis. *A. replica* Prefabricated laboratory copy of an implant fixture or abutment that is combined with an impression coping prior to casting of an impression. The replica will then be cast within the stone model. *Customizable a.* An implant abutment that may be modified (trimmed) intra- or extra-orally to allow placement of a definitive restoration. *Custom made a.* An implant abutment that has been made to order to fit an underlying implant fixture. *Healing a. (temporary abutment)* An abutment designed to be connected to an underlying implant fixture which sits transmucosally to allow healing of the soft tissues prior to the placement of a definitive abutment and restoration. *Implant a.* That part of an implant that supports a prosthesis.

ac *Ante cibum.* Before meals.

acanthosis Increase in the number of cells of the prickle cell layer of stratified epithelium, seen typically in eczema and psoriasis.

accelerator (promoter) Substance used in small quantities to increase the rate of a chemical reaction. *A. catalyst. See* catalyst.

access A way in, a means of approach. *A. cavity.* Coronal opening into a pulp cavity required for effective shaping, cleaning and filling of the pulp space during root canal treatment. *Surgical a.* Preparation of hard and soft tissue to allow entrance to, visualization and adequate instrumentation of a treatment site.

accessory Additional, subordinate to, contributing to the main function. See also *A. (lateral)root canal. A. point. See* root canal filling point.

accommodation Adjustment, e.g. changes in the eye pupil as a result of fluctuating levels of illumination.

accretion 1. Gradual deposition of material on a surface, e.g. plaque and calculus on teeth. 2. Adherence of parts normally separated.

acellular 1. Free from cells. In medicine a vaccine may be described as acellular if it contains no cells. 2. Not characterized by a cellular structure. An organism which is not divided into cells, often referred to as unicellular or single-celled.

acesulfame-potassium Intense sweetener with approx. 130 times the sweetness of sucrose. Commonly used in low calorie soft drinks. *See* sweetener.

acetone Inflammable, colourless liquid used as an organic solvent and having a characteristic odour (peardrops).

acetylsalicylic acid (aspirin) Mild analgesic with anti-fever and anti-inflammatory properties. May be combined with other analgesics. Some 7% of the population may exhibit gastric reactions to it, giving rise to nausea, vomiting, pain and gastric haemorrhage. Pure aspirin tablets should not be taken when the stomach is empty. Soluble aspirin tablets (BP) 300 mg are less irritant but paracetamol (q.v.) is preferred. *A. burn.* Opaque, wrinkled,

sloughing burn produced within 30 minutes if aspirin tablet remains on the mucous membrane of the mouth.

ache A continuous dull pain.

aciclovir (acyclovir) An antiviral drug of some use against the herpes viruses. The treatment is primarily symptomatic and only effective if started at the onset of the infection. Trade name Zovirax.®

acid Corrosive substance having a sharp sour taste and capable of neutralizing bases with the formation of salts. Turns blue litmus red. *A. etching. See* etching. *A. bath.* Acid solution, generally 50% hydrochloric or sulphuric acid, used to cleanse the surface of a metal casting of its oxide coating. The process is known as *pickling*. The casting is placed in the acid in a test tube and heated. Boiling should be avoided because of the acid fumes evolved.

acid etchant Liquid or gel form, typically 37% phosphoric acid, used in bonding resins to tooth structure. Modifies and roughens dentine and enamel surfaces.

acid–pumice-microabrasion 'Abrasive' technique using a strong acid (hydrochloric or phosphoric) and pumice for controlled removal of surface enamel to improve the aesthetics of teeth with dental opacities and hypoplasia. Often used to treat dental fluorosis.

acidic Pertaining to an acid.

acidifier Chemical compound, usually acetic acid, used in the processing of photographic and radiographic film to maintain the acidity of the fixing and stop-bath solutions (q.v.).

acidogenic theory Most commonly accepted theory on the aetiology of dental caries, postulated by W. D. Miller in 1890. According to Miller, plaque bacteria metabolize refined carbohydrates to produce acid which demineralizes enamel.

acidulated Rendered acidic in reaction.

acidulated phosphate fluoride (APF) Sol, gel or foam preparation professionally applied to cleaned teeth, usually for 4 minutes in a tray, to reduce dental caries incidence.

acini Plural of acinus.

acinus A small, sac-like dilatation, as found in excretory glands, which clusters round and opens into the branches of a gland duct.

acquired immune deficiency syndrome See AIDS.

acromegaly Condition marked by unusual enlargement of the body extremities and of the jaws. Due to hyperfunction of the pituitary gland growth hormone.

acrylic Referring to synthetic resins derived from acrylic acid and used in the manufacture of medical and dental prostheses. *A. denture. See* denture. *A. resin. See* resin. *A. trimmer.* Rotary instrument used to remove and shape acrylic resin. Manufactured in various shapes and may be of steel or an abrasive material having a wide pore structure (pumice-like).

ACTH (adrenocorticotrophic hormone) See corticotrophin.

actinomycosis Disease caused by *Actinomyces bovis* or *israelii* affecting cattle and, less commonly, humans. Affects the jaws but may also affect the tongue, lungs or intestines. Characterized by chronic suppurative inflammatory lesions discharging thick yellow pus containing sulphur crystals. Also known as '*wooden*' or '*lumpy*' jaw.

activator 1. Agent rendering chemicals capable of reacting with others. 2. Myofunctional removable orthodontic

appliance constructed to lie in contact with all or part of the teeth in both dental arches. It does not fit firmly to the teeth and provides its activation by displacing muscles in and around the mouth from their natural resting position, e.g. Fraenkel, monobloc and Andresen appliances (q.v.).

active eruption Normal movement of an erupting tooth into the oral cavity.

acu- Prefix signifying relationship to sharp or needle.

acupuncture Puncturing the tissues at certain specific areas of the body with fine stainless steel needles in order to relieve pain, allow escape of fluids and act as a counter-irritant. Used in China to relieve pain during surgical operations and thought to act on the autonomic nervous system.

acute 1. Describes a condition of severe rapid onset and short duration. Opposite to chronic. 2. Describes intense symptoms such as sharp and severe pain.

acute ulcerative gingivitis (AUG); acute necrotizing ulcerative gingivitis (ANUG); necrotizing ulcerative gingivitis. See gingivitis.

adamantinoma See ameloblastoma.

Adcortyl in orabase® See triamcinolone acetonide dental paste.

Addison's anaemia See pernicious anaemia.

adenitis Inflammation of a gland.

adenocarcinoma Malignant epithelial tumour arising from glandular structures. Also applies to tumours with a glandular growth pattern.

adenoids See gland.

adenoma Benign epithelial tumour derived from glandular tissue. See also adenocarcinoma.

adenomatous Relating to an adenoma.

adhesion 1. Action of sticking to, by molecular attraction of certain dissimilar molecules, by viscosity of surface or by grasping. 2. In surgery, the abnormal joining of two normally separate parts by new tissue produced as a result of inflammation. 3. In dentistry, the force which retains an upper denture in place without the use of adhesive gums or mechanical aids such as 'suction' cups.

adhesive Substance causing surface attachment. *Tray a.* Prevents impression materials lifting from impression trays, thus causing distorted models. *Denture a.* Used to retain ill-fitting dentures, e.g. gum tragacanth (q.v.). *Dentine a.* Resin based adhesive used to bond restorative materials to tooth substance. *Orthodontic a.* Used to bond orthodontic brackets to enamel.

adhesive bridge. *See* bridge.

adipose Fat. Fatty. *A. tissue.* Connective tissue with a predominance of fat cells, which serve as both an insulating layer and energy store.

ADJ Amelo-dentinal junction.

adjunct That which is an accessory or is additional.

adjustable articulator *See* articulator.

adjustable axis face-bow Face-bow (q.v.) with adjustable arms, used in conjunction with an adjustable articulator, to record the retruded hinge axis (q.v.). Also known as *kinematic face-bow, hinge axis locating face-bow* or *hinge bow.*

adjustment Process of modifying a state. In dentistry, an alteration made to a denture. *Occlusal a. (or equilibration)* Selective grinding of teeth in order to remove premature contacts and occlusal interferences and to establish a stable occlusion.

adjuvant Substance added to a drug to assist the action of the main ingredient.

adolescence Period of time during growth which precedes puberty and continues until adulthood. Altered patterns of behaviour are seen which are associated with a change in hormones which also produces physical changes.

ADR Adverse drug reaction.

adrenal glands *See* suprarenal gland.

adrenaline *See* epinephrine.

adsorption Phenomenon in which the atoms or molecules of a foreign substance are held on the surface of a liquid or solid material.

adult Grown to full size or maturity.

adumbration Poor edge definition of an image on a radiographic film due to cross-over X-rays. *See also* penumbra.

adventitia Outermost layer of tissue forming the coat of an organ. *Tunica a.* Outer coat of arteries and veins.

–aemia Suffix referring to blood.

aerobe Organism, usually a micro-organism which requires oxygen to survive.

aerobic Characterized by the presence of, in the case of an environment, or requirement for, in the case of an organism, oxygen.

aerodontalgia Toothache caused by the reduction in ambient pressure during high-altitude flying and due to the expansion of gas within the pulp chamber of a tooth.

aerosol 1. Suspension of matter in a gas, e.g. saliva and water in air generated by a turbine handpiece. 2. The container itself or the substance in it which is under pressure and can be released as a fine spray.

aesthesia The capacity of feeling, sensing or perceiving.

aesthetic dentistry Term used to describe the treatment techniques used to improve the position and symmetry of the teeth, jaws and face in order to improve the appearance, as well as the function of the teeth, mouth and face.

aetiology Study of the cause and history of disease.

AFD (anode-to-film distance) *See* FFD (focus-to-film distance).

afferent Conveying towards a centre. Relating to sensory nerves which conduct sensory impulses to the brain from receptor nerve endings—internal and external. Also applied to blood and lymph vessels returning their contents to the heart or blood vessels.

affinity Attraction. The tendency of substances to react together and form a new compound.

agar Extract from seaweed, used in the form of a jelly as a culture medium for micro-organisms and for duplicating techniques in the laboratory.

agate Very hard gemstone. Used to make spatula blades which are resistant to abrasion.

agent Any power, principle or substance producing a chemical, physical or biological effect.

agglutination Clumping together of particles or cells suspended in a fluid.

aggressive periodontitis *See* periodontitis.

agranular Without granules.

AIDS (acquired immune deficiency syndrome) A person with AIDS is defined as: 'A person with a disease that is indicative of an underlying cellular immune deficiency, but who, at the same time, has no known underlying cause for cellular immune deficiency nor any other cause of reduced resistance associated with a disease' (definition given by R.C.W. Dinsdale in "Viral Hepatitis, AIDS and Dental Treatment", British Dental Journal Publications, 1985). *See also* herpes.

air Colourless, odourless, gaseous mixture forming the earth's atmosphere. Consists of about one part of oxygen together with four parts of nitrogen and small amounts of other elements. *A. motor.* Drill motor, driven at medium speeds by compressed air and coupled directly to a conventional handpiece having no driving cable. *A. rotor.* Handpiece incorporating an air-driven high-speed rotor. *A. syringe.* See syringe. *A. turbine. See* a. rotor.

airway 1. Route for the passage of air into and out of the lungs. 2. Nasal or oropharyngeal tube inserted into an unconscious patient's airway to maintain it patent and unobstructed.

AJC Acrylic jacket crown. *See* crown, jacket.

ala A wing-like process, e.g. the ala of the nose. *A.nasi.* The cartilagenous wing of the nostril.

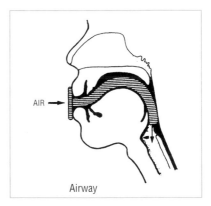

Airway

alae Plural of ala.

ala-tragal line (Camper's line)
Imaginary line running from the inferior border of the ala of the nose to the superior border of the tragus of the ear. Used as a reference plane in orthodontics, radiography and prosthetics, when determining the occlusal plane.

Albers–Schönberg disease *See* osteopetrosis.

alcohol More correctly termed *ethyl alcohol* or *ethanol*. Contains 95% alcohol and 5% water. Obtained by the action of yeast on sugar solutions, particularly glucose and grape sugar. In dentistry, used as a solvent, surgical antiseptic and during cavity toilet (q.v.). *Absolute a.* Alcohol containing no more than 1% water. *Denatured a.* Ethyl alcohol to which certain denaturants have been added to render it unfit for human consumption or to adapt it for industrial uses.

–algia Suffix meaning pain.

alginate Salt of alginic acid (obtained from seaweed) which, when mixed with water in the recommended proportions, forms an irreversible hydrocolloid (q.v.) gel used for dental impressions.

alginate impression material *See* impression material, irreversible hydrocolloid.

align 1. To bring into line. 2. In orthodontics and prosthetics, to move teeth into their correct position so as to conform to the correct occlusal plane and arch form.

alimentary tract (or canal) Tubular passage through which food passes from the mouth, oesophagus, stomach, small and large intestines and rectum during the processes of digestion, absorption and excretion.

alkali Compound that is very soluble in water, producing a caustic or corrosive

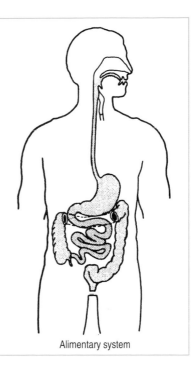

Alimentary system

solution which neutralizes acids to form salts. In aqueous solution, alkalis dissociate with the formation of hydroxyl (OH) ions. Alkali turns red litmus blue.

allelograft *See* graft.

allergic Relating to allergy.

allergy Abnormal or exaggerated reaction to a normally harmless substance introduced into the body or applied to its surface. A condition of hypersensitivity.

allograft *See* graft.

alloy 1. Product formed by the fusion of two or more metals that are mutually soluble in the liquid state. 2. Product of the fusion of several metals, usually supplied as shavings and mixed with mercury. *Admixed amalgam a.* Alloy containing particles of different composition. *Encapsulated a.* Proportioned

7

quantities of alloy and mercury separated in a capsule, the mercury being contained beneath a foil which is broken to allow mechanical mixing, so producing a standard property amalgam. *High copper amalgam a.* Alloy with increased copper content to reduce corrosion. *Lathe cut amalgam a.* Alloy cut on a lathe so as to produce irregular-shaped particles to be mixed with mercury. *Silver tin a.* Contains silver, tin and small quantities of copper and zinc. *Spherical amalgam a.* Alloy in the shape of spherical beads. *Zinc free amalgam a.* Absence of zinc minimizes the adverse effects of contamination by moisture and saliva. Amalgam alloy may be presented in lathe cut or spherical forms. The mercury is generally triple distilled for the sake of purity and it is important that the proportion of mercury to alloy is correct in order to obtain the best amalgam properties. A proportioner may be used to obtain the correct amounts of each, and may be adjusted to suit the operator but now generally supplied preproportioned in encapsulated form. Mercury should not be handled nor left exposed because of the poisonous properties of its vapour.

alopecia A reversible hair loss.

alum *See* potassium aluminium sulphate.

alumina Substance added to porcelain to produce increased strength. *A. (aluminous) porcelain.* Dental porcelain to which is added a significant amount of recrystallized alumina, in order to increase the strength of the final restoration.

aluminium oxide Abrasive sometimes used as a polishing agent and now also added to dental porcelain and cement powders to increase the strength of the final restoration.

alveolar Relating to an alveolus. *A. bone.* The bone of the alveolar process that supports and surrounds the teeth. *A. crest.* Most coronal portion of the alveolar bone. *A. margin.* Coronal aspect of the bone which forms the tooth sockets. *A. mucosa.* Mucosa covering the base of the alveolar process and the floor of the mouth. It is loosely attached to the periosteum of the bone and is movable. *A. process.* Portion of the maxilla or mandible which contains the sockets of erupted teeth and the crypts of the developing teeth. *A. ridge.* Residual ridge in which alveolar bone remains after the loss of the teeth. *A. septum.* Partition of the bone separating individual alveoli of multirooted teeth.

alveolectomy Partial or complete excision of the alveolar process of the maxilla or mandible.

alveoli Plural of alveolus.

alveolotomy Trimming and moulding of the outer plate of the alveolar process following septal alveolectomy in order to achieve the more aesthetic placing of a denture.

alveolus Structure with a sac-like dilatation. *Dental a.* One of the sockets in the alveolar process of the maxilla or mandible which retains teeth by means of the periodontal ligament fibres. Term sometimes incorrectly used to describe the alveolar process. *Pulmonary a.* Small air sac situated in the lungs, having single-celled walls across which the exchange of oxygen and carbon dioxide gases takes place during respiration.

alveoplasty A general term used to describe the surgical reshaping of the alveolar ridges.

Alvogyl® A sedative dressing material used in the management of dry socket. Among its active ingredients are iodoform and eugenol.

amalgam Mercury-containing alloy which becomes a soft silvery paste on mixing and later hardens. *See also* alloy. *A. carrier.* Metal or plastic instrument used to convey amalgam, in its plastic state, to the mouth and deposit it into a prepared tooth cavity. Sometimes called an *amalgam gun.* After use excess amalgam should be expelled immediately from the nozzle to prevent blockage when it has set hard. *A. condenser.* 1. Hand instrument used to condense amalgam in a cavity preparation. 2. Engine-driven device which mechanically condenses amalgam. *A. core.*

Amalgam restoration, usually retained by pins, post or adhesives, designed to support another restoration. *A. plugger.* Double-ended hand instrument having round- or oval-shaped ends which may be serrated or plain. Used to plug and condense amalgam into a cavity preparation. *A. tattoo.* Brown or black area of pigmentation caused by the accidental implantation of amalgam in the oral tissues.

amalgamation Mixing together of alloy and mercury to form amalgam. *See also* trituration.

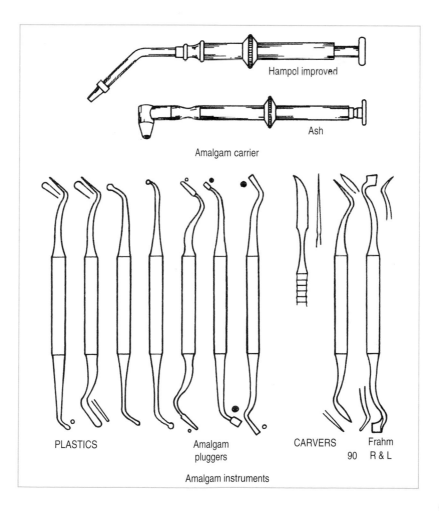

Hampol improved

Ash

Amalgam carrier

PLASTICS   Amalgam pluggers   CARVERS   Frahm
                                                      90   R & L

Amalgam instruments

amalgamator Electrically driven mechanical device, often with a built-in proportioner, used to amalgamate alloy and mercury in a capsule. A timing clock controls the mixing time. Should stand in a shallow plastic tray to trap any mercury spillage. Now superseded by the introduction of pre-encapsulated amalgam. Commonly relates to the mechanical device that mixes encapsulated dental amalgam (materials).

Ambu bag® Portable apparatus having a semi-collapsible bag, used for pressure ventilation. Its facepiece is placed over the patient's mouth and face, and the bag gently squeezed 15–20 times/minute (or in time with the recovering person's breathing) in order to introduce air into the lungs. Usually connected by an inlet tube to an oxygen cylinder fitted with a reducing valve.

ambulant Able to walk.

ameloblast Ectodermally derived cell primarily responsible for the formation of enamel (amelogenesis).

ameloblastoma Neoplasm of tissues of the type characteristic of the tooth

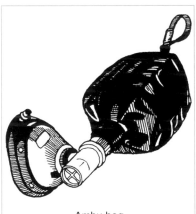

Ambu bag
(By courtesy of Ambu International, PO Box 215, Copenhagen, DK 2600)

enamel organ, but which does not advance to become formed enamel. Also called *adamantinoma*.

amelo-dentinal junction (dentino-enamel junction) Junction between tooth enamel and dentine.

amelogenesis Formation of enamel. *A. imperfecta.* Hereditary condition resulting in the formation of imperfect enamel characterized by either hypoplasia of the tooth enamel (the teeth becoming worn down to the level of the gingivae and stained dark brown) or hypocalcification of the enamel, which becomes pitted, chalky and stained, sometimes having areas in which the enamel is absent.

amino acid Substance derived from the breakdown of protein foods during digestion and concerned with growth and repair.

amnesia Loss of memory.

amoeba A single-celled micro-organism belonging to the animal kingdom capable of locomotion and engulfing food by forming cell extensions known as pseudopodia.

amoeboid Resembling an amoeba in form or method of locomotion.

amorphous Having no definite shape or form. Devoid of molecular crystallinity or stratification.

amoxicillin (Amoxyl®**, Penbritin**®**, Vidopen**®**)** Rapidly absorbed broad-spectrum antibiotic. Dispensed in tablet form or in sachets to be dissolved in water.

Amoxyl® *See* amoxicillin.

ampere (A) The ampere is that constant current which, if maintained in two straight parallel conductors of infinite length, of negligible circular cross-section, and placed one metre apart in vacuum, would produce between these conductors a force equal to 2×10^{-7} newton per metre of length.

amphetamine A drug which produces a feeling of boundless energy and speeds up body activities by stimulating the nervous system—'pep pill'.

amphotericin (Fungilin®) An antifungal agent used to treat oral fungal infections.

ampicillin Semi-synthetic, broad-spectrum penicillin in tablet form. May cause rashes, and is active against many Gram-negative organisms.

ampoule Small glass vessel in which a specified dose of a drug is sealed in a sterile condition, e.g. one containing a drug for intramuscular injection.

amputation Complete or partial removal of a limb. *Root a.* The surgical removal of a root of a tooth.

amyl nitrite Clear, yellowish, inflammable liquid sealed in a small gauze-covered ampoule. When the ampoule is crushed, the vapour is inhaled to relieve spasms such as angina pectoris (q.v.). It is a vasodilator and heart stimulant. Is subject to substance misuse.

amylase (ptyalin) Enzyme secreted by the parotid and submandibular salivary glands and the pancreas. It breaks starch down into smaller molecules.

amyxorrhoea Deficiency or lack of mucous secretion.

an- *See a-.*

anachoresis Blood-borne infection in which micro-organisms are attracted towards certain local lesions while the rest of the body appears to remain immune from these organisms.

anaemia Condition caused by a deficiency of blood or red blood cells, a lack of haemoglobin in the red blood cells or

an excess of white blood cells. The skin and mucous membrane become pale and the symptoms are weakness, headaches and lack of energy. It is a symptom of a number of other diseases and conditions. *See also* pernicious anaemia.

anaerobe Organism, usually a micro-organism, which can only survive in the absence of oxygen.

anaesthesia Loss of feeling or sensation in some part of the body due to nerve impulse blockage by mechanical means or by the use of drugs. *General a.* Anaesthesia of the whole body with complete loss of consciousness produced by injection or inhalation of an anaesthetic or analgesic drug. *Local a. See* analgesia, local.

anaesthetic 1. Relating to anaesthesia. 2. Agent which produces anaesthesia. *Inhalation a.* Anaesthetic agent in the form of a gas or vapour administered via the respiratory tract, e.g. nitrous oxide. Premedication, in the form of narcotic drugs, is usually given prior to an anaesthetic. *Intravenous a.* Method used to render a patient unconscious by introducing an anaesthetic solution directly into a vein by injection, e.g. propofol.

anaesthetist Medical specialist who administers anaesthetics and analgesics.

analgesia Absence of pain sensation while the patient remains conscious yet without necessarily losing the sense of touch and pressure. *Audio a.* Analgesia produced by listening to sound. *Block a.* Injection of an analgesic solution in such a position that it effectively blocks the transmission of nerve impulses along a pathway remote from its receptor endings, e.g. the mandibular (inferior dental) nerve block. Also known as *conduction analgesia. Epidural a.* Produced by injection of analgesic solution into the space surrounding the spinal cord external to the dura mater. *Infiltration a.* Method of producing analgesia in a localized area by injecting analgesic solution which seeps or diffuses through the tissues to affect nerve endings at the site, as opposed to applying the solution to a nerve trunk. *Intra-osseous a.* Analgesia obtained by injection of analgesic solution into alveolar bone adjacent to a tooth. *Local a.* Induced localized numbness of body tissues and absence of pain sensation. *Refrigeration a.* Method of relieving pain by lowering the temperature of the tissues, e.g. by spraying ethyl chloride onto a site to be anaesthetized. *Regional a.* Removal of pain perception from an area of the body, rather than from the whole body, by the use of analgesic drugs. *Relative a.* State of sedation induced by the inhalation of a regulated mixture of oxygen and nitrous oxide gas through a nose-piece accompanied by semi-hypnotic suggestion. The patient remains conscious and able to co-operate throughout a surgical or restorative procedure. In addition, analgesic solutions may be injected locally if required. *Surface* or *topical a.* Numbness produced by the topical application of an analgesic paste, e.g. Xylocaine® paste.

analgesic Drug used to produce analgesia. May be in the form of solutions for injection (formerly termed local anaesthetics), pastes, sprays or lozenges. These drugs block the conduction of impulses from nerve receptors to the brain. Other analgesics reduce pain sensation by acting upon the brain without causing loss of consciousness, e.g. aspirin, codeine, ibuprofen, dihydrocodeine (DF118®), paracetamol, pethidine. *A. solution.* Acts locally to block the passage of pain impulses along nerve pathways to the brain. May be used as spinal or epidural injection and to provide analgesia in dental and other surgery. Dental analgesic

solutions are manufactured in 1.8 and 2 ml glass cartridges. The main constituent is isotonic Ringer's solution (q.v.) containing *lidocaine*—the analgesic agent— *buffer salts* and traces of *antiseptics*. To these may be added a vasoconstrictor such as epinephrine or octapressin. The solutions may contain 2–4% of the analgesic agent.

anaphylactic shock Acute allergic reaction characterized by a sudden general circulatory collapse which may be severe and sometimes fatal. Treated by injections of epinephrine, antihistamine and hydrocortisone.

anaphylaxis Hypersensitive state of the body to injection of certain foreign proteins. May lead to anaphylactic shock and can prove fatal if not treated immediately.

anastomosis A joining together. In anatomy, the direct or indirect communication of blood vessels without an intervening capillary network. In surgery, the artificial connection between two tubular organs which are normally separate.

anatomical crown That part of a tooth normally covered by, and including, the enamel.

anatomical impression tray *See* impression tray.

anatomical root That part of a tooth normally covered by, and including, the cementum.

anatomical tooth Artificial tooth whose crown simulates the morphology of a natural tooth.

anatomy The study of the structure of living organisms. In medicine, the study and description of the form and structure of the human body.

ANB angle The angle between the points A, N and B in cephalometrics. Used to define the skeletal pattern of the individual. The average ANB angle is 3 degrees (Class I) plus or minus 2 degrees. Angles less than this are described as skeletal Class III and angles greater as a skeletal Class II.

anchorage Collective term for those areas resisting any forces applied to move certain teeth. Such areas may include other teeth, when the anchorage is intra-oral, or they may be extra-oral such as orthodontic headgear. *Orthodontic a.* Resistance to unwanted tooth movement during orthodontic treatment. *Extra-oral a.* Type of orthodontic anchorage with apparatus using the top or back of the head or neck to achieve anchorage – headgear, cervical headgear or halo. *Reciprocal a.* Type of orthodontic anchorage in which the movement of two or more teeth is balanced against the movement of one or more opposing teeth.

Andrews' 6 keys to occlusion A definition of optimal occlusion as defined by Andrews. The 6 keys are: 1) molar relationship: the distal surface of the distobuccal cusp of the upper first permanent molar occludes with the mesial surface of the mesial-buccal cusp of the lower second permanent molar; 2) crown angulation (mesial-distal tip): the gingival portion of each crown is distal to the incisor portion and varied with each arch tooth type; 3) crown inclination (labial-lingual, buccal-lingual): anterior teeth (incisors) are at sufficient angulation to prevent overeruption. Upper posterior teeth – lingual tip is constant and similar from canine to second premolar and increased in the molars. Lower posterior teeth – lingual tip increases progressively from the canines to the molars: 4) no rotations; 5) no spaces; 6) flat occlusal planes.

Andrews' straight wire A particular prescription of a pre-adjusted edgewise appliance designed to use a straight arch wire. The brackets incorporate the tip, torque and 'in-out' that is normally bent into the arch wire so simplifying fixed orthodontic appliances.

aneurysm Balloon-like swelling of the wall of a blood vessel, usually an artery, through a defect, injury or disease of the vessel. Aneurysm of the aorta may lead to its rupture and sudden death.

aneurysmal bone cyst Lesion of bone that appears radiolucent radiographically and is composed of giant cells and sinusoidal vascular tissue.

Anexate® *See* flumazenil.

angina An oppressive sensation, discomfort or suffocating pain. *A. pectoris* (also known as *cardiac a.* or *a. of effort*). Literally angina of the chest. Severe substernal pain and a sense of oppression, often extending into the neck and left arm, produced by an inadequate blood supply to the myocardium. The pain is commonly brought on by exertion or stress. It can be prevented or relieved by drugs such as glyceryl trinitrate. If drug treatment proves ineffective the obstructed segment of the coronary artery may be bypassed with venous or arterial grafts. *See also* cellulitis (or *Ludwig's angina*) and necrotizing ulcerative gingivitis (or *Vincent's angina*).

angioma Benign tumour composed of blood or lymphatic vessels.

angioneurotic oedema (Quincke's oedema) Allergic condition producing a generally transient enlargement of tissues, accompanied by itching and commonly affecting the eyelids, cheeks, lips or tongue. Caused by a localized vascular change that allows the rapid escape of fluid into the tissues.

angle In anatomy, a corner. *A. board.* Apparatus for positioning the patient's head during oblique or temporomandibular joint radiography. *A. of the eye.* The outer or inner corner of the eye. *A. of the mandible.* That part of the mandible formed by the junction of the ramus and the body. *A. of the mouth.* The point where the upper and lower lips join. *A. osteotomy.* Excision of a segment of mandible from the region of the angle, either unilaterally or bilaterally, for the correction of prognathism. *Cavosurface a.* Angle formed between the surface of a tooth and a cavity wall. *Line a.* Angle formed at the junction of two tooth surfaces or of two cavity walls.

Angle Edward Angle, credited for being the father of modern orthodontics, developed modern fixed appliance treatment and defined Angle's occlusion.

Angle's classification of malocclusion The American orthodontist's (Edward Angle) classification, based on the mesial position of the lower first molars relative to the upper first molars. The upper first molar's mesiobuccal cusp occludes with the mesiobuccal fossa of the lower first molar. The orthodontic classification is now more related to the position of the upper and lower incisor teeth. *See also* malocclusion.

angular cheilitis Condition characterized by dryness, burning, chapping or ulceration of the angle of the mouth. Attributable to candidal and/or staphylococcal infection in association with haematinic deficiency, vitamin B complex deficiency, loss of vertical dimension and saliva drooling.

angulation In radiography, the direction in which central X-rays and the cone of the X-ray machine are directed towards the teeth and the radiographic film.

anhydrous Dry. Containing no water.

ankyloglossia Tongue tie. The complete or partial binding of the tongue to the floor of the mouth or alveolar ridge due to an abnormally short lingual fraenum that limits tongue movement.

ankylosis Immobility and fixation of a joint due to disease, trauma or surgery. *Dental a.* Solid fixation of a tooth owing to fusion of cementum and alveolar bone, the periodontal ligament being obliterated. *False a.* Inability to open the mouth due to trismus rather than to disease of the temporomandibular joint.

annealing Low temperature heat treatment of metals to relieve internal stresses.

annular Ring shaped.

anode Electrically positive electrode of a battery or appliance, such as an X-ray apparatus, towards which the negatively charged electrons move.

anodontia Developmental absence of some or all teeth.

anodyne A pain-relieving drug.

anomaly Irregularity. One not fitting into a group.

anorexia Partial or complete loss of appetite.

anosmia Partial or complete loss of smell.

anoxia Insufficiency or lack of oxygen, characterized by a bluish complexion (cyanosis).

anoxic Pertaining to or characterized by anoxia.

ANS *See* anterior nasal spine.

antagonist One who opposes another. 1. In anatomy, any muscle which opposes and neutralizes the effect of another muscle. 2. In pharmacology, a drug which counteracts the action of another drug.

3. In dentistry, a tooth in one jaw which occludes with a tooth in the other jaw.

ante– Prefix meaning before, either in time or place.

antenatal Before birth.

anterior Situated before or in front of another object. *A. bite plane.* Platform of acrylic resin in the anterior region of a removable appliance on which the lower teeth occlude, thus preventing posterior tooth contact. *A. guidance. See* guidance. *A. nasal spine (ANS).* The top of the anterior nasal spine as seen in a lateral skull radiograph. *A. occlusal projection. See* standard occlusal projection. *A. open bite.* Occlusion in which the lower teeth are neither overlapped in the vertical plane nor occlude with the upper incisors when the posterior teeth are in occlusion. *A. protected articulation. See* articulation. *A. tooth. See* tooth.

anterior open bite *See* anterior.

antero- Prefix meaning before.

anthrax Acute infectious disease of cattle, sheep, goats and other herbivores caused by the spore forming bacterium *Bacillus anthracis.* Transmitted to humans by direct contact with infected animal material such as wool or hides or by inhalation of spores which can remain dormant for many years. Infection is most commonly cutaneous via cuts or abrasions, causing inflammation in 1-2 days followed by ulceration with associated necrosis lasting some 10 days. Mortality is about 20% if untreated and rare following appropriate antibiotic therapy. A pulmonary form resulting from inhalation of, usually, spores causes a much more serious condition which is normally fatal. An intestinal form, caused by ingestion of infected material, causes acute inflammation of the intestinal tract, vomiting of blood and severe diarrhoea which is fatal in as much as 60% of cases. Anthrax is now rare in the UK.

anti- Prefix meaning against or opposing.

antibacterial Any substance that destroys or inhibits the growth of bacteria.

antibiotic 1. Destructive of life. 2. Drug derived from a micro-organism which prevents the growth of, or destroys other micro-organisms, e.g. penicillin. Some antibiotics are more effective than others against specific organisms and the choice may be decided by sensitivity tests. They may be administered orally, topically, by intramuscular or intravenous injection or intravenous infusion. Should be given in advance of dental treatment in cases with a history of rheumatic fever and subacute bacterial endocarditis. Their action is bacteriostatic or bactericidal. Accidentally discovered by Sir Alexander Fleming in 1929. *Bactericidal a.* One that kills bacteria. *Bacteriostatic a.* One that suppresses the growth or reproduction of bacteria. *Broad-spectrum a.* One that is effective against a wide range of pathogenic bacteria.

antibody Protein substance produced by the lymphatic system cells in response to the presence of an antigen to which it is antagonistic. An antibody produced against a specific antigen (e.g. bacteria, pollens or foreign red blood cells) is the basis of both allergy (q.v.) and immunity (q.v.).

anticoagulant Drug used to prevent or retard the clotting of blood especially in the treatment of coronary thrombosis, e.g. warfarin, heparin or sodium citrate.

anticonvulsant Drug used to reduce the incidence or severity of convulsions in epilepsy, e.g. phenytoin (Epanutin®).

antidepressant Drug used to reduce the symptoms of depression, e.g. fluoxetine (Prozac®).

antidote Drug that counteracts the effect of poison.

anti-emetic Drug that reduces the incidence and severity of vomiting and nausea.

antiflux Material applied to the surface of a metal in order to confine the flow of the solder during soldering, e.g. graphite.

antifungal 1. Destructive to fungi. 2. Drug used to destroy micro-organisms such as *Candida albicans* which cause infections typified by angular cheilitis (q.v.) and denture stomatitis, e.g. nystatin and amphotericin.

antigen Substance which, under suitable conditions, stimulates an immunological response and reacts with antibodies.

antigenic Relating to an antigen. Derived from ANTIbody GENerator.

antihistamine Drug that inhibits the effect of histamine in the body. Used to control allergic reactions such as hay fever, pruritus and urticaria. Some antihistamines are strongly anti-emetic and are used to alleviate motion sickness. A common side-effect is drowsiness and they are sometimes used to promote sleep.

antihypertensive drug Drug used to reduce the high blood pressure of patients suffering from hypertension, e.g. propranolol.

anti-Monson curve *See* reverse curve.

antioxidants Substances which, when present at low concentrations relative to those of an oxidizable substrate, will significantly delay or inhibit oxidation of that substrate. Thought to protect the body against damage by free radicals, for example, during the pathogenesis of periodontal disease.

antipyretic Agent that prevents or reduces a fever, e.g. aspirin.

antiseptic Chemical that is sufficiently non-toxic to living tissue yet destroys or prevents the growth of pathogenic microbes, e.g. alcohol, acridine dyes, hexamine.

antisialogogue Substance that arrests or reduces salivation.

antitetanus serum (ATS) Serum given as precautionary injection to provide immunity to tetanus. May give rise to anaphylactic shock (q.v.), hence a test dose is first tried.

antitoxin Antibody produced by the body as a reaction to the toxins produced by bacterial invasion.

antiviral Drug used to treat virus infection, e.g. aciclovir.

antral Pertaining to an antrum. *A. fistula.* *See* oro-antral fistula. *A. packing.* Placing of a pack, usually consisting of materials such as ribbon gauze soaked in Whitehead's varnish or paraffin/flavin emulsion, to support the floor of a fractured orbit or part of the zygoma and to reduce haemorrhage. *A. puncture.* *See* antrostomy. *A. washout.* Irrigation of the interior of the antrum.

antritis (maxillary sinusitis) Inflammation of the antrum.

antrostomy Surgical procedure in which an opening is made through the inferior meatus of the nose into the maxillary antrum in order to secure drainage and enable the sinus to be washed out.

antrum General anatomical term for a cavity or chamber within a bone. *A. of Highmore.* *See* maxillary antrum or sinus. *Frontal a.* Situated in the frontal bone.

ANUG Acute necrotizing ulcerative gingivitis. *See* gingivitis.

anxiolytic Able to prevent or allay anxiety, tension and panic as experienced by some patients prior to dental treatment. *A. drugs* 'Sedative' drugs such as midazolam, diazepam and temazepam when given in low doses. In higher doses these drugs act as hypnotics (q.v.).

aorta Main and largest artery arising from the left ventricle of the heart and which transports oxygenated blood to the general circulation.

apatite Inorganic mineral substance. A calcium phosphate found in teeth and bone. Soluble in soft drink acids and carbohydrate fermentations, but when treated with certain fluoride solutions the resulting fluoro-apatite is not susceptible to acid destruction and caries.

apertognathia *See* open bite.

aperture 1. An opening or orifice. 2. In radiography, the opening in the tube head. *See* exit port.

apex 1. General anatomic term for the top of a body, organ or part, or the pointed end of a conical object. 2. That part of a tooth root furthest from the crown. *Anatomical/radiographic a.* The external tip of a dental root. *Physiological a.* Synonyms: apical constriction, cement-dentine junction. Internal narrowing of a root canal close to the root apex, to which instruments and filling materials are extended during root canal treatment. *A. locator.* Electronic device to measure canal length during root canal treatment (*see also* electronic apex locator).

apexification More correctly termed *root-end closure induction.* Process whereby an immature, open permanent tooth apex is induced to continue root formation, to form a closed apex or to produce a calcific barrier across the root canal. Typically

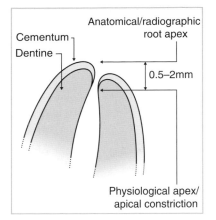

Anatomical/radiographic root apex

Cementum

Dentine

0.5–2mm

Physiological apex/ apical constriction

achieved by repeated canal dressing with non-setting calcium hydroxide paste. Increasingly achieved with MTA cement. *See* apexogenesis.

apexogenesis Treatment designed to preserve vital pulp tissue in the apical part of a root canal in order to complete formation of the root apex (*see also* apexification).

APF *See* acidulated phosphate fluoride.

aphagia Inability to swallow.

aphasia Speech disorder due to brain damage or illness.

aphtha Small whitish painful ulcer occurring in the mouth, either singly or in crops. Usually recurrent.

aphthae Plural of aphtha.

aphthous Relating to aphthae. *A. stomatitis. See* stomatitis. *A. ulcer.* Ulcer having a duration of 10–14 days and for which there is no accepted cure. Topical steroid preparations may be used to reduce the extent of ulceration. Chlorhexidine gluconate has been shown to promote the healing of aphthous ulcers.

apical Referring to the tip or apex of the tooth root and its immediate surroundings. *A. abscess. See* abscess. *A. curettage.*

apical

A

17

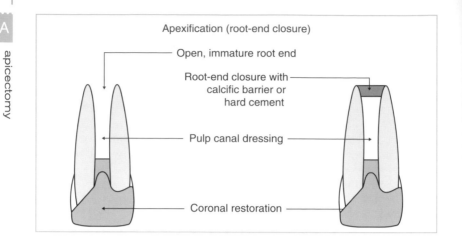

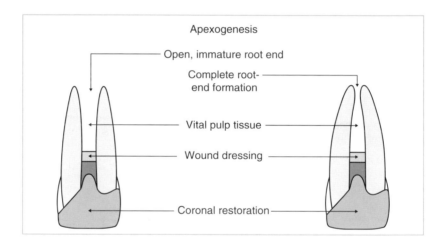

Surgical removal of chronic inflammatory tissue surrounding the apex of a tooth. *A. cyst. See* cysts of dental origin. *A. elevator. See* elevator. *A. foramen. See* foramen. *A. granuloma.* Chronic inflammatory lesion at the apical third of a tooth root.

apicectomy More correctly root-end surgery. Surgical procedure to remove the apex of a tooth root together with some of the surrounding tissues. Usually accompanied by root-end cavity preparation and filling (see retrograde root filling). Synonyms for apicectomy: *apicoectomy (USA), root-end resection.*

aplasia Failure of an organ or structure to develop.

aplastic Relating to aplasia.

apnoea Temporary cessation of breathing.

apogee In medicine, the most severe stage of the climax of a disease.

appliance Device used to perform a particular function. In orthodontics, a device bonded or attached to the teeth used to effect or prevent movement of the teeth and associated structures. *Andresen a.* Acrylic myofunctional device to produce tooth movement and influence growth. Also known as a *monobloc activator. A variation is the medium opening activator (MOA). Bass a.* A myofunctional appliance. *Begg a.* Fixed, multibracket appliance: see Begg technique. *Bimler a.* A myofunctional appliance. *Bionator a.* A myofunctional appliance. *Craniofacial a.* A device used to immobilize jaw fractures. *Edgewise a.* Fixed, multi-banded appliance which uses a rectangular archwire ligated to brackets in order to achieve orthodontic tooth movement. *Extra-oral a.* Apparatus using the top or back of the head or neck for anchorage—a headgear, cervical gear or halo. *Fixed a.* Orthodontic device cemented or attached to the teeth. *Fraenkel a.* An orthodontic myofunctional appliance: see Fraenkel. *Herbst a.* A fixed myofunctional appliance. *Johnson twin wire a.* An orthodontic fixed appliance using twin archwires. *Myofunctional a.* A removable orthodontic appliance that functions by muscular action in order to try and influence growth of the jaws, e.g. Andresen, Fraenkel. *Orthodontic a.* Device used to apply forces to the teeth and their supporting structures to produce changes in the relationship of the teeth and their positions. Used to carry out active or passive phases of orthodontic treatment. *Pre-adjusted a.* When the fixed appliance bracket slot is machined to incorporate the tip, torque and 'in-out' that was conventionally bent into the archwire, so simplifying fixed orthodontic technique. *Rickett's a.* A pre-adjusted edgewise appliance. *Twin block a.* A two-piece myofunctional appliance.

applicator Small ball-ended hand instrument used to apply medicaments and cements.

approximal (proximal) Situated close together. *A. cavity.* Cavity involving a mesial and/or distal surface of a tooth. *A. surface.* Adjacent surfaces of teeth in the same dental arch. Usually the mesial surface of one tooth and the distal surface of the next. In the case of the two central incisors, the mesial surfaces of each tooth. Also called *interstitial* or *interproximal surfaces.* The adjectives 'proximal' and 'interproximal' are deprecated.

apron spring Orthodontic fine wire spring, wound on a heavy gauge wire or bow and suspended beneath it to produce a force to move teeth.

aqua Latin word meaning water.

aqueous Watery. Prepared with water.

arch Structure or structures having a regular curved form. *A. bar fixation.* Surgical technique for immobilizing a fractured mandible or maxilla, by bending a metal bar to conform to the buccal and labial surfaces of the teeth and attaching the bar to the teeth by soft stainless steel wire ligatures passed around the necks of the teeth. *Dental a.* Bow-shaped arrangement of the mandibular and maxillary teeth.

archwire In orthodontics, a length of fine wire contoured to the dental arch and fitting into brackets or other orthodontic attachments on the buccal or labial aspects of the teeth.

arcon articulator *See* articulator.

area A limited space.

areola 1. Any small space in a tissue. 2. Reddish round ring around an inflammatory lesion on the skin. 3. Brownish or pink area around the nipple of a breast. 4. That part of the iris surrounding the pupil of the eye.

areolae Plural of areola.

areolar Relating to or resembling an areola.

Arkansas stone Especially hard stone used for sharpening metal instruments such as excavators and enamel chisels.

armamentarium The instruments, materials and equipment necessary to carry out an operation.

arrhythmia Any variation from the normal rhythm of the heart.

arrow head clasp *See* Adams' clasp.

arterial Pertaining to an artery or arteries.

arteriole A minute arterial branch.

arteriosclerosis Group of diseases associated with thickening and loss of elasticity of artery walls. Hardening of the arteries results in a reduced blood flow which may impair the efficiency of any organ.

arteritis Inflammation of small vessels and minute arteries.

artery Vessel through which blood passes from the heart to the body. It has three coats: an inner (tunica intima) consisting of one cell thickness; a middle coat (tunica media) containing elastic tissue; and an outer coat (tunica adventitia) containing fibrous tissue. An artery, when divided, spurts bright red blood and does not collapse. Larger arteries can be felt to pulsate in time with the heart beats. *Alveolar a.* Posterior superior to the upper jaw and teeth, posterior inferior to the lower jaw and teeth. *A. forceps. See* forceps. *Buccal a.* To the cheeks. *Carotid a.* (internal and external). Main artery to the head arteries. *Coronary a.* Supplies the heart muscle. *Dental a.* Anterior, posterior and inferior; supply the jaws and teeth. *Facial a.* To the face. *Labial a.* (inferior and superior) To the lower and upper lips. *Lingual a.* To the tongue. *Maxillary a.* (external and internal) To the maxilla.

Nasopalatine a. To the palate. *Sublingual a.* To the tongue. *Submental a.* To the mylohyoid muscle, the submandibular and the sublingual salivary glands and the skin around the chin.

arthritic Relating to arthritis.

arthritis Inflammation of a joint. *Osteo a.* Chronic inflammation of a joint occurring mainly in old age, mostly in males, affecting one or several joints and producing pain, stiffness, deformity and lack of joint function. Generally resulting from old injury, trauma and disease. The condition is visible on radiographs. *Rheumatoid a.* Inflammatory disorder of the connective tissue affecting multiple joints. Of unknown cause, it commences in early adult life and is more prevalent in females. Common sites are finger and foot joints which become stiff, swollen and painful. Also found in the temporomandibular joint. Its course is not steady, with periods of remission.

arthro- Prefix denoting a relationship to a joint or joints.

arthrodesis Surgical fusion of a joint.

arthrography The technique of examining a joint, such as the TMJ, by means of radiography.

arthroplasty The surgical reconstruction of a joint by the use of a prosthesis.

arthrotomy Surgical incision or opening into a joint.

articaine (carticaine, Septanest®) An amide local anaesthetic that is used in dental local anaesthesia. It is presented as a 4% solution with epinephrine (adrenaline) as a vasoconstrictor at a concentration of 1:100,000 or 1:200,000.

articular Concerning a joint. *A. cartilage.* Protective cover of cartilage over bone surfaces forming a joint. *A. system.*

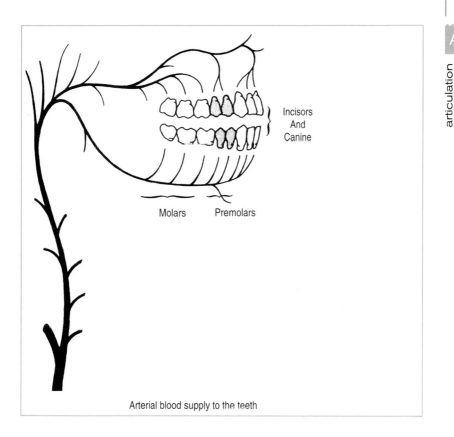

Incisors
And
Canine

Molars   Premolars

Arterial blood supply to the teeth

Body system concerned with the joints and bones of the locomotory system.

articulate 1. Capable of expressing oneself clearly. 2. To join, to unite by joints. 3. In dentistry, to place the teeth in their correct relationship with respect to each other.

articulated Connected by a joint.

articulating paper Strip of paper coated with pigment used for marking areas of contact between opposing teeth.

articulation 1. The enunciation of words to produce speech. 2. The point or type of contact between two skeletal elements. 3. In dentistry, the contact existing between opposing teeth of the maxilla and the mandible while the mandible is moving. *Anatomical a.* The rigid or movable function of two or more bones. *Anterior protected a.* A protected arrangement of the teeth in which the vertical and horizontal overlap of the anterior teeth disengages the posterior teeth in all mandibular excursive movements. *Balanced a. See* occlusion. *Canine protected a.* An arrangement of the canine teeth that prevents posterior tooth contact or lateral eccentric mandibular movements. *Edge-to-edge a.* Articulation of the anterior teeth along their incisal edges. *Free a.* Condition where the dental articulation is not obstructed by any cuspal interference. *Functional a.* The tooth contacts occurring between the maxillary and mandibular teeth during mastication and deglutition.

articulator Mechanical device to which models of the upper and lower arches are attached and which reproduces recorded positions of the mandible in relation to the maxilla. Assists in the study of occlusion and the construction of prostheses and restorations. *Adjustable a.* Articulator used by the dental technician, which can be adjusted to accommodate the many positions and movements of the mandible relative to the maxilla as recorded in the mouth. *Anatomical a.* Articulator which attempts to reproduce the normal movements of the jaw during mastication. *Arcon a.* An articulator which differs from the usual anatomical articulator in that the condylar analogue is in the mandibular portion of the articulator and the condylar track in the maxillary component. *Hinge* or *plane line a.* Articulator with a simple hinge joint preventing any lateral or sliding movement. *Plasterless a.* A fixed plate articulator that allows models to be grasped, controlling the correct occlusion without the need for plasterwork. *Semi-adjustable a.* An articulator that allows adjustments that reproduce mandibular movements in a sagittal plane only.

artificial Not natural. *A. respiration.* Process of forcing air—with or without added oxygen—into and out of the lungs in order to start the natural cycle of breathing, or to stimulate it when it has failed. Any obstruction of the airway must first be removed. *A. stone.* High-strength model and die material, based on calcium sulphate, used during the construction of crowns and special prostheses. *A. saliva DPF.* An oral spray useful in saliva deficiency and dry mouth (xerostomia). Trade names Luborant®, Glandosane®, Saliva Orthana®.

asbestos A fibrous, non-flammable silicate mineral previously used in casting operations in the laboratory and in certain dressings. Inhalation of asbestos dust causes lung inflammation therefore use now restricted and controlled.

ascorbic acid (vitamin C) Water-soluble vitamin essential for maintaining the integrity of cell walls and healthy connective tissue. Used to promote wound healing and to prevent scurvy (q.v.). Taken in tablet form. Present in many fruits, especially citrus fruits and vegetables, it is an essential element of the diet.

asepsis Free of infectious micro-organisms.

aseptic Free from infectious or septic material. Sterile. *A. technique.* Method of work, involving the use of sterile instruments, employed to reduce the possibility of introducing infectious micro-organisms

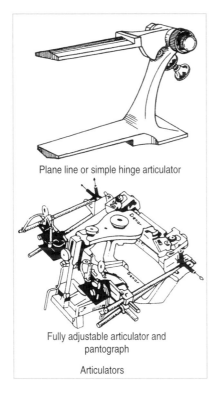

Plane line or simple hinge articulator

Fully adjustable articulator and pantograph

Articulators

into the tissues or bloodstream during a surgical procedure.

aspartame Intense sweetener with approx. 180 times the sweetness of sucrose. Commonly used in low calorie soft drinks. *See* sweetener.

aspect The direction in which an object faces.

asphyxia Suffocation. Life-threatening condition caused by the failure of oxygen to reach the lungs, due to obstruction or damage to any part of the respiratory system.

aspirate To withdraw fluids from the body by means of syphonage apparatus.

aspirating syringe *See* syringe.

aspiration 1. Withdrawal by suction (a negative pressure) of air, fluid or debris from any cavity of the body. 2. The act of drawing in breath.

aspirator Apparatus producing a high volume, low vacuum suction. When fitted with an *a. tip*, it may be used to remove fluids, blood, saliva and debris from the mouth, and to assist in keeping the operator's mouth mirror clear.

aspirin *See* acetylsalicylic acid.

assay Testing or determination of the purity of a metal.

asthma Allergy condition causing difficulty in breathing. Attacks may be brought on by hypersensitivity to foreign substances or emotional upsets.

astringent 1. Drug which shrinks tissues and/or arrests or restricts secretion, discharge or haemorrhage. 2. In dentistry, agent used to contract gingival tissue away from a crown preparation in order to facilitate impression taking.

asymmetrical Unable to be divided into two equal parts. Not equally balanced.

ataxia Failure to co-ordinate muscles, resulting in irregular jerky movements. Staggering.

atheroma Disease of an artery when its lumen is narrowed by cholesterol deposits which later become fibrotic and calcified.

atomizer Device which breaks down and projects liquids in the form of a fine spray.

atonic Weak. Referring to muscles without normal tone.

atria Plural of atrium.

Atridox® *See* controlled delivery device.

atrium (auricle) Semantically, an 'entrance hall' or 'vestibule'. In anatomy, a cavity into which one or more cavities open. One of the two upper chambers of the heart which pump blood through the heart valves into the ventricles.

atrophic Relating to atrophy.

atrophied Relating to atrophy, shrunken.

atrophy Wasting, emaciation. Diminution in size and function due to lack of use, disease or destruction of the nerve or blood supply to the tissues.

atropine Drug extracted from the plant belladonna. Used with premedication before surgery to inhibit respiratory and gastric secretions and to assist in relaxing muscles.

attached gingiva That part of the gingiva which is attached to the underlying bone and cementum of the teeth.

attachment 1. The means by which two objects are fastened to each other. 2. Colloquialism for a precision attachment (q.v.). 3. Deprecated term describing any clasp, crown or inlay used to attach a partial prosthesis to a natural tooth. *New a.* A reunion of connective tissue with a root surface deprived of its periodontal ligament.

attenuation In radiology, the process by which a beam of radiation is reduced in energy when it passes through matter.

attrition Loss of tooth substance or of a restoration as a result of mastication or of occlusal or approximal contact between the teeth.

atypical Not typical. Not conforming to the expected type. *A. facial pain.* A deep, unilateral aching pain. Often described as a burning pain and usually of unknown aetiology.

audioanalgesia *See* analgesia.

audit The systematic appraisal of the implementation and outcome of any process in the context of prescribed targets and standards. *Clinical a.* The process by which medical and dental staff collectively review, evaluate and improve their practice. This includes (a) the access of patients to care (appointments, investigations, admissions, waiting times), (b) the process and outcome of care and (c) the administrative and financial constraints relevant to clinical practice.

auditory Concerned with hearing.

AUG (acute ulcerative gingivitis) *See* gingivitis.

Augmentin® *See* co-amoxiclav.

aura Premonition or warning of an impending attack such as a person suffering from epilepsy might experience.

aural Concerning the ear.

auricle *See* atrium.

auriculotemporal syndrome *See* Frey's syndrome.

auscultation An aid to diagnosis by listening and interpreting sounds produced within the body.

auto transplant To transplant a body part within the same individual. Commonly used in association with auto transplantation of teeth within a patient.

autoclave *See* sterilizer.

autogenous Self-generated. *A. graft. See* graft. *A. vaccine.* Vaccine made from organisms already infecting the patient.

autograft *See* graft.

auto-immune disease Any disease believed to be caused, in part, by a hypersensitivity reaction of the host tissues.

auto-immunity Akin to allergy, where certain factors within the body tissues develop autogenic properties, so causing the formation of antibodies.

automatic amalgam condenser Powered handpiece used on amalgam which has just been packed into a prepared cavity, in order to attain condensation and adaptation. It produces a series of percussions variable in speed.

automatic mallet Hand-operated spring-loaded mallet used to condense gold foil; a rarely used technique.

autonomic Self-governing, functionally independent. *A. nervous system.* Independent body system which is self-controlling and cannot be consciously governed. Concerned with body functions such as glandular activity, digestion and the activity of involuntary muscles. These activities continue during sleep.

autopolymerizing resin *See* resin.

avascular Having no blood supply.

avitaminosis Disease resulting from lack of vitamins, e.g. rickets (vitamin D deficiency) or scurvy (vitamin C deficiency).

avulsion Traumatic removal of a tooth from its socket.

axial Relating to an axis.

axis Central line around which a body may rotate. *Condylar a. See* intercondylar a. *Hinge a. See* transverse horizontal a. *Intercondylar a.* A hypothetical line joining the rotation centres of the condyles. *Longitudinal a. See* sagittal a. *Sagittal a.* An imaginary anteroposterior line about which the mandible may rotate through a frontal plane. *Terminal hinge a. See* transverse horizontal a. *Transverse horizontal a.* (Hinge a., Terminal hinge a.) An imaginary line about which the mandible rotates on its condyles during opening and closing without any sideways movement. *Vertical a.* A hypothetical line around which the mandible rotates in the horizontal plane.

axon Elongated process of a nerve cell or neurone which links up with another through its dendrites. It is an extension of the nerve cell body and conducts nerve impulses away from the cell.

AZT Azidothymidine (Retrovir®). A drug used to lengthen the median incubation period of HIV virus (q.v.).

bacillary Relating to bacilli or other rod shaped forms.

bacilli Plural of bacillus.

bacillus A rod shaped bacterium. Previous use as a suffix to define a disease causing micro-organism, e.g. typhoid bacillus, tubercle bacillus and tetanus bacillus, is now archaic terminology. *Bacillus.* A genus of bacteria characteristically Gram positive and spore forming, ubiquitous in nature and commonly found in soil. Some species are pathogenic, e.g. *B. cereus* (food poisoning) and *B. anthracis* (anthrax).

background radiation Radiation that is always present, arising from natural sources.

backing Metal component of a crown, bridge or denture designed to protect a tooth coloured facing (usually of porcelain).

backscatter That portion of scattered radiation that is deflected at an angle greater than 90° from the central X-ray beam.

bacteraemia Condition in which bacteria are present in the blood stream. The condition may be transient, intermittent or continuous. In rare cases a bacteraemia may develop into a septicaemia or an endocarditis. In dentistry, many dental procedures can cause a low grade, transient bacteraemia which is not normally a significant hazard.

bacteria Single celled prokaryotic micro organisms belonging to the taxonomic kingdom Monera. They are ubiquitous with some species capable of living in extreme environmental conditions. Many are symbiotic or pathogenic in plants and animals but most are not normally harmful to humans although they may cause disease under certain conditions. *Pathogenic b.* are overtly harmful. Some bacteria can exist for years in a dormant state as *spores* which enable survival in unfavourable conditions. Spores are significantly more resistant to heat and chemical disinfectants than the normal, vegetative, form of bacteria.

bacterial endocarditis (sub-acute) Condition now generally known as *infective endocarditis.* Inflammation of the lining membrane of the heart, especially that of the heart valves, and generally associated with *Streptococcus viridans*, which may have been released into the bloodstream. Inflammatory changes result in deposits of fibrin and blood platelets (called vegetations) on the heart valve surfaces. Antibiotics are mandatory when patients with a history of this condition undergo dental treatment involving the possible release of bacteria into the bloodstream, e.g. extractions, scaling, trauma or surgery to the gingival tissues.

bactericidal Destructive to bacteria.

bactericide Physical, chemical or biological agent that destroys micro-organisms.

bacteriology The scientific study of bacteria.

bacteriostat An agent which inhibits the growth and multiplication of bacteria.

bake Process by which porcelain restorations are hardened by heating at electrically controlled temperatures generally in a vacuum furnace, the vacuum reducing the possibility of air bubbles. The porcelain is first baked to a biscuit (q.v.) state and then glazed at a higher temperature.

balance 1. A condition of equilibrium. 2. Apparatus to accurately weigh materials and metals such as gold.

balanced occlusion *See* occlusion.

balancing contacts *See* non-working side contacts.

balancing extraction Extraction of a tooth, following the removal of one from the contralateral side or opposite arch, in order to balance space loss, prevent drift from the midline and hopefully preserve symmetry of the dental arch.

balancing side Side opposite to the working side (q.v.) of the natural or artificial dentition.

balsam (Peru balsam) Aromatic herbal gum used in Whitehead's varnish, in some zinc oxide-eugenol cements and in root canal sealers.

band A stainless steel metal ring formed to the circumference of a tooth, most commonly used to retain orthodontic brackets on molar teeth. *B. contouring pliers. See* pliers. *B. pusher* (or *driver*). Instrument used to adapt and place a stainless steel band on a tooth. *B. seater.* Flat-bladed instrument used to push bands onto a tooth by biting force. *B. splitting pliers. See* pliers. *Matrix b. See* matrix band. *Orthodontic b. See* orthodontic band. *Preformed b.* Seamless stainless steel band manufactured in varying sizes and shapes in order to fit intimately around the crowns of teeth involved in fixed appliance orthodontic treatment.

bar In prosthetics, a metal segment of greater length than width that is used to connect two parts of a removable partial denture. A bar attached to two or more teeth or roots in order to support and retain a complete or partial denture, e.g. *B. attachment.* A bar joining two or more roots, teeth or implant superstructures and supporting or retaining a prosthesis. *B. connector.* In prosthetics, a bar joining two or more parts of a partial denture. Dolder bar (q.v.), lingual bar (q.v.). *See also* connector.

barbed broach Endodontic hand instrument with barbs pointing towards the handle. Used mainly for removal of vital pulp tissue, cotton wool and other materials from the pulp space. Synonym: nerve broach.

barbiturate One of a group of general anaesthetic, sedative, hypnotic and tranquillizing drugs which affect the brain centres without causing loss of consciousness. Designed to lessen anxiety before operations (premedication). Prescribed in tablet form. When taking these drugs, the patient should not drink alcohol or drive a vehicle, e.g. pento-barbitone.

barrel That part of a syringe which holds the cartridge of solution to be injected.

basal The base portion. In physiology, refers to the lowest possible level. *B. bone.* See bone. *B. cell carcinoma.* See rodent ulcer. *B. metabolic rate (BMR).* Measurement of the rate at which foods are digested and modified for tissue building and repair, and waste products are produced by the body.

basal cell carcinoma Carcinoma of the basal cells of the skin or epidermis. Rare before middle age and usually found on the face, especially in fair-skinned people persistently exposed to hot sun. Treatment is by excision or radiation.

base 1. The foundation on which something is attached or rests. 2. The principal ingredient of a compound. 3. In chemistry, a substance which contains a hydroxyl group—OH, e.g. sodium hydroxide. 4. In dentistry, that part of a removable prosthesis in contact with the tissues and which supports the artificial teeth. *B. metal alloy.* Alloy containing cobalt, chromium and nickel, in varying quantities. Used in conservative and prosthetic dentistry as an inexpensive alternative to the noble metal alloys. *Cavity b.* See cavity. *Metal b.* The swaged or cast metallic portion of a denture base (q.v.) onto which is attached the resin portion of the denture and the artificial teeth.

baseplate 1. Temporary foundation on which an occlusal rim is built or on which a trial denture is set up. Consists of a combination of waxes and resins

or acrylic. 2. The acrylic resin part of a removable orthodontic appliance, fitting to the necks of standing teeth and the mucosa, and securing in position any springs, wires or clasps.

basion Central part of the anterior margin of the foramen magnum (q.v.).

basket crown Cast-metal three-quarter crown used as a temporary restoration for a fractured or malformed tooth.

basophil One of the five types of white blood cells having a granular cytoplasm and a nucleus of two or three lobes occupying about half of the cell and containing histamine and heparin. Little is known about these cells, which are not very motile.

Bass appliance See appliance.

bayonet forceps See forceps.

BCG Abbreviation for bacille Calmette–Guérin. The base of an immunizing vaccine against tuberculosis.

bd Abbreviation of Latin phrase 'bis dic', twice a day. Used in prescription writing.

BDHA British Dental Hygienists' Association.

beam diameter Maximum diameter of the X-ray beam of radiation measured at the cone end of the apparatus.

beam guiding instrument (position indicating device or PID) Apparatus used in intra-oral radiography to align the X-ray beam onto a film held in a film holder. In the paralleling technique, the apparatus ensures that the central beam strikes the teeth at right angles to their long axis and the film at right angles to its plane.

beam size The dimensions of the X-ray beam at the cone end of the apparatus.

beechwood creosote Antiseptic and mildly analgesic liquid consisting of a mixture of cresol, guaicol and other phenols, previously used for the disinfection of the necrotic radicular pulp primarily in non-vital pulpotomies in the primary dentition. This technique is no longer commonly used.

Begg technique Fixed orthodontic technique developed by Dr P. R. Begg and first described in the 1950s. Uses light wires (and hence light forces) in a modified ribbon arch attachment.

Bell's palsy *See* palsy.

benign Describes a tumour that is not malignant, e.g. papilloma. It does not destroy the tissues from which it originates, nor spread to other parts of the body. Generally recurrence is unlikely following excision.

Bennett angle Angle formed by the sagittal plane and the path of the advancing condyle during lateral mandibular movement, as viewed in the horizontal plane.

Bennett movement (or shift) Lateral shift of the condyles and articular discs during a lateral excursion of the mandible.

benzocaine Analgesic used topically in the form of lozenges, sprays or pastes to relieve the pain of ulcers in the mouth, prior to local anaesthetic injections and to facilitate the taking of impressions in those patients who are inclined to retch.

benzodiazepines A group of drugs useful as anxiolytics (q.v.), hypnotics (q.v.) and anticonvulsants. They have fewer side-effects than barbiturates and are less dangerous in overdosage. However, dependence and tolerance to their effect occur and, thus, they should not be prescribed indiscriminately.

benzoyl peroxide Catalyst for chemically/self/auto-curing fissure sealants.

benzylpenicillin (penicillin G) The first of the penicillins. Injected intramuscularly, to provide a rapid, high concentration in the bloodstream from which it is soon excreted.

beriberi A deficiency disease associated with an imbalance between the intake of carbohydrates and thiamine (vitamin B_1).

betametasone (Betnesol®) A corticosteroid sometimes used in the management of inflammatory conditions of the oral mucosa. It is taken either as a tablet or by dissolving the tablet in water to use as an oral rinse.

Betnesol® *See* betametasone.

bevel The angle that one line makes with another when not at right angles. In dentistry, the inclined edge or surface of a cutting instrument or cavity preparation.

bi- Prefix meaning two or, exceptionally, indicative of the presence of hydrogen in a molecule, e.g. bicarbonate.

bicuspid 1. The mitral valve of the heart situated between the atrium and the ventricle. 2. Premolar tooth, i.e. having two cusps.

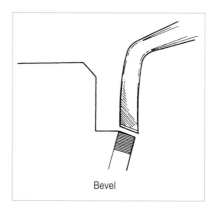

Bevel

bifid tongue Developmental defect resulting from the incomplete fusion of portions of the tongue along the midline.

bifurcation Division into two branches. Division where one structure divides into two, such as the junction of the two roots of the lower molar teeth or where a blood vessel divides into two.

bilateral Occurring on two sides.

bile Liquid product of the liver, golden brown in colour and stored in the gallbladder. It breaks down and assists in the absorption of fats, aids digestion and prevents putrefaction of the contents of the intestines.

bimaxillary Strictly, pertaining to the left and right maxilla. Loosely used (particularly in orthodontics) to describe an affectation, relationship or connection between the maxilla and the mandible. *B. protrusion.* Forward projection or prognathism of both jaws, the alveolar processes and the teeth, beyond normal limits in relation to the cranial base.

binangled Describes hand instruments, such as some enamel chisels, in which the shank has two angles. The cutting edge is placed at right angles to the long axis of the handle.

bio- Prefix meaning life.

biochemistry The study of the chemistry of living organisms and the substances involved in their metabolism. Physiological chemistry.

biofilm A collection of micro-organisms which excrete extracellular polymeric substances, or sticky polymers, which hold the biofilm together. The biofilm is attached to either an inert or living surface. Examples are the slime inside a water pipe and dental plaque.

biological width Collective term to describe the overall dimension of the junctional epithelium and dento-gingival connective tissue attachment. Range 2-4 mm in health.

biology The study of the structure, function and organization of living organisms.

biomaterials Synthetic, pharmacologically inert and non-toxic substances designed for implantation and incorporation in the human body.

bionator *See* appliance.

biopsy Microscopical study of a piece of tissue which has been removed from the body in order to decide whether a pathological condition exists. Employed as an aid to diagnosis. *Excisional b.* Complete removal of a lesion for histological examination. *Incisional b.* Partial removal of a lesion for histological examination.

BIPP *See* bismuth iodoform paraformaldehyde paste.

bird beak pliers *See* pliers.

biscuit In dentistry, describes the state of porcelain after it has been baked in a furnace once before being glazed. *See also* bake.

bisect To cut into two parts.

bisecting angle technique In radiology, technique in which the beam of radiation is directed perpendicularly towards an imaginary line which bisects the angle formed by the plane of the film and the long axis of the tooth. *See* Appendix 10.

bisection Division into two parts by cutting. Also called *hemisection.*

bis-GMA (Bowen's resin) Bisphenol-A-glycidyl methacrylate. Short polymer commonly associated with dental restorative materials and dentine adhesives. It is an extremely viscous liquid and is thinned with diluent monomers

29

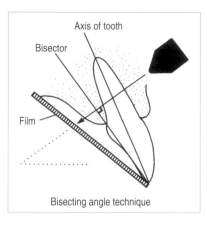

Axis of tooth

Bisector

Film

Bisecting angle technique

such as TEGDMA (triethylene-glycol dimethacrylate).

bismuth iodoform paraformalde-hyde paste (BIPP) Yellow paste previously used as a dressing following some surgical procedures.

bite 1. Loose term for occlusion. 2. Registration of the occlusion by the use of wax or other material. 3. In orthodontics, term describing various classifications of occlusion. *Anterior open b.* Occlusion where the mandibular incisors are not overlapped in the vertical plane by the maxillary incisors and do not occlude with them when the posterior teeth are in occlusion. *B. block.* Deprecated term commonly used to describe a block of wax used to determine the occlusal relationship of the jaws during the construction of a prosthesis. The preferred term is *occlusal rim. B. guard.* Deprecated term for occlusal overlay appliance (q.v.). *B. plane.* Acrylic resin orthodontic appliance covering all of the upper teeth and retained by wire clasps. *B. raising appliance.* Deprecated term for occlusal overlay appliance (q.v.). *B. registration material. See* wax, bite. *B. rehabilitation. See* rehabilitation. *B. wax. See* wax. *B. wing radiograph.* Intra-oral radiograph showing both upper and lower teeth in occlusion on the same film. The film is held in position by a holder or tab, on which the patient closes the teeth during exposure. The developed radiograph shows the presence of caries, overhanging edges of restorations, calculus and the level of the alveolar bone crests. *Check b.* (or *check record*). Thin wax rim used to record an occlusion. Often has a thin soft metal foil embedded in it. Warmed before use and chilled afterwards. *Cross-b.* Uni- or bilateral malocclusion involving one or more teeth in each dental arch. *Edge-to-edge b. See* articulation. *Open b.* Condition in which some teeth do not occlude when others are in occlusion. *Posterior open b.* Condition where some of the posterior teeth do not meet on occlusion.

black copper cement Zinc phosphate type of cement containing black copper oxide which gives the cement its characteristic black colour. Formerly used in the restoration of deciduous teeth and in the cementation of metal splints and orthodontic bands.

black hairy tongue (nigrities) *See* tongue.

black lead *See* graphite.

Black's classification of cavities Historical classification of tooth cavities according to the site of origin of the carious process. *Class 1:* Any simple occlusal, palatal or lingual cavity in molar or premolar teeth such as carious pits and fissures. *Class 2:* SIMPLE—Any mesial or distal carious cavity in molar and premolar teeth. COMPOUND—Simple cavity but also involving another surface. *Class 3:* Cavity in the mesial or distal surfaces of canines and incisors but not involving the incisal angle. *Class 4:* Cavity in the mesial or distal surfaces of canines or incisors also involving the incisal angle. *Class 5:* Cavity in the

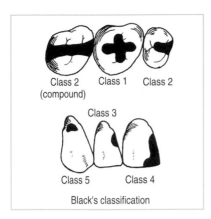

Class 2 Class 1 Class 2
(compound)

Class 3

Class 5   Class 4

Black's classification

gingival third of the labial, buccal, lingual or palatal surface of any tooth. Does not classify recurrent or root surface lesions.

Blake's universal gingivectomy knife *See* periodontal instruments.

blanch To become pale or lose colour, due to fear, cold, strong emotion or as a result of illness.

bland Mild, soothing; not irritant.

bleaching Removal of stains or colour by chemicals. In dentistry, the elimination or reduction of discoloration of the crown of a tooth by the temporary application of bleaching agents such as hydrogen peroxide. The process may be accelerated by the action of heat or ultra-violet light.

bleeder Lay term for a haemophiliac. Often used to describe a patient with an abnormal bleeding time (q.v.).

bleeding Lay term for haemorrhage. *Bleeding on Probing Index (BoP). See* Index, Bleeding on Probing.

bleeding time Time taken for oozing of blood to cease following a finger prick—normally 3–4 minutes.

blind abscess *See* abscess.

block *See* analgesia.

blood Red sticky fluid which circulates through the heart and blood vessels, carrying nutrient materials and oxygen to all body tissues and waste products and carbon dioxide away from the tissues. There are millions of corpuscles (blood cells) floating in the blood plasma. The red cells (erythrocytes) contain haemoglobin which gives the blood its red colour. They carry oxygenated blood together with an antigen known as the rhesus factor. Erythrocytes are formed in the bone marrow of children and certain long bones in the adult. The life of an erythrocyte is normally 4 months, after which it is destroyed in the liver or spleen, its iron content being saved for further use. The white cells (leucocytes), which are far fewer in number, are concerned with the body's defences against invading micro-organisms. Their number increases considerably in the presence of infection. Blood platelets (thrombocytes) are concerned with the blood clotting mechanism. *B. count.* Calculation of the number of blood cells per cubic millimetre, using a microscope to view a sample drop. *B. group system.* System of classification of the various inherited types of human blood. In a blood transfusion, the blood group of the recipient must be of the same blood group, or a compatible group, as that of the donor, so as to prevent a severe and possibly fatal reaction. There are four main human blood groups: A, B, AB and O. Group AB is a universal recipient from all of the other groups. *B. plasma.* Fluid portion of the blood. Consists mostly of water (92%), containing proteins, salts, hormones, waste products, nutrients, clotting agents and antibodies. *B. pressure.* Pressure maintained in the circulation, by the pumping action of the heart, the elasticity of the vessel walls, the viscosity and volume of the blood, and the capillary resistance. *B. serum.* Clear, yellowish fluid which separates from the blood when clotting takes place. Blood plasma from which fibrinogen has been removed during the clotting process. *B. vessels.* Composed of arteries, veins and capillaries. The smaller arteries are called *arterioles* and the smaller veins *venules.*

BLS Basic life support.

blunt dissection Separation of tissues by the use of a blunt instrument.

BMR *See* basal metabolic rate.

BNF British National Formulary. A compendium of all the drugs available for prescription in the United Kingdom including useful appendices covering drug interactions and prescribing for medically compromised patients.

Bocosan® *See* sodium perborate.

boiling-out Term used in the construction of dentures. The action of placing a flask (q.v.) in boiling water in order to separate it into two halves and thus enable the dental technician to wash out the melted wax, leaving the denture teeth embedded in the plaster.

bolus Rounded mass of solid or semi-solid food, formed by the action of the tongue, teeth and palate, during mastication, and ready to be swallowed.

bonded crown Jacket crown in which porcelain is fused to a platinum–gold

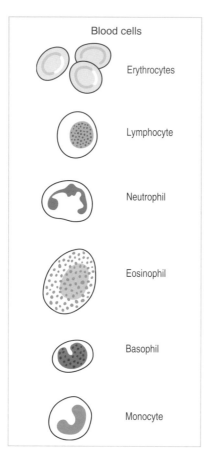

Blood cells

Erythrocytes

Lymphocyte

Neutrophil

Eosinophil

Basophil

Monocyte

Individual's blood group	Blood group of people from whom individual can receive blood	Blood group of people to whom individual can give blood
A	A, O	A, AB
B	B, O	B, AB
AB	A, B, AB, O	AB
O	O	A, B, AB, O

matrix which forms the fitting surface of the restoration.

bonded retainer *See* retainer.

bonding Binding together, e.g. porcelain to gold or other metal, or certain filling materials to tooth enamel. *B. resin. See* resin bonding.

bone Dense connective tissue impregnated with calcium salts and forming the skeleton. It has an outer, harder layer—*compact b.*, and an inner network—*cancellous b.*, containing red bone marrow. Microscopic study reveals systems of small canals (haversian canals) containing blood vessels, a small amount of delicate connective tissue, nerve filaments and lymphatics. The outer aspect of bone is covered by a thin layer of fibrous tissue called *periosteum*, which provides a rich blood supply to the underlying bone. Bone provides attachment for the muscles of the body to allow movement, protects the soft organs such as the brain, eyes, lungs, etc. and supports the body. New red blood cells are produced from bone marrow. *Alveolar b.* Tooth-bearing portion of the bone of the jaw, forming the alveolar process. Develops with the eruption of the teeth and is resorbed when the teeth are lost. *Basal b.* That part of the maxilla or mandible which underlies the alveolar process. *B. chisel.* Bone cutting instrument which has a flat blade with a square bevelled end. *B. cutting forceps. See* forceps. *B. nibbling forceps. See* forceps. *B. file.* Hand instrument, mostly double ended, with serrated cutting blades. Used to smooth irregular bone edges. *B. gouge.* Hand instrument similar to a bone chisel but having a hollowed-out blade similar to a Coupland chisel (q.v.). *B. graft.* Transplantation of healthy bone to replace missing or diseased bone. *B. rasp.* Hand instrument

similar to a b. file, having a large number of independently formed teeth on its blade. Used to smooth irregular bone. *B. shears.* Similar to bone cutting forceps. *Bundle b.* Bone lining the tooth socket into which are inserted Sharpey's fibres (q.v.). *Cancellous b. (the medulla).* Spongy, honeycomb-like bone which lies within the outer shell of compact bone (cortex). *Compact b.* Harder outer shell of bone sometimes called *cortical b. Skeletal b.* Basal bone of the skeleton on which other types of bone may be developed, e.g. alveolar bone. *Spongy b.* Inner part of bone composed of cancellous, spongy or porous bone (the medulla).

Bonjela paste® *See* choline salicylate dental paste.

BoP Bleeding on probing.

borax Common name for sodium tetraborate. Used in fluxes for soldering, or to retard the setting time of plaster of Paris.

borborygmus Gurgling and rumbling sound made by flatus moving in the intestine.

border A bounding line, edge or surface. *B. moulding.* Shaping of an impression material by the manipulation of the soft tissues adjacent to the borders of an impression. *B. movement.* Movement of the mandible along the extremity of its range in any direction. *B. seal. See* seal.

Botox® *See* botulinum A toxin.

botulinum A toxin (Botox®, **Dysport**®**)** A toxin used to counter the effects of excessive muscle activity. It has been used to reduce hypertrophy of the muscles in the facial region such as masseter. It has also been used in aesthetic surgery to reduce wrinkles.

bounded saddle That portion of a prosthesis which is limited by a natural tooth at each end.

bow Orthodontic wire bent to the shape of the dental arch in the incisor region. May be labial or lingual. Usually has U-loops for adjustment of the tension of the bow.

Bowen's resin *See* Bis-GMA.

box That part of a compound cavity, excluding the occlusal portion, which has four cavity surfaces. *B. tray. See* impression tray.

boxing (of an impression) Provision of a wall, usually of wax, to form a box around an impression to reduce time and effort in subsequently trimming and shaping plaster models. It is attached to the perimeter of the impression to contain the cast material until it has set.

boxing out In orthodontics, a recess created on the fitting surface of a removable appliance to allow for the movement of an active spring.

B-point Orthodontic cephalometric landmark defined as the position of the deepest concavity on the anterior profile of the mandibular synthesis.

BPE Basic periodontal examination.

bracing Resistance to the horizontal components of masticatory forces. *B. arm.* That portion of a partial denture designed to resist the action of lateral displacing force. Sometimes known as a *lateral resistive arm*.

bracket Metal, plastic or ceramic orthodontic component welded to an orthodontic band or cemented directly onto a tooth. Archwires or other orthodontic wires may be attached to it. *B. removing pliers. See* pliers. *B. table.* A swing table forming part of a dental unit (q.v.).

bradycardia Condition in which there is an abnormally slow heart beat.

brain That part of the central nervous system contained in and protected by the skull. It consists of the cerebellum (q.v.), the cerebrum (q.v.) and the brainstem—the medulla oblongata, midbrain and the pons varoli. The brain and spinal cord are enclosed in three membranes called the meninges and are made up of grey matter (q.v.) and white matter (q.v.).

brazing Method of joining metals (often confused with soldering) by drawing, by capillary action, a molten filler metal into the space between the surfaces of two metals held in close apposition.

bridge (fixed prosthesis) Prosthesis which replaces one or more clinical crowns of missing natural teeth. It is soldered or otherwise attached to one or more retainers such as a metal wing, crown or gold inlay, themselves cemented to abutment teeth roots or implants. It is not intended to be removed by the patient. *Adhesive b.* Generic term for a bridge dependent upon adhesive technology to allow metal wing(s) to be bonded to a minimally prepared retainer(s) (*see* Maryland b and Rochette b). *B. retainer.* Restoration cemented to an abutment tooth which provides retention for a bridge. *B. span.* That part of a bridge between two abutments. *B. unit.* Individual part of a bridge such as a pontic or a retainer. *Cantilever b.* A bridge in which the pontic has a bridge retainer or retainers at one end only. *Fixed-fixed b.* One piece bridge, the pontic or pontics being integral with the retainers at both ends. *Fixed-movable b.* The pontic (that part which replaces the missing tooth or teeth) is integral with a bridge retainer at one end only. At its other end it has a limited degree of movement controlled by the retainer at that end. Often called *fixed-free b.* (deprecated). *Maryland b.* A modification of the Rochette bridge where the fitting surface of the framework is electrolytically etched in order to enhance

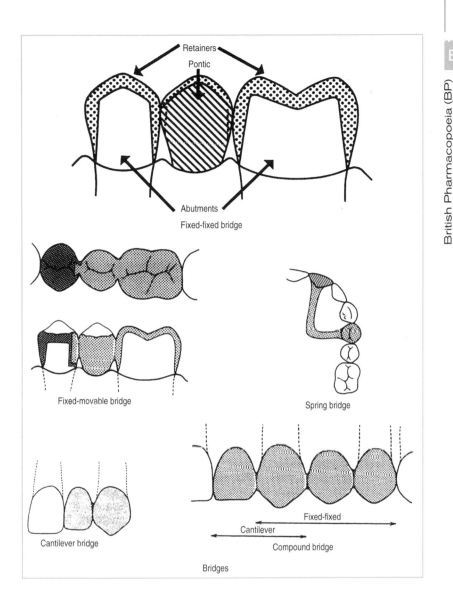

Retainers
Pontic
Abutments
Fixed-fixed bridge

Fixed-movable bridge

Spring bridge

Cantilever bridge

Fixed-fixed
Cantilever
Compound bridge

Bridges

the metal-composite-etched enamel bond. *Rochette b.* Type of small fixed bridge with perforated retainers at each end which are bonded by composite cements to neighbouring teeth following etching. Used to support or replace loose incisors for a limited period. *Spring cantilever b.* The remote pontic is integral with one end of a bar adapted to the underlying mucosa. *Temporary b.* Bridge made of temporary materials which is placed into position on bridge preparations during the period in which the definitive bridge is being constructed by the dental technician.

British Pharmacopoeia (BP) Authoritative list of drugs in general use, published under the auspices of the General Medical Council by HM Stationery Office. It lays down the strict standards for drugs and their dosage.

bronchial asthma Asthma (q.v.) resulting in gasping for breath because of spasm of the muscular walls of the bronchi. Often occurs in members of the same family. The cause is obscure and includes such factors as allergies to dust, pollens, face powders, certain foods and drugs, bronchial infections and mental distress.

bronchiole Smallest branch of the bronchus which terminates in the alveoli (or air sacs) of the lungs.

bronchitic Inclined to or suffering from bronchitis.

bronchitis Inflammation of the bronchi. May be acute or chronic.

bronchospasm Difficulty in breathing caused by spasm of the muscular walls of the bronchus, as in asthma or whooping cough.

bronchus Any part of the air passages from where the trachea bifurcates into right and left bronchi to the bronchioles in the lungs.

Browne's tube Small glass sterilizer control tube containing a red liquid which changes to green on reaching a certain temperature. This change indicates that the correct temperature has been reached, but is not proof of sterilization. The green spot tube is used in a dry heat sterilizer (q.v.), the black or yellow spot in steam sterilizers (q.v.).

bruise Discolouration of the tissues due to haemorrhage into them. A contusion.

bruxism The involuntary grinding or clenching of teeth. Often associated with stress or anxiety and frequently triggered by occlusal irregularities. Sequelae

to bruxism may include abnormal tooth wear patterns, joint or neuromuscular problems and periodontal breakdown.

buccal Term denoting the surfaces of premolars and molars facing towards the cheeks. Pertaining to or adjacent to the cheeks. *B. inlay. See* skin grafting vestibuloplasty. *B. retractor. See* retractor. *B. segment classification.* Anteroposterior relationships of the jaws classified according to the relationship of the lower molar teeth to the upper molar teeth, with particular reference to the first molars. *See* Angle's classification. *B. spring.* Orthodontic wire spring working from the buccal aspect of a tooth. *B. sulcus.* Fold in the oral tissues, by mucous membrane and bounded externally by the cheeks and internally by the teeth. *B. tube.* Tube usually attached to the buccal aspect of an orthodontic appliance in the molar region, through which a wire may pass.

buccinator muscle The cheek muscle. A thin flat muscle on the side of the face between the maxilla and the mandible.

buffer salt Chemical substance which, when present in a solution, allows only a slight change in reaction when an acid or alkali is added. Included in local analgesic solutions to maintain the acid/alkali balance compatible with blood and tissue cells.

bulbous Having the appearance of a bulb. Relating to a swelling.

BULL Buccal of upper; lingual of lower (cusps).

bulla Large vesicle or blister formed in or under the mucous membrane and containing a clear fluid.

bundle bone *See* bone.

bupivacaine (Marcain®) A long-acting amide local anaesthetic agent. When used as a regional block anaesthetic in dentistry it can provide up to 8 hours of local anaesthesia and is useful in the management of post-operative pain.

bur Rotary milling tool with sharp blades of various shapes, designed to fit into handpieces. Term also used for small rotary diamond instruments. Consists of a cutting portion (the head), the shaft which attaches the bur to the handpiece and a generally tapering shank which joins the head to the shaft. Burs of various shapes and sizes are used to prepare cavities and trim restorations. They may have long smooth shanks to be used in straight handpieces, or latch type with shorter shafts. They are made of steel and some may have hardened blades made of tungsten carbide (*TC b.*). There are also smaller, smooth shaft burs which are retained in the head of high-speed handpieces by friction grip (*FG b.*). There are three main types: 1. *Fissure b.* Cylindrical or tapered with flat or rounded ends and their blades may be cross-cut, e.g. *flat fissure b., X-cut fissure b., round-ended fissure b., tapered fissure b.* 2. *Inverted cone b. Round* or *(rosehead) b.* 3. In addition there are *Curson cavity* and *restoration finishing b.* of various shapes. *Wheel b., end-cutting b.* which has its cutting blades at its end only, used for cutting and smoothing shoulder preparations (q.v.). *Diamond b.* Round, cylindrical, tapered and a variety of other shapes. *Finishing b.* These burs

ØSchaft ØShank Øde tige Øde mango	Lange Length Longueur Longitud mm	inch	
2,35 mm	70,00.	2,75	Straight extra-long
2,35 mm	55,00–65,00	2,17–2,56	long
2,35 mm	44,50–50,00	1,75–1,97	standard
2,35 mm	25,00–38,00	0,98–1,50	short
2,35 mm	34,00	1,34	Contra-angle extra-long
2,35 mm	26,00–28,00	1,02–1,10	long
2,35 mm	21,00+22,00	0,83+0,87	standard
2,35 mm	16,00	0,63	miniature
1,60 mm	25,00	1,00	Friction grip extra-long
1,60 mm	21,00	0,83	long
1,60 mm	19,00	0,75	standard
1,60 mm	16,00	0,63	short

Bur dimensions

have smaller and more numerous blades, made in various shapes and sizes, e.g. round, flame, barrel, pear. *Miniature b.* Range of burs made to be used in miniature handpieces. *See also* Appendix 8.

Burkitt's tumour or lymphoma A rapidly growing malignant lymphosarcoma originally described in East African young children. It affects the jaws and the viscera and may be due to a virus.

burn Injury to tissues caused by sun, chemicals, friction, flame, heat, electricity or radiation.

burning mouth A burning sensation that affects the oral mucosa associated with a number of pathological conditions such as lichen planus, sensitivity reactions, geographic tongue and pernicious anaemia. The burning sensation can affect otherwise clinically normal oral mucosa and is then labelled '*burning mouth syndrome*'.

burnisher Hand instrument with rounded edges, used to polish or burnish the surface of metallic restorations by rubbing, e.g. *ball, beavertail, fishtail-shaped. Engine-driven b.* are also available.

burn-out 1. Elimination, by heat, of a wax or acrylic pattern from an investment which has set hard to form a mould into which a molten metal may be cast. *See also* 'Lost wax' process. 2. In radiography, an area of film with excessive blackening due to a relative overpenetration of the X-ray beam.

butt joint Joint in which two flat surfaces are brought together without overlapping.

button Excess metal remaining at the end of a sprue (q.v.) after casting.

BW Bitewing radiograph

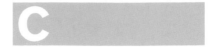

cachectic Pertaining to cachexia.

cachet Flat, rice-paper capsule used to enclose a drug of unpleasant taste.

cachexia Condition associated with chronic diseases characterized by general body decline, loss of weight and generalized weakness.

CAD/CAM Computer aided design/computer aided manufacture.

Caffey's disease (infantile cortical hyperostosis) Disease characterized by abnormal thickening of cortical bone, particularly the clavicles and the mandible.

cajuput *See* oil of cajuput.

calciferol Vitamin D_2. *See* vitamin.

calcific barrier Barrier or bridge of calcific material which may gradually form over an exposed pulp, or an open root-end in response to treatment. *See also* direct pulp cap, apexification. Synonym: dentine bridge.

calcification Process whereby calcium salts are deposited in specialized tissue. The condition may be normal, as in the formation of teeth or bone, or abnormal, as in hyperparathyroidism. Acids formed by plaque, and acid etchants, decalcify enamel tissue—a reverse process to calcification. *See* Appendix 2 for ages of calcification.

calcifying epithelial odontogenic tumour Uncommon neoplasm arising from odontogenic epithelium, and characterized by sheet-like arrangements of epithelium. Clinically it behaves like an ameloblastoma with regard to age, sex and distribution.

calcination To heat a substance in order to drive off any water, so leaving a calcined, dry powder, e.g. plaster of Paris.

calcium Greyish-white chemical element found in bones, teeth and blood. A metal which forms salts such as c. oxide and c. carbonate. A daily average of 500 mg is required in a normal diet; more is required during fevers, pregnancy, lactation and growth. Present in dairy products. The parathyroid glands secrete a hormone which regulates the calcium content of the blood at a constant level. *C. carbonate (chalk).* Salt of calcium which, when finely ground, is used as an abrasive in toothpastes and polishing agents. *C. hydroxide.* Salt of calcium used to encourage the formation of reparative dentine. The powder may be mixed with water to form a paste, or it may be obtained ready mixed in tubes. It is placed in deep cavities as a seal and a protective lining, or in direct contact with the pulp in endodontic procedures (*see* apexification). *C. sulphate.* Salt of calcium obtained by calcining naturally occurring gypsum. It yields two forms of hemihydrate: the alpha-hemihydrate forms the basis of artificial stone and the beta-hemihydrate forms plaster of Paris (POP). Both are used in the construction of dental models and as investing material.

calculus A stone. Generic term for any concretion occurring accidentally in the body. In dentistry, formerly known as *tartar* (lay term) or *calcarous deposit* and consisting of a hard deposit of mineralized plaque attached to the teeth. Depending on its location, relative to the gingival margin, it is described as *supragingival c.* or *subgingival c.* and, rarely, as *sub-* or *supra-marginal c.* In medicine, calculi may occur in any

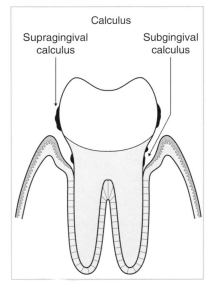

Calculus

Supragingival calculus   Subgingival calculus

reservoir organ or their passages, e.g. *biliary c.* (or gallstones), *renal c., salivary c.,* etc.

Caldwell–Luc operation Surgical procedure in which an opening is made above and posterior to the upper canine tooth through the maxillary sinus wall to either remove a displaced tooth/root or to effect drainage of the sinus and allow irrigation.

calibration 1. Determination of the diameter of a tube or cylindrical object. 2. Graduated marking of a measuring instrument from a given standard.

calipers Two-armed instrument, often with a scale attached, used for measuring length and, in special forms, the internal and external diameters of cylindrical bodies.

callus 1. Repair tissue which is deposited around the fractured ends of bones. A rudimentary type of new bone, soft at first, which in time hardens to prevent movement of the fractured ends of a bone. 2. Localized hyperplasia of the horny layer of the epithelium which has been subjected to pressure or friction.

calvaria Skull-cap, cranial vault or concha of cranium. The top of the skull made up of the frontal, parietal and occipital bones.

Camper's line *See* ala-tragal line.

camphorated paramonochlorophenol (CMCP) Medication used as a root canal dressing since the 19th century.

canal Narrow tubular passage.

canaliculus Extremely narrow tubular passage in bone. A minute canal through which tissue fluid and metabolites may pass.

cancer Malignant growth arising from epithelial cells. The term is commonly used to describe all malignant growths.

cancerous Relating to cancer.

cancrum oris Gangrenous stomatitis that may spread to the facial tissues. May occur in severely debilitated children.

candela (cd) The SI unit of luminous intensity and defined as the luminous intensity, in a given direction, of a source that emits monochromatic radiation of frequency 540×10^{12} hertz and that has a radian intensity in that direction of $1/683$ watt per steradian.

candelilla wax *See* wax.

Candida Genus of yeast-like fungi which causes candidiasis (moniliasis or thrush). *Candida albicans* is the most common aetiological agent, but numerous other *Candida* species may be implicated.

candidiasis Moniliasis or thrush. Acute or chronic infection due to the species *Candida*. Generally involves mucous membranes, as in oral thrush or as in vulvovaginitis, but may also affect the skin, heart or lungs.

canine Single cusped tooth having a relatively long root and a pronounced cingulum in the permanent dentition. In the primary dentition it lies distal to the lateral incisor and mesial to the first primary molar in each quadrant. In the permanent dentition it lies distal to the lateral incisor and mesial to the first permanent premolar in each quadrant. It is intended to tear and cut food. The permanent maxillary canine is the longest tooth. The crown of the lower canine is usually tilted lingually. The primary canines begin to calcify before birth, and erupt at about 18 months. Calcification is usually complete by 2½ years and the root starts to resorb at 7 years of age before being shed at 12 years. The permanent canines commence to calcify at 4–5 months and are complete on eruption at the age of 10–12. *C. eminence.* Ridge of bone on the maxilla covering the root of the canine. *C. fossa.* Depression on the external surface of the maxilla distal to the canine eminence. *C. guidance.* Directional guidance provided by the upper canine during lateral excursions of the mandible. *C. protected articulation. See* articulation.

cannula 1. Glass, polythene or metal tube, or a blunt needle used to effect communication between a body cavity and the exterior. 2. Teflon®-coated plastic needle used for administering intravenous drugs and fluids.

cantilever bridge *See* bridge.

cap A protective covering. Colloquialism for a full or partial replacement of a natural crown. *C. splint.* A cast-metal or acrylic resin splint fitting accurately over the crowns of natural teeth and cemented in place to immobilize a fractured jaw. *Skull c. See* skull.

capillary Very small blood vessel of single cell thickness, forming a connection between arterioles and venules.

Capillaries are found in dense networks all over the body and facilitate the exchange of nutrients, waste products and other substances, between the fluid in the vessels and the surrounding tissue cells through their semipermeable walls. The walls of capillaries consist of a single layer of epithelial cells known as endothelial cells which part at their junctions to allow leucocytes to pass through them during the process of inflammation.

capillary haemorrhage Haemorrhage from a capillary vessel or vessels, indicated by oozing.

capnograph (carbon dioxide analyser) An instrument for measuring the level of carbon dioxide in expired air.

capnophilic Bacteria which grow best in or may require for growth carbon dioxide at a concentration higher than that normally found in air.

capping 1. The technique of covering an exposed pulp to protect against irritants and to encourage healing. 2. Colloquialism for crowning. *See* cap.

capsular Relating to a capsule surrounding a joint.

capsule 1. The ligament surrounding a joint as in the case of the temporomandibular joint. 2. The container in which filling materials may be mixed mechanically. *C. vibrator.* Mechanical apparatus used to mix restorative materials in a capsule.

capsulorrhaphy Surgical repair of a joint capsule by suturing; to repair a laceration or to prevent a dislocation.

capsulotomy Surgical opening of a joint capsule.

Carabelli cusp Accessory cusp situated on the mesiopalatal aspect of some maxillary permanent first molars and deciduous second molars.

carat 1. The carat of an alloy refers to the parts of gold in an alloy in 24 parts, e.g. a 22 carat gold has 22 parts of gold and 2 parts of other metals, 24 carat being pure gold. *See also* fineness. 2. Measure of weight for precious stones (1 carat = 200 mg).

carbamazepine An anticonvulsant drg used in the management of trigeminal neuralgia. Trade name is Tegretol®.

carbohydrates Starch, cellulose and sugar types of food which produce energy and heat. A compound of carbon, hydrogen and oxygen, the hydrogen and oxygen usually being in the same proportion as in water, i.e. 2 : 1. They are classified as mono-, di-, tri-, poly- and heterosaccharides, and provide an immediate source of energy from food after being broken down by digestion. The monosaccharides (simple sugars) include glucose (also called dextrose) and fructose (also called levulose). Galactose is digested lactose. The disaccharides include sucrose, maltose and lactose. Most fruits and vegetables contain some natural sugars. The starches are found in wheat, rice and potatoes.

carbolic acid Caustic, poisonous distillate of coal tar, or synthetically produced, used as an antiseptic and disinfectant. Pure carbolic (phenol) was once used to destroy the bacteria associated with carious cavities.

carbolized resin Sedative and antiseptic dressing used for the relief of pain due to an exposed pulp. Consists of a mixture of phenol, resin alcohol and, sometimes, zinc oxide and cotton wool fibres.

carbon dioxide Odourless, colourless gas which emerges as an end-product of respiration. It is carried by the carbonates in the blood plasma and leaves the body via the lungs and out into the atmosphere. In its solid condition (*c. d. snow*) it may be used as an escharotic and as a method of testing the vitality of teeth. Carbon dioxide is an important factor in the physiology of respiration. Any increase in the blood stimulates the nervous system to increase the breathing rate, controlled by the respiratory centre of the brain. This action increases the supply of oxygen and the elimination of carbon dioxide until the amount of carbon dioxide in the blood returns to normal.

carbon monoxide Colourless, poisonous gas (as given off by car exhausts). Prevents the normal exchange of carbon dioxide and oxygen during respiration, and is readily absorbed by the red blood cells to form carboxyhaemoglobin.

carborundum Abrasive powder containing silicon carbide bonded with clay or other material. Used in rotary grinding instruments.

carbuncle Staphylococcal infection of a sweat gland or hair follicle. Larger than a boil, it has several abscess cavities within a localized area and multiple drainage sinuses.

carcinogen Agent that induces cancer, e.g. tobacco tar.

carcinogenic Capable of producing a carcinoma.

carcinoma *See* cancer.

carcinomatous Relating to a carcinoma.

cardi- Prefix meaning of the heart.

cardiac Pertaining to the heart. *C. arrest*. Cessation of the heart beat and hence failure to supply oxygenated blood to the brain centres. It is accompanied by cessation of respiration. The blood circulation must be restored within 2 minutes to prevent brain cell damage. *C. failure*. May be of slow or sudden onset and is not to be confused with cardiac arrest. Due to disease, the heart output is insufficient to maintain normal blood circulation. *C. muscle*. Specialized muscle tissue, supplied by the coronary arteries, which forms the walls of the heart.

cardiovascular system System circulating blood throughout the body and consisting of the heart and blood vessels.

caries 1. In medicine, the decay or death of bone. 2. In dentistry, *dental c.* Disease (said to be the most common human affliction) resulting in the demineralization, cavitation and breakdown of calcified dental tissue by microbial activity. *Approximal c. (proximal or interstitial c.)* Dental caries beginning in the mesial or distal surface of a tooth, usually just below the contact point. *Arrested c.* Dental caries whose progress has become static. *C.-free or immune.* A patient who shows no evidence of dental caries. *C.-prone.* A person who in spite of good oral hygiene exhibits a generally increased rate of dental caries. *Early childhood c.* Dental caries involving maxillary primary incisors within months after their eruption, which spreads rapidly to involve other primary teeth. Previously known as rampant caries or nursing bottle caries. *Incipient c.* The very first stage of the disease process where the carious lesion is just coming into existence. *Interstitial c. See* approximal c. (preferred term). *Proximal c.* See approximal c. (preferred term). *Radiation c.* A caries-like destruction of tooth substance following radiation therapy. The condition is associated with xerostomia (q.v.). *Rampant c.* A type of caries that may appear suddenly and become widespread rapidly. *Recurrent c.* Dental caries

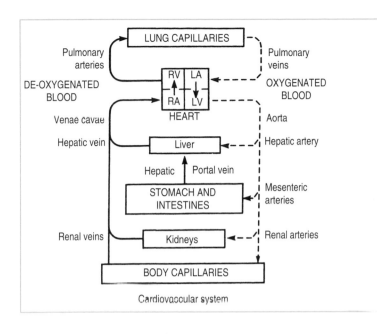

Cardiovascular system

that extends either beneath or beyond the margins of a restoration, due to the accumulation of debris resulting from inadequate cavity restoration. *Residual c.* Dental caries allowed to remain on the floor of a prepared cavity, generally because its removal would lead to pulp exposure. *Root c,* Dental caries seen in older persons particularly where the supporting tissues have receded. The lesions occur in the cementum and are probably due to increased debris stagnation because of neglectful oral hygiene and decreased salivation.

cariogenic (cariogenicity) Clinical term used to describe the caries-producing potential of a food or drink.

carious Describes a tooth affected by caries.

carnauba wax *See* wax.

carotid artery Principal artery on each side of the neck carrying oxygenated blood to the brain and head, by its internal and external branches.

carrier Person who harbours the microorganisms of a disease, can act as a source of infection but is asymptomatic, e.g. typhoid, paratyphoid and serum hepatitis B.*Amalgam c.* Instrument for transporting amalgam to a prepared tooth cavity.

cartilage Tough, flexible and slightly elastic connective tissue consisting of specialized cells (chondrocytes) in a matrix of collagenous fibres and chondromucoid. Depending on the types of fibre present in the tissue, cartilage is differentiated into *hyaline, elastic* or *fibro-cartilage*. It has few blood vessels, receiving its nourishment from surrounding tissues. Rings of cartilage support the trachea and strengthen the walls of the bronchi to keep them patent. At birth many bones are composed mainly of cartilage, which is gradually replaced by bone.

cartilaginous Consisting of cartilage.

cartridge syringe *See* syringe.

carve To shape or model a filling material in its plastic condition, e.g. amalgam, wax.

carver Hand instrument with a blade or nib used to contour the surface of filling materials in their plastic state, waxes, models and patterns, e.g. Ward's, Frahm's, Le Cron's.

carving wax *See* wax.

case control study A study or trial in which individuals with a particular disease or condition (cases) are compared with another group of individuals from the same population without the disease or disorder (controls).

cassette In radiography, a metal, light-proof holder of various sizes for radiographic film. Used extra-orally. Contains a pair of intensifying screens, the unwrapped film being placed between them in a darkroom. A marker may be required to indicate whether the film relates to the patient's right or left side.

cast 1. Reproduction obtained from an impression of oral or facial tissues, usually in plaster of Paris, which may be strengthened by the addition of other substances. 2. To make a cast or casting, using an impression as a mould, in a heated investment material. *C. crown.* Partial or full veneer crown cast entirely of a metal alloy. *Diagnostic (study) c.* A cast made especially for study, diagnosis and treatment planning. *Investment c.* A cast made of a refractory material that will withstand high temperatures without disintegrating. *Master c.* The accurately made cast on which dental restorations and prostheses are fabricated. *Study c. See* diagnostic c.

casting 1. Shape, usually in metal, which has been formed in a mould. 2. Process of forcing molten metal into a mould to form a casting. *C. gold. See* gold. *C. machine.* Mechanism which injects, by centrifugal force (q.v.), molten metal into a prepared preheated die by means of pressure, vacuum or centrifugal action. *C. ring.* Metal tube containing a refractory investment material which forms a mould for casting of metal inlays, crowns, appliances and metal prostheses. *C. shrinkage. See* shrinkage. *C. wax. See* wax.

CAT scan (computed axial tomography) An X-ray procedure which reproduces a reconstructed image of a transverse section of the body.

catalyst Substance which accelerates or retards a chemical reaction without itself undergoing any change.

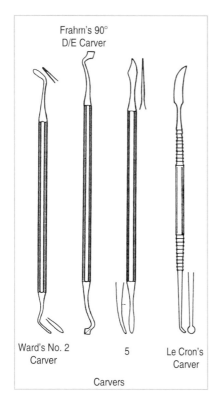

Frahm's 90°
D/E Carver

Ward's No. 2
Carver

5

Le Cron's
Carver

Carvers

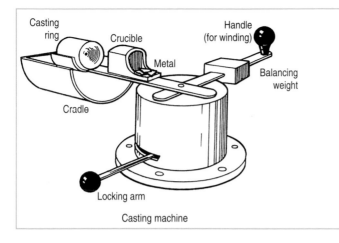

Casting ring

Crucible

Handle (for winding)

Metal

Balancing weight

Cradle

Locking arm

Casting machine

catalytic Causing catalysis (change in the speed of a reaction).

catgut Absorbable thread, prepared from the submucous layer of sheep's intestines and used for deep suturing.

catheter A hollow tube, inserted into any body canal such as a vein, artery, etc. It is used to infuse or withdraw materials into or out of the body.

cathode 1. Conductor which repels electrons and negative ions in electrolysis, in gas discharge tubes and thermionic radio valves. 2. Negative electrode of an X-ray tube.

causal Relating to a cause or causes.

causalgia Burning intense pain that sometimes occurs after injury of a sensory nerve.

caustic Substance which corrodes or destroys tissues, e.g. zinc chloride.

cauterization Local destruction of tissues by chemicals or heat.

cautery Apparatus to remove unwanted or diseased tissues by the use of a heated wire or iron. Superseded by the electric cautery or the use of very high-frequency electric currents.

cavernous sinus One of the paired cavities within the sphenoid bone at the base of the skull, through which arteries and veins pass. *C. s. thrombosis.* Acute inflammatory infection, with thrombus formation, within the cavernous sinus. Often caused by infection in the oral cavity draining into the sinus.

cavitation Process in which the hard tissues of a tooth crown are undermined by caries, causing them to cave in and form a cavity.

Cavitron® *See* ultrasonic scaler.

cavity In dentistry, a condition caused by caries, trauma, abrasion, erosion or attrition, resulting in the loss of hard tissue. Refers to such cavities only and should not be applied to a tooth preparation. *C. base.* Cement lining placed in the depth of a tooth preparation to protect the pulp from thermal and chemical irritation, or trauma. *C. floor.* Floor of a tooth preparation on which a restoration is placed. *C. liner.* A material, that may have adhesive properties, applied to the walls of a tooth preparation. Intended to seal the ends of the dentinal tubules and so protect them from irritants and the effects of

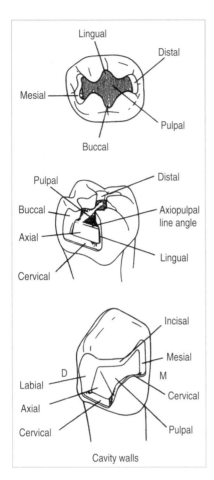

Lingual

Distal

Mesial

Pulpal

Buccal

Pulpal

Distal

Buccal

Axiopulpal
line angle

Axial

Lingual

Cervical

Incisal

Mesial

Labial

D

M

Cervical

Axial

Cervical

Pulpal

Cavity walls

micro-leakage. *C. lining material.* Used as a lining beneath a restoration, to insulate the tooth against thermal or chemical irritation. May be used to reduce the bulk of a large restoration, e.g. zinc phosphate cement, zinc carboxylate cement and quick-setting zinc oxide cements. *C. preparation (tooth preparation).* Removal of diseased and weakened tooth tissue and the shaping of sound tooth tissue to permit the placing and retention of a temporary or permanent restoration. *C. sub-base.* Material placed in the depth of a preparation

before the insertion of a cavity base. May contain calcium hydroxide to promote the formation of reparative dentine. *C. toilet.* Cleaning and removal of debris, and the drying of a tooth preparation by irrigation, spray and then compressed air. *C. wall.* One of the enclosing sides of a prepared cavity. *Compound (complex) c.* Cavity involving two or more surfaces of the clinical crown, i.e. disto-occlusal or mesio-occlusal cavity.

cavo-surface line angle *See* outline.

cavo-surface margin *See* outline.

CD (controlled drug) Preparations subject to prescription requirements of the Misuse of Drugs Regulations 1985.

CDS Community Dental Service.

cefalexin (cephalexin) Semi-synthetic antibiotic administered orally and active against Gram-positive and Gram-negative infections.

cell 1. In biology, the basic structural unit of living organisms comprising cytoplasm bounded by a membrane. Eukaryotic cells have a complex internal structure comprising the endoplasmic reticulum, mitochondria and a nucleus which contains genetic information associated with protein. Other specialist organelles may be present depending on the type of cell. Eukaryotic cells reproduce by mitosis (q.v.) and are classified according to shape (e.g. columnar, squamous), function (e.g. secretory, nervous), arrangement (e.g. stratified), special features (e.g. ciliated), presence in a particular tissue (e.g. cartilage cells) or cytoplasmic inclusions (e.g. fat cells). Prokaryotic cells possess no internal membrane structure, organelles or nucleus. Genetic information usually comprises a single chromosome with no associated protein and is free in the cytoplasm. 2. In electricity, an apparatus for producing electrical energy by the chemical action of its components.

cellular Composed of cells.

cellulitis Diffuse inflammation of connective and subcutaneous tissues. Characterized by oedema, pain, redness and interference with function. Usually occurs in the loose tissues under the skin, such as in the neck. Also known as *Ludwig's angina*.

celluloid strip. *See* strip.

cellulose acetate Material used in the manufacture of matrix strips and crown forms.

Celsius Inventor of the centigrade temperature scale in which there are 100° Celsius between the melting point of ice (0°C) and the boiling point of water (100°C) recorded at sea level. In temperature measurements the term Celsius is now preferred.

cement 1. Any substance which sets to a hard mass on being mixed with water or other medium. 2. In dentistry, term covering materials used for luting, lining and as a permanent (e.g. silicate, glass-ionomer) or temporary (e.g. zinc phosphate, zinc oxide, etc.) filling. The components are mixed in their correct proportions to provide a plastic mass which sets in due course. *See also* black copper cement, silicate cement, zinc oxide/EBA cement, zinc oxide-eugenol cement, glass-ionomer cement, zinc phosphate cement, zinc polycarboxylate cement.

cementation Process of cementing a restoration in place by the use of a luting agent or cement.

cementoblast Cell concerned with the formation of cementum.

cementocyte Cell found in the cellular layer of cementum. Somewhat stellate-shaped cell with radiating thin processes.

A product of cementoblast cells which have remained in the newly formed cementum.

cemento-enamel junction Line formed between the cementum and enamel at the anatomical neck of the tooth.

cementogenesis Formation of cementum by cementoblast cells.

cementoid Layer of matrix which has not yet calcified on the forming surface of cementum.

cementoma Generally benign proliferation of odontogenic connective tissue in the mandible or maxilla which produces cementum or cementum-like tissue. Often associated with the apices of teeth.

cementosis Laying down of cementum.

cementum Thin, calcified, bone-like tissue covering the tooth root and providing attachment for Sharpey's fibres (q.v.). *Primary c.* Acellular innermost layer of the cementum, that is later covered in the apical portion by cellular *secondary c.*

centigrade 1. Consisting of 100 divisions. 2. Scale measuring temperature in degrees Celsius (q.v.).

central Related to, or situated at a centre; not at the periphery. *C. bearing device.* Mechanical device, used intra-orally, to record the position of the mandible in selected jaw positions. *C. nervous system.* That part of the nervous system which co-ordinates and controls the activities of the body. It comprises the brain and the spinal cord. *C. ray.* Central ray of the beam of radiation emitted by an X-ray machine. *C. sterile supply department (CSSD).* Central sterilization premises found in hospitals.

centric Relating to, or situated at the centre. *C. jaw relation; c. relation. See* retruded jaw relation. *C. occlusion. See* occlusion.

centrifugal force Outward force exered by a revolving body. In dentistry, the principle is used when introducing a paste into a root canal with a spiral root canal filler and in a casting machine.

centrifuge Device for separating, by centrifugal force, components of different densities in a liquid.

cephalometric analysis Analysis of measurements of the skull taken from lateral and anteroposterior radiographs of certain fixed points of the skull. In orthodontic diagnosis various tracings are drawn from lines joining recognized points and their angles of intersection are measured. *See* Appendix 10.

cephalometric radiograph A lateral skull radiograph taken with the patient placed in a cephalostat (q.v.). This positions the patient with their head oriented at 90° to the X-ray beam at a distance of 5ft from the tube. The film is placed 15 inches from the head. This is a standard under which all cephalometric radiographs are taken worldwide. It ensures that radiographs taken at different centres are directly comparable.

cephalometric tracing Tracing, on drafting paper or film, of selected structures from a cephalometric radiograph (q.v.).

cephalometrics The technique of obtaining a cephalometric radiograph (q.v.) and preparing a series of cephalometric tracings (q.v.) from which measurements can be made for the purpose of orthodontic diagnosis and/or anthropometric evaluation. *See* Appendix 10.

cephalosporins Semi-synthetic broad-spectrum antibiotics originally derived from the micro-organism *Cephalosporium acremonium*. The cephalosporins have a similar structure to the penicillins but have absolute indications for their use.

cephalostat (craniostat) Apparatus used to hold the head steady and at a standard angle during radiological examinations, thus ensuring precise, reproducible relationships between the X-ray tube, the subject and the film.

ceramics General term for dental porcelain work.

cerebellum That smaller part of the brain lying below the cerebrum known as the hindbrain. Concerned with balance, co-ordination of fine movements and posture.

cerebral Relating to the cerebrum.

cerebrospinal rhinorrhoea Leakage of cerebrospinal fluid from the nose, sometimes seen as a result of facial skeleton fractures.

cerebrum Largest part of the brain, divided into a left and a right hemisphere. Contains the centres of the higher functions of the brain. Interprets impulses received from sensory organs throughout the body, such as sight, sound, touch, pressure, temperature and smell. Also connected with memory, reasoning and emotion.

cermet Metal reinforced glass ionomer cements. Use now largely superseded.

cervical 1. In anatomy, relating to the neck or to the cervix or to a more constricted area of an organ. 2. In dentistry, the area where the tooth crown joins the root. *C. line.* Line around a tooth marking the junction of the enamel of the crown and the cementum of the root. *C. margin.* That part of a preparation, or of a restoration, closest to the neck of a tooth. *C. wall.* Cavity surface bounded by the cavity floor and the cavosurface angle, and further qualified by its position, e.g. mesial, distal, etc. 3. In radiography, *c. burn out* or *c. radiolucency* is the radiolucency seen at the margin of a tooth and sometimes mistaken for caries. 4. In orthodontics, *c. strap* or *neckstrap* is a type of headgear that fits around the neck only.

chalk *See* calcium carbonate.

chancre Primary lesion of syphilis, generally situated at the site of infection.

channel slice preparation Tooth preparation for a cast-metal restoration in which the walls are tapered or sliced and tapering grooves are cut to increase retention.

chart In dentistry a visual record or diagram of a patient's dentition and dental state.

charting Recording of clinical details of a patient's dentition and surrounding tissues, personal details and medical history. Most dental charts have a diagrammatic representation of the teeth which is divided into quadrants. The Zsigmondy–Palmer or Chevron charting system is widely used in Europe and in the UK National Health Service. *See* Appendix 3.

Cheatle's forceps *See* forceps.

check record Method of verifying a previously taken interocclusal record (q.v.) by repeating the procedure. Sometimes referred to as a *check bite*.

cheek teeth Collective (lay) term for molars and premolars.

cheilitis *See* angular cheilitis.

cheiloplasty Surgical procedure to correct congenital or traumatic lip deformities.

chelating agent Material able to sequester metallic ions. Endodontics: liquid or gel containing EDTA which may decalcify root canal walls, ease instrument entry and remove smear layer.

chelation In dentistry, chemical sequestration of calcium ions from tooth tissue.

cheloid *See* keloid.

chemical fog Fog, or darkening of the whole or part of a radiograph, due to deterioration of the processing solutions.

chemotaxis The migration of cells in response to some chemical stimulus.

chemotherapy Use of chemical compounds in the treatment of diseases.

cherubism Appearance of a child who is suffering from multilocular cysts of the jaws and thus has an expanded face likened to that of a cherub.

chicken pox (varicella) Mild infectious disease of childhood with an incubation period of 14 days. Slight fever accompanies irritating transparent vesicles over all the body which later dry to become scabs. The patient is free from infection when all scabs have shed.

children's dentistry *See* paedodontics, paediatric dentistry or children's dentistry.

chin cup An orthodontic appliance used to attempt to restrict development of the mandible in growing children.

china clay Naturally occurring hydrous aluminium silicate used as a filler in certain dental materials.

chip syringe Instrument, now rarely used, consisting of a rubber bulb attached to a nozzle and used to blow away debris and to dry cavities during operative procedures.

Chirocaine® *See* levobupivacaine.

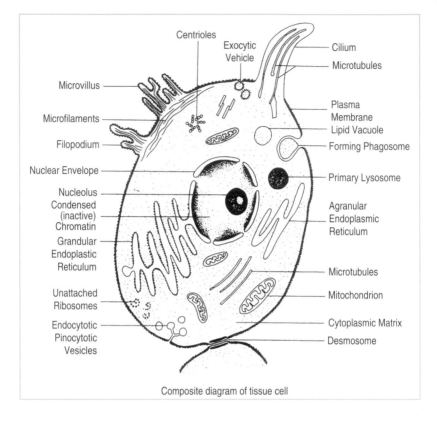

Centrioles

Exocytic
Vehicle

Cilium

Microtubules

Microvillus

Microfilaments

Filopodium

Plasma
Membrane
Lipid Vacuole

Forming Phagosome

Nuclear Envelope

Nucleolus
Condensed
(inactive)
Chromatin

Grandular
Endoplastic
Reticulum

Primary Lysosome

Agranular
Endoplasmic
Reticulum

Microtubules

Mitochondrion

Unattached
Ribosomes

Endocytotic
Pinocytotic
Vesicles

Cytoplasmic Matrix

Desmosome

Composite diagram of tissue cell

chisel Hand instrument used to remove hard tissues such as enamel or bone by chipping, cleaving or paring. The bevelled blade may be in line with the handle or at an angle to it. *Bone c.* Single-ended chisel with longer handle and a square end which can be struck by a mallet. *Coupland c.* Bone hand chisel or gouge with hollowed out blade attached to a pear-shaped hollow octagonal handle. Obtainable in several widths. *Enamel c.* Usually single ended, except for marginal trimmers.

chloramphenicol Broad-spectrum antibiotic produced from a bacterium or synthetically. Has serious side-effects and is now rarely used. Trade name: Chloromycetin®.

chlorhexidine Antiseptic used in an aqueous or alcoholic solution on skin surfaces, worktops and to disinfect instruments. Inhibits bacterial plaque when used as a mouthwash in a 0.2% strength three times daily. Also incorporated in a toothpaste.

chloroform Colourless, volatile liquid with a characteristic smell and taste. Previously used as an inhalation anaesthetic. In dentistry, used as a solvent for gutta percha. *See* chloropercha.

Chloromycetin® *See* chloramphenicol.

chloropercha (archaic) Root canal sealer created by dissolving gutta percha in chloroform.

cholecalciferol Vitamin D_3.

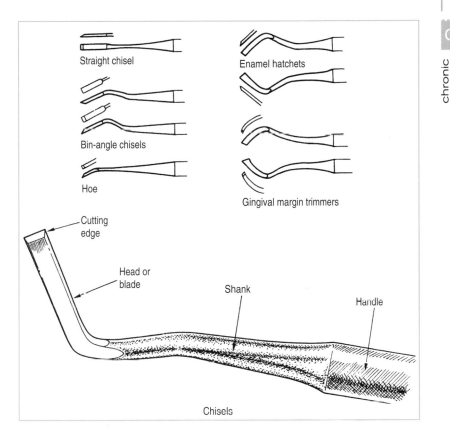

Straight chisel

Enamel hatchets

Bin-angle chisels

Hoe

Gingival margin trimmers

Cutting edge

Head or blade

Shank

Handle

Chisels

cholesterol crystals Small yellowish crystals sometimes found in cyst cavities.

choline salicylate dental paste Anti-inflammatory, analgesic paste containing a soluble salicylate which may be applied to the affected mucosa three to four times daily. Trade names: Bonjela®, Teejel®, Pyralvex®.

chondroma Benign tumour of cartilage.

chorea Involuntary jerky movement, particularly affecting the face and limbs, due to disease of the basal ganglia in the cerebrum.

Christmas disease Hereditary bleeding akin to haemophilia but due to a deficiency of a different blood coagulation factor—the Christmas Factor or Factor IX.

chrome cobalt *See* cobalt chromium.

chromium Metal which is very resistant to corrosion. Used as an alloy in fixed and removable prostheses. *C. oxide.* Fine polishing agent.

chromosome One of the 46 thread-like structures in the human cell nucleus that carry genetic information along their length in the form of genes. During cell division, chromosomes divide and distribute themselves equally in daughter cells. They contain DNA (q.v.) and RNA (q.v.).

chronic Of slow onset and long duration.

chronic

51

chronic periodontitis *See* periodontitis.

chuck Adjustable tool for holding rotary instruments. Used on a lathe or by hand. Also used in turbine handpieces to retain friction grip burs (q.v.).

chyle Milky emulsion of fats and lymph found in the intestine during digestion.

chyme Partially digested food as it passes from the stomach into the intestine where it is converted into chyle.

cicatrix *See* scar.

cilia Plural of cilium.

ciliated Describes epithelium which has become specialized to present cilia.

cilium 1. Microscopic, hair-like filament projecting from some epithelial cells. Its whip-like action sweeps away foreign bodies. Found in the respiratory tract. 2. An eyelash.

cingulum Bulge or ridge found on the palatal or lingual aspects of incisor and canine teeth, near to their cervical margins.

circulation In medicine, the movement of blood propelled through the body by the action of the heart.

circulatory system *See* cardiovascular system.

circumferential wiring Technique used in mandibular jaw fracture cases to immobilize the bone fragments. Stainless steel wire is passed round the lower border of the mandible from within the mouth under an anaesthetic. The ends are then tied over a splint or existing denture.

circumoral Around or close to the mouth.

circumzygomatic wiring (archaic) Immobilization of a fractured maxilla by percutaneous wiring over the zygomatic arch and down into the mouth.

Citanest® *See* prilocaine hydrochloride.

clamp Surgical instrument designed to compress an organ or tissue thus preventing the escape of contents, e.g. a blood vessel or the cut end of the intestine. In dentistry, *see* rubber dam clamp.

clasp A metal holding device such as is used for partial dentures and orthodontic appliances, in the form of a cast-metal arm or wire which acts as a direct retainer and stabilizer by contacting and surrounding, or partially surrounding, an abutment tooth. *Adams' arrowhead c.* Clasp of stainless steel wire used to retain removable orthodontic appliances and consisting of a buccal wire connecting two arrowhead formations to fit into the mesio- and distobuccal undercuts. The wire is continuous over the occlusal surfaces, to be held in place in the base-plate by several bends. *Circumferential c.* Clasp which is continuous around a tooth. *Gingivally approaching c.* (*Roach c.*) Denture-retaining clasp, the arm of which passes adjacent to the soft tissues and approaches its point of contact on a tooth from the gingival margin. *Occlusally approaching c.* Clasp originating on the occlusal side of a survey line and ending in the infrabulge area. *Orthodontic c.* Component, made of non-staining, springy metal, of orthodontic appliances which contacts and partially surrounds a tooth to provide retention and stability. *Reciprocal c.* Clasp arm, or other extension, of a partial denture, used to oppose the action of laterally displacing forces. *Roach c. See* gingivally approaching c.

clearance USA terminology - to remove calculus from the teeth. *See* scaling. *Full c.* UK terminology - the act of removing all teeth from a patient's mouth. *Upper c.* The act of removing all the upper teeth.

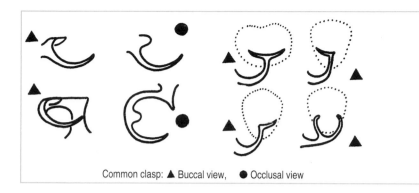

Common clasp: ▲ Buccal view, ● Occlusal view

Lower c. The act of removing all the lower teeth.

cleft Fissure or elongated opening which occurs due to failure of parts to unite during development. *C. lip (harelip).* Congenital condition (sometimes involving the maxillary bone) in which there is a developmental defect along the normal lines of fusion of the lip tissues, causing a cleft or fissure. May be uni- or bilateral and is frequently associated with cleft palate. Gives rise to feeding problems. Treatment is by orthodontic therapy and/or surgery. *C. palate.* Lack of fusion along the normal developmental lines of the palate. May be partial or complete and may include a cleft lip. Gives rise to feeding, dental and speech problems.

cleidocranial Relating to the head and the clavicle. *C. dysostosis. See* dysostosis.

cleoid Carving or excavating instrument whose blade resembles a pointed spade.

clicking Noise arising from the temporomandibular joint heard by the patient and the practitioner during excursions of the mandible.

clindamycin An antibiotic useful against penicillin-resistant Staphylococci and in the management of bony infections. It is also used in dentistry as prophylaxis against infective endocarditis in patients allergic to penicillin. Trade name Dalacin C®.

clinical audit *See* audit.

clinical crown *See* crown.

clinical dental technician Member of the dental team who, in addition to the remit of a dental technician, is able to provide clinically a range of removable dental appliances and complete dentures, without prior review by a dentist.

clinical root That portion of the anatomical root attached to the alveolar bone by the periodontal ligament.

clinical trial Planned experiment designed to assess the relative efficacies of treatments in human subjects by comparing predetermined outcomes in groups of participants treated with test (usually new) treatments with those of comparable groups of subjects receiving control (standard) treatments, often involving a placebo; *see* placebo. The groups may be established through randomization.

closed fracture *See* fracture.

Clostridium tetani Anaerobic, Gram-positive, spore-forming, rod-shaped bacteria. *C. tetani* spores are common in soil and the faeces of many animals, e.g.

horses, cattle, sheep, chickens, dogs and cats. Infection occurs via a wound but only in very low levels of oxygen which permit the spores to germinate (puncture wound). Aetiological agent of tetanus. Patients should be warned to avoid contact with soil, especially manure-containing soil, immediately following oral surgery.

closure Act of closing or bringing together two parts. *Flask c.* Closing together of the two halves of a metal flask during the construction of a denture.

clot Semi-solid mass or lump, usually of a soft slippery nature. In medicine, a coagulated mass of blood.

clotting The act of forming a clot. A defensive body mechanism to arrest haemorrhage. Blood vessel injury promotes the formation of a fine meshwork of fibrin fibrils from the fibrinogen of the blood plasma. Erythrocytes and thrombocytes become trapped in the fibrils to form a soft plug at the site of injury. This action, together with several other factors, causes the blood flow to lessen or cease. The soft plug solidifies to become a clot.

CMCP Camphorated para-monochlorophenol (q.v.).

CNS Central nervous system.

CO Centric occlusion.

coagulant Substance which assists the coagulation of blood.

coagulate To become clotted or to cause coagulation.

coagulation Formation of a blood clot. The process in which many coagulation factors of the blood clotting process interact to result in the formation of an insoluble fibrin clot. *C. time.* Time taken for shed blood to coagulate—normally 4–8 minutes.

co-amoxiclav (Augmentin®) A broad-spectrum antibacterial drug useful in the management of severe infections. It is a mixture of amoxicillin and clavulanic acid that is administered orally or by injection.

cobalt Chemical metallic element used to form many alloys and pigments. *C. chromium.* Alloy of cobalt and chromium used in the construction of some partial dentures and other prostheses. The alloy is hard, resistant to corrosion and has a high melting point.

cocci Plural of coccus.

coccus Spherical-shaped bacterium. Staphylococci occur in clusters resembling a bunch of grapes (Greek *staphyle*). Streptococci occur in chains (Greek *streptos*), e.g. *Staphylococcus aureus, Streptococcus pyogenes.*

codeine Drug derived from morphine and used as an analgesic and in allaying irritating coughs.

codeine compound tablet (BP) Analgesic tablet containing aspirin, phenacetin and codeine.

coffin spring Heavy gauge wire placed posteriorly between two separated sections of a removable orthodontic appliance to exert pressure causing expansion or contraction.

cohesion Property exhibited by some materials whereby their constituent molecules are attracted to each other and resist separation.

cohesive gold foil Gold foil which is freed from surface contamination by heating, thus making it possible to condense by pressure welding.

coil Object wound in a spiral. *C. spring winder.* Orthodontic instrument consisting of a sleeved spindle around which a fine stainless steel wire is wound to form a coil spring.

col Small depression in the interdental gingiva below the interproximal contact area between the buccal and lingual papillae.

cold curing resin *See* resin, autopolymerizing.

cold sore *See* herpes labialis.

collagen White protein fibres in the skin, bone, cartilage and other connective tissues of the body—the principal components of connective tissue. *C. fibres.* Found in connective tissue, the most common tissue in the body. They do not stretch. Bundles of collagen fibres found deep in the mucogingival complex are grouped according to their position: 1. OBLIQUE—the majority group running obliquely downwards from the socket wall to the cementum of a tooth root; 2. TRANSSEPTAL; 3. CIRCULAR; 4. LONGITUDINAL; 5. ALVEOLO-GINGIVAL; 6. DENTO-GINGIVAL.

collagenous Relating to collagen.

collapse State of extreme prostration due to defective heart action, haemorrhage or severe shock.

collar 1. A band that encircles any neck-like structure. 2. In dentistry, a narrow metal band that fits over an abutment or forms part of a post and core construction.

collateral 1. Secondary or accessory. 2. A small branch.

collet That area of a prosthesis which serves as a collar round the neck of a tooth.

collimation Literally, making parallel. In radiography, the action of restricting the size of the X-ray beam by means of a collimator.

collimator Diaphragm or tube lined with an X-ray absorbing material

designed to restrict the size of the X-ray beam.

colloid Material in which particles remain uniformly in suspension, e.g. silicate cement, hydrocolloid impression materials.

colloidal State of dispersion between a gel and a sol.

collutorium, collutory A mouthwash or gargle.

colour coding Grading of small instrument sizes by colour as recognized by the International Standards Organization (ISO). The smallest sizes are indicated by white markings graduating through yellow, red, blue, green to black.

coma Complete unconsciousness and collapse in which all reflexes are absent and the patient cannot be aroused.

comatose In a state of coma.

commensal *Adj:* A relationship between two different organisms in which one benefits and the other is unaffected. *Noun:* An organism participating in a relationship with another organism in which one benefits while the other is not harmed.

comminuted Broken into small fragments. *C. fracture. See* fracture.

comminution Reduction into small particles.

communicable diseases *See* infectious diseases.

community dentistry (dental public health) That branch of dentistry that is concerned with the prevention and control of dental diseases and the promotion of oral health.

compact Dense.

compactor 1. A condenser; an instrument that aids the process of joining or packing a material, e.g. in gold foil restorations. 2. In endodontics, a small, engine-driven instrument, akin to a Hedstroem file but with reverse flutes, used to feed in, plasticize and compact gutta percha in a root canal. Sometimes called a *McSpadden Compactor®* after its inventor.

compatible Capable of existing in harmony with another person or drug.

compensating curve Curvature of the plane of dentures made to compensate the effects of the movements of the condyles of the mandible and to obtain a balanced occlusion.

compensating extraction Removal of a tooth from one quadrant following the extraction of a tooth from the opposing quadrant in order to preserve buccal occlusion and prevent the development of a malocclusion.

competent lips Lips which provide a seal when the mandible and the facial muscles are at rest.

complete denture Denture replacing the entire maxillary or mandibular dentition.

complex cavity *See* cavity, compound.

complex composite odontome *See* odontome.

complication Additional pathological condition which develops during the course of a disease.

compomer (polyacid-modified resin composite) Resin composites containing fluoroaluminosilicate glass to facilitate release of fluoride.

composite Substance made up of separate parts. *C. odontome. See* odontome. *C. resin. (c. filling material).* Resin-based filling material consisting of an organic polymer resin matrix such as methyl

methacrylate or polymer precursors such as BIS-GMA, to which has been added an inert inorganic filler material such as quartz, aluminium silicate or glass. Polymerization (q.v.) of the matrix may be initiated by chemical catalysts or visible light. *Microfilled c. resin* contains submicron filler particles, less heavily filled, highly polishable. *Hybrid c. resin* conventional and submicron filler particles combined.

composition 1. In chemistry, the proportion of the components forming a mixture, or the elements forming a compound. 2. In dentistry, obsolete name for *impression compound. See* impression material.

compound 1. In pharmacology, to mix two or more substances intimately together, as with drugs. 2. In chemistry, a substance of constant composition formed by the union of two or more different atoms of different elements and held together by valency bonds. 3. *See* impression material. *C. cavity. See* cavity. *C. fracture. See* fracture.

compression bone plate See plate.

Computed axial tomography *See* CAT scan.

concentric Having a common centre.

concha of cranium *See* calvaria.

concrescence Fusion of two normally separate parts.

concretion 1. Mass formed of parts pressed together. 2. A calculus or deposit in a body cavity.

concussion Limited period of loss of consciousness caused by injury to the head. In dentistry, minor injury to a tooth in which the tooth is not displaced or mobile and there is no rupture of periodontal ligament fibres.

condensation Compaction of material into a smaller space to increase density. In endodontics, to compact filling material into a root canal. *Cold c.* Compaction of materials by pressure alone. *Warm (thermoplastic) c.* Compaction of material after warming to improve material flow and adaptation.

condenser In dentistry, a hand instrument designed to pack restorative materials into a prepared tooth cavity. *Automatic* or *mechanical c.* Instrument designed to supply a controlled force during the condensation of restorative materials such as amalgam or gold foil. May be spring activated or pneumatically or electrically controlled.

condensing osteitis Localized, chronic, low-grade inflammation in which abnormally dense bone is produced. Associated with the apices of non-vital teeth or with the site of the apex after extraction of the tooth.

conditioned reflex action Response to an unnatural stimulus which is acquired during life. May be changed by experience and is the basis of human habits, e.g. eye blink, knee jerk.

conduction anaethesia or **analgesia** *See* analgesia, block or regional.

condylar Relating to or involving a condyle. *C. axis. (Transverse c. axis)* Imaginary line drawn through the condyle of the mandible about which it rotates. *C. guide.* That part of an anatomical articulator which attempts to guide the replica condyles into the true condylar path known as the *c. track. C. path.* Path travelled by the mandibular condyle during any mandibular excursions.

condyle Rounded articular surface at the end of a bone involved in a joint. *C. of the mandible.* Knob-shaped process on the superior aspect of the posterior border of the ramus of the mandible. It has a narrow neck expanding upwards into a head which is relatively narrow anteroposteriorly and wide from side to side. It is smooth on the articular surface. Together with the condyle on the opposite side of the head, it forms the hinge part of the temporomandibular joint system, fitting into the glenoid fossa of the temporal bone. The lateral pterygoid muscle is attached to its neck anteriorly.

condylectomy Surgical removal of the whole of the condyle of the mandible.

condyloid Resembling a condyle.

condylotomy Sectioning of the condylar neck of the mandible without removal of the condyle.

cone In radiography, that part of the X-ray apparatus which determines the minimum anode-to-film distance and indicates the direction of the central axis of the X-ray beam. Cones may be short or long, tubular or conical, and may be fitted with filtration or collimation devices. *See also* collimation, collimator.

confidence interval The range of values between which the true value for an effect, e.g. an intervention, occurs. A 95% confidence interval gives the two values between which the true value occurs in 95% of cases.

confluent Merging together, joining.

congenital Existing at the time of birth, inherited. *C. epulis of the newborn.* Benign tumour of soft tissue of the mandibular or maxillary area, present at birth.

conical Cone shaped. *C. tooth. See* tooth.

coning off Radiological term for an error in directing the central ray of the X-ray beam to the best advantage. It produces a blank area on the processed film with a typical curved margin.

connector That part of a removable partial denture that joins components on one side of the arch to those on the other side. *Minor c.* The connecting link between the major connector or the body of the partial denture and other units of the denture such as clasps, occlusal rests or indirect retainers. *See also* labial bar, lingual bar, Kennedy bar, palatal bar.

conscious Being awake and aware of one's surroundings.

consciousness The state of being conscious.

conscious sedation *See* sedation.

consent Approval by patient prior to examination and treatment. To be valid, consent should be informed, i.e. the patient must understand the treatment to be carried out, any risks, aftercare and precautions necessary. Written consent is always preferable. Special care is needed when obtaining consent from children under the age of 16 years and special needs patients.

conservative dentistry In the UK the term is restricted to that part of restorative dentistry which concerns itself with the restoration of individual teeth and includes endodontics, crowning and fixed bridgework. However, the dividing line between conservative and prosthetic dentistry is ill defined and, generally speaking, removable prostheses depending for their retention on precision attachments are considered to be within the province of conservative dentistry, while those relying on clasps for retention and stabilization belong to the field of prosthetic dentistry. *See also* endodontics, operative dentistry, prosthetic dentistry.

constrictor That which causes constriction or shrinking.

consultant Hospital-based specialist in medicine or dentistry who accepts complete responsibility for a patient's treatment.

consultation A meeting of persons to decide a course of action. In dentistry, a visit by a patient seeking advice on a specific dental and/or oral condition. It should include a full examination (q.v.), a careful assessment of the findings and a formulation and presentation of a treatment plan (q.v.) to the patient, preferably as a written report.

contact 1. Touching together. 2. Person who has been in close association with another suffering from an infectious disease. *C. area.* The area of crown contact between two adjacent teeth, sometimes referred to as a *c. point. C. surface. See* approximal surface. *Initial c.* First touching of upper and lower teeth when the jaws are closed. *Occlusal c.* Contact of the upper and lower teeth when the jaws are closed normally. *Premature c.* Initial contact of teeth which causes a deviation of the jaws on closure. *See* premature occlusal c.

contagion A substance or agent which mediates the passing of an infectious disease from one person to another.

contagious Relating to a disease capable of being passed from one person to another.

contaminate To pollute or infect.

contiguous In contact or very close.

continuous loop wiring *See* wiring.

contour 1. A boundary or outline. 2. To sculpt or carve a material or restoration to a desired shape. 3. *C. lines of Owen.* Microscopic lines sometimes seen in dentine representing co-incidence of the secondary curves of the dentinal tubules or accentuated deficiencies of mineralization.

contra- Prefix meaning opposed to or against.

contra-angle Instrument having two or more off-setting angles along its shank in order to bring the working end closer to the long axis of the handle.

contraction Becoming smaller or shorter.

contra-indication Any factor in a patient's history that makes it unwise to carry out a certain treatment plan.

contralateral side The side opposite to the working side.

contrast 1. To show opposing qualities in an object or situation. 2. In radiography, the varying density appearing on a radiograph. *C. medium*. Radio-opaque substance which, when introduced into air- or fluid-filled structures, allows them to be seen.

controlled delivery device Method of applying an antimicrobial or antibiotic to a periodontal pocket. An adjunctive treatment method for periodontal disease. Designed to provide drug delivery for over 24 hours. Examples include PerioChip® – 2.5 mg of chlorhexidine in a gelatine matrix; Atridox® – 10% doxycycline in a polymer vehicle.

controlled drugs *See* Misuse of Drugs Act.

contusion A bruise. Discoloration and swelling of the skin following injury.

convenience form Shaping of a cavity preparation to allow access and to facilitate the manufacture and insertion of a restoration.

convex Curved, as the outside of a circle or sphere.

convulsion State of violent involuntary muscle contraction.

copal Resin obtained from tropical trees and used in a solvent as varnish.

coping Thin, cast-metal cap, without external undercuts, that is fitted over a preparation. *Implant impression c*. A removable close fitting attachment for an implant fixture or abutment. Usually held in place via a screw or by friction, they allow an accurate impression of an implant fixture or abutment to be recorded prior to construction of the definitive restoration *See* implant. *Transfer c*. Base metal or resin cap used to obtain precise relative locations during the taking of impressions of multiple preparations.

copolymer Polymer made up of two or more different monomer units.

copper Red-coloured malleable metal. *C. amalgam*. Amalgam containing mainly copper and mercury and made plastic by heating, just prior to use, and trituration. *C. band. See* c. ring. *C. ring*. Thin-walled copper tube used to contain and support impression material. Supplied in graded and numbered sizes. May be softened by annealing (q.v.). Can also be used as a temporary crown or matrix band. *C. ring impression*. Impression of a tooth preparation using a copper ring to contain the impression material. An overall impression may be necessary to demonstrate the contact areas to the technician. *C. sulphate*. Blue crystalline substance used in solution to permit the deposition of copper in plating techniques. In powdered form has been used in the treatment of periodontal pockets.

core Correctly shaped and well-retained substructure to a partial or full veneer crown. May be part of a post and core system and may be cast or prefabricated. A core may also be constructed of a plastic material adhered to remaining tooth tissue or retained physically. *C. porcelain*. Opaque porcelain laid on the platinum matrix which provides a strong and optically uniform base for jacket crown construction.

cornu Synonym for pulp horn (q.v.).

cornua Plural of cornu.

coronal 1. Relating to or belonging to the crown of the head. 2. *C. or frontal plane*. Any plane passing longitudinally through the body from side to side, dividing the body into dorsal and ventral parts. 3. In dentistry, relating to the crown of a tooth as opposed to the root. *C. seal*. Protection against the ingress of fluids and micro-organisms from the mouth.

coronary Encircling, as of a vessel, nerve or tooth. *C. arteries*. Arteries supplying the heart muscle. The earliest branches from the aorta. Narrowing or blocking of these arteries may give rise to severe pain—angina (q.v.). *C. thrombosis*. Blockage of the coronary arteries by a thrombus (q.v.).

coronoid process Pointed bony process on the anterior superior margin of the ramus of the mandible. It provides attachment for the temporal muscle which assists in closing the mouth.

coronoidectomy Surgical removal of the coronoid process of the mandible.

coronoidotomy Sectioning of the coronoid process of the mandible.

corpuscle Blood cell.

Corsodyl® mouthwash *See* chlorhexidine.

cortical plate Hard bone covering the inner and outer surface of the alveolar process.

corticosteroid Hormone produced by the adrenal glands or their synthetic substitutes. Widely employed in the treatment of many conditions in steroid therapy, e.g. prednisolone, hydrocortisone. Used topically in the mouth for recurrent aphthae.

corticosteroid therapy Treatment of diseases by corticosteroid hormones.

corticotrophin (ACTH) Adrenocorticotrophic hormone secreted by the anterior pituitary gland which stimulates the adrenal glands to produce cortisol steroids. Synthetic adrenal steroid in the form of hydrocortisone or prednisone may be injected or applied in jelly form as an anti-inflammatory agent.

cortisol (hydrocortisone) The natural hormone of the adrenal gland. Used as an anti-inflammatory drug.

corundum Mineral form of aluminium oxide powder used as an abrasive in polishing.

coryza An inflammation of the mucous membrane of the nose and nasopharynx often accompanied by a nasal discharge, e.g. condition caused by the common cold.

cosmetic dentistry Lay term to describe conservative dental procedure aimed at improving the aesthetics of the patient's dentition and general facial appearance.

Costen's syndrome *See* temporomandibular joint dysfunction.

co-trimoxazole (Septrin®) An antibacterial drug. It is a mixture of trimethoprim and sulfamethoxazole.

cotton wool (absorbent cotton) Material prepared from purified cotton from which natural waxes and seeds have been removed so that it will absorb moisture.

counter-die The reverse of a die.

counter-irritant Agent used to disguise the effect of, or relieve a previously existing irritation.

Coupland chisel *See* chisel.

cover screw A generic term used to describe a screw fixed to the exposed surface and internal thread of an implant fixture or implant abutment. It is placed to avoid tissue ingress or packing of debris inside the implant.

COX 2 inhibitors COX is an abbreviation for cyclo-oxygenase, which is an enzyme involved in the inflammatory process. There are a number of forms of this enzyme (COX 1, COX 2 and COX 3 have been recognized to date). Inhibition of COX 1 causes side-effects such as gastro-intestinal irritation. Non-specific COX inhibitors such as aspirin produce gastric side-effects. The COX 2 inhibitors do not have this disadvantage. Long term use of COX 2 inhibitors is limited as they do produce cardiovascular problems.

CPITN Community periodontal index of treatment needs. *See* index.

CPR Cardiopulmonary resuscitation.

cracked tooth syndrome Name given to the acute pain sometimes experienced by patients whilst chewing. The cause is difficult to locate and is commonly due to a vertical tooth fracture or split extending across the marginal ridge, through the crown and into the pulp chamber. It may become visible by the use of disclosing dyes and by transillumination.

cranial Relating to the skull or cranium. *C. nerves.* Twelve pairs of nerves arising from the brain to the base of the skull, as opposed to the spinal nerves arising from the spinal cord. They are conventionally numbered in Roman numerals as follows: I, olfactory; II, optic; III, oculomotor; IV, trochlear; V, trigeminal; VI, abducent; VII, facial; VIII, auditory; IX, glossopharyngeal; X, vagus; XI, accessory; XII, hypoglossal. *C. vault. See* calvaria.

craniofacial dysjunction fracture *See* Le Fort III fracture.

craniofacial dysostosis *See* dysostosis.

craniomandibular fixation *See* fixation.

craniostat *See* cephalostat.

cranium That part of the skull which encloses the brain as distinct from the face.

crater Bowl-shaped cavity or hollow surrounded by an elevated edge.

crazing Pattern of minute hair-like cracks on the surface of porcelain and acrylic polymers.

creep To slowly change shape, as do heated metals and ceramics under load. Amalgam restorations may flow or creep under heavy masticatory forces.

crenulation Shrivelling of cells caused by any surrounding hypertonic fluid. Cellular fluid leaves the cell in an attempt to dilute the surrounding solution.

crepitus Grating sound heard when fragments of fractured bone are moved against each other.

cresol Yellowish liquid obtained from coal tar and containing a small percentage of phenol. Sometimes used as an antiseptic and as a disinfectant. In combination with formaldehyde solution, formocresol (q.v.) is used in root canal therapy as a devitalizing agent and antiseptic.

crest Narrow elongated ridge generally used in the description of bones, e.g. the nasal crest of the maxilla, but sometimes used to describe soft tissue, e.g. gingival crest (q.v.).

cretinism Retardation of mental and physical development. A type of congenital hypothyroidism.

The Cranial Nerves

I. OLFACTORY	Concerned with the sense of smell.
II. OPTIC	Concerned with vision.
III. OCULOMOTOR	Concerned with eyelid and eye movements.
IV. TROCHLEAR	Concerned with oblique movements of the eyeball.
V. TRIGEMINAL	
a. OPHTHALMIC	Supplies the eyeball, conjunctiva, lacrimal gland, skin of forehead, eyelids and nose, mucous membrane of nose and paranasal sinuses, dura mater.
b. MAXILLARY	Supplies middle part of face, upper lip, and lower eyelid; maxillary teeth and gingiva; soft palate and roof of mouth, maxillary sinus and mucous membrane of nasopharynx.
c. MANDIBULAR	Supplies the muscles of mastication, lower part of face, mandibular teeth and gingiva, anterior two-thirds of tongue, mylohyoid muscle, cheek, skin of temporal region, temporomandibular joint and external ear.
VI. ABDUCENT	Concerned with eye movements.
VII. FACIAL	*Motor part*: Muscles of facial expression, scalp, external ear, buccinator, stylohyoid, platysma.
	Sensory part: Anterior two-thirds of tongue, soft palate and part of pharynx.
	Parasympathetic part: Salivary, nasal and lacrimal glands.
VIII. AUDITORY	Concerned with hearing.
IX. GLOSSOPHARYNGEAL	Supplies tongue and pharynx, palatine tonsil, and fauces.
X. VAGUS	*Motor part*: Laryngeal and pharyngeal muscles and to heart, lung and alimentary tract.
	Sensory part: From heart, lungs and alimentary tract.
XI. ACCESSORY	Muscles of larynx and pharynx.
XII. HYPOGLOSSAL	Supplies muscles of the tongue and floor of the mouth.

crevice Narrow opening or fissure. *Gingival c. See* gingival.

crevicular epithelium *See* epithelium.

crevicular fluid *See* gingival crevicular fluid.

crib Round wire clasp fitting round a tooth to provide retention for a prosthesis. Both ends of the wire are secured to the baseplate of a removable orthodontic appliance or a denture. *See* Adams' clasp.

cribriform Perforated, sieve-like.

cricothyrotomy *See* tracheostomy.

cristobalite Form of silica used with plaster of Paris as a refractory in investment materials.

criteria Plural of criterion.

criterion Standard by which matters may be judged.

CRO Centric relation occlusion.

crossbite Malocclusion of anterior or posterior teeth in which the labiolingual or buccolingual relationship of opposing teeth is the reverse of normal, i.e. a reverse horizontal overlap. Can be isolated to a single tooth or a segment of teeth.

cross-infection *See* infection.

cross-linking Creates chemical bonds between molecular chains in a polymer, making the resin stronger and more rigid.

cross-sectional study Observational study of a population at one point in time. Often used to assess the prevalence of a disease or disorder in a population.

cross-striations Lines seen under the microscope which cross enamel prisms and are thought to indicate their daily growth.

Crouzon's disease *See* dysostosis, craniofacial.

crowding Malocclusion resulting from the disproportion in the combined mesiodistal dimension of the teeth and the size of the maxilla or mandible, leading to a displacement from the dental arch.

crown 1. That part of a tooth covered by enamel. 2. Replacement (restoration) of part or all of the clinical crown, cemented into place. May be made of metal, plastic, porcelain or a combination of these. Classified by extent, method of construction and materials used. *Anatomical c.* That portion of the tooth normally covered by, and including, the enamel. *Basket c.* Cast-metal crown, with or without a facing, used as a restoration for fractured or malformed anterior teeth. *Cast c.* Metal veneer crown, full or partial, and constructed by the casting process. *Clinical c.* Anatomical term for that part of a tooth which is visible above the gingival margin at any stage of eruption. *C. lengthening.* A surgical procedure sometimes required to increase crown length and thus improve artificial crown retention. *C. scissors. See* scissors. *Dowel c.* Crown with a prefabricated post. *Full veneer c.* Extracoronal restoration which covers the entire clinical crown of a tooth. *Jacket c.* Full veneer crown completely covering the prepared tooth and having a cervical shoulder. Constructed of porcelain or resin (*see* temporary c.) and cemented into place. *Partial veneer c. (three-quarter c.).* Cast-metal extracoronal restoration covering most of the surfaces of the clinical crown of a tooth. *Polycarbonate c.* Preformed opaque tooth-coloured crown for temporary/provisional treatment available in a range of sizes usually for anterior teeth. *Porcelain bonded c.* Cast-metal crown to which porcelain has been bonded externally. *Porcelain jacket c.* Full veneer porcelain crown possessing a shoulder at its

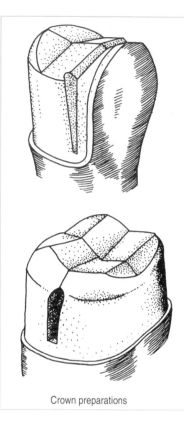
Crown preparations

being cemented to the tooth and the outer part fixed over it. Used in bridgework when there are problems concerning parallelism of the abutment teeth. *Temporary c.* Full veneer crown made of aluminium, resin, stainless steel or acrylic resin to protect a tooth preparation and the soft tissues surrounding it. It is easily removed, maintains the occlusion and is placed in position while a permanent restoration is being constructed. *Temporary post c.* Temporary crown that incorporates a post. *Three-quarter c. See* partial veneer c.

cruciform Shaped like a cross.

cryo- (kryo-) Prefix denoting cold, freezing or frost.

cryosurgery Surgical technique in which tissue is destroyed by freezing.

cryotherapy Use of extremely low temperatures in the treatment of disease.

crypt Small blind recess or pocket. *Dental c.* Cavity in the alveolar bone in which a tooth develops before eruption.

CSSD Central sterile supply department.

CT (computed tomography) *See* CAT scan.

cubital Relating to the elbow.

culture 1. To grow micro-organisms. 2. *Noun.* The micro-organisms resulting from growth, usually in artificial media. *C. medium.* Substance used to cultivate micro-organisms, e.g. broth, agar, serum.

cure 1. To restore to health. 2. In dentistry, the process whereby an acrylic resin is polymerized and thus hardened.

curettage Instrumenting the walls of a bony cavity by curette to remove chronically inflamed tissue and bone.

curette Spoon-shaped instrument used to remove tissue by scraping, e.g.

gingival margin. *Post c.* Crown retained by a metal post. *Preformed metal c.* Crown form constructed from stainless steel, but often also containing chromium, made available in a range of sizes for primary and permanent molar teeth. Used for permanent restoration of primary teeth with extensive caries or following pulp therapy and semi-permanent restoration of permanent molar teeth with hypoplasia, tooth surface loss or other dental defects (e.g. amelogenesis imperfecta). *Shell c.* Full veneer crown made from plate metal. *Strip c.* Preformed transparent crown form used with composite resin for temporary/provisional treatment of anterior teeth and restoration of fractured incisors. *Telescopic c.* Two-part crown, the inner part

Mitchell's trimmer (q.v.), Volkmann's spoon (q.v.). *See also* periodontal instruments.

curing time The time necessary to attain a full cure in a thermosetting plastic or rubber.

curve To bend without any angles. An arch. That which is bent. *C. of Monson.* Occlusal curve on which artificial teeth are set up. All of the cusps should touch a curve of 102 mm in radius whose centre is at a smooth point between the eyebrows (glabella). *C. of Spee.* Curve running from the condyle of the mandible along the superior surface of all mandibular teeth to the central incisors, having an arc of 6.5–7 mm when seen from the lateral skull view. *C. of Stephan.* Graph illustrating the 24-hour rise and fall of plaque acidity during and between meals, especially the increased rise due to intake of refined carbohydrates—particularly sweets and sweet drinks—between meals.

Cushing scalers *See* scalers.

cusp 1. A pointed projection. 2. Protrusion or eminence usually arising from the occlusal surface of a posterior tooth and canines. *C. angle.* Angle made by the slopes of a cusp with a plane at right angles to the long axis of the tooth. *C. capping.* The inclusion of cusp(s) in the cavity preparation and their restoration to functional occlusion with a restorative material. *C. of Carabelli. See* Carabelli cusp. *C. height.* The distance between the tip of a cusp and its base plane.

cuspal interference Unwanted contact of any cusp with an opposing tooth which may deflect or prevent the normal occlusion of the rest of the teeth.

cuspid *See* canine (preferred name).

cuspidor Spittoon generally fitted with a water-flushing device.

custom tray *See* impression tray, special.

cutaneous Relating to the skin.

cuttle Polishing agent made of ground cuttle fish bone and consisting mainly of calcium carbonate.

CVA Cardiovascular accident.

cyanoacrylate adhesive Rapid-setting acrylate-based adhesive employed in household, industrial and medical applications. Applications in dentistry include wound closure and retrieval of fractured instruments from root canals.

cyanosed Relating to cyanosis.

cyanosis Bluish appearance of the skin and mucous membranes caused by insufficiency of oxygen in the blood.

cyanotic Showing the symptoms of cyanosis.

cyclamate Intense sweetener with approx. 50 times the sweetness of sucrose. *See* sweetener.

Cyklokapron® *See* tranexamic acid.

cylindroma Malignant salivary gland neoplasm.

cyst 1. Prefix denoting a bladder. 2. Abnormal cavity in the tissues lined by well-defined epithelium and containing fluid or a semifluid material. *Apical or radicular c.* Cyst of inflammatory origin associated with the apical region of a pulpless tooth. *C. lining membrane.* Soft tissue lining of a cyst, usually composed of epithelium. *C. pack.* Pack of ribbon gauze impregnated with antiseptic, bismuth iodoform paraform paste or Whitehead's varnish. Inserted postoperatively into a cyst cavity. *C. plug.* Plug of material such as acrylic resin used postoperatively to keep open a cyst cavity, allowing it to heal from the base upwards. *Dermoid c.* A congenital cyst containing elements of ectodermal origin and found in skin, floor of the mouth and the upper neck. *Multilocular c.* Cyst with several adjoining cavities. *Residual c.* Cyst left behind following the removal of a pulpless tooth from which it arose. *Sebaceous c.* Benign retention cyst of a sebaceous gland which secretes sebum. May occur almost anywhere in the body. A single cyst cavity. *Unilocular c.* Single cyst cavity in bone. *See also* median palatine cyst.

cyst of dental origin Cyst arising from proliferation of ectodermal tissue present in the formation of teeth. *Dentigerous c.* Cyst arising from the follicle surrounding the developing tooth. *Developmental c.* Cyst arising from abnormal development tissues. *Eruption c.* Cyst arising from the follicle of an erupting tooth.

cytological examination A microscopic examination of cells obtained from a smear of a suspected lesion.

cytology The study of the structure and function of cells.

cytoplasm Jelly-like protoplasm that surrounds the nucleus of a cell and is contained within the cell wall.

cytotoxic Any substance or drug that is harmful to cells. *C. drug.* Drug used to treat cancerous growths (e.g. vinblastine). Destroys cancer cells more readily than normal cells.

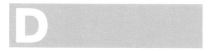

dactyl- Prefix denoting the fingers or toes.

Dakin's solution *See* sodium hypochlorite.

Daktarin® *See* miconazole.

dam *See* post dam, rubber dam.

dangerous drugs Certain controlled drugs defined by an Act of Parliament which specifies certain requirements in the writing of prescriptions for these drugs, e.g. opiates, cocaine, etc.

dappen pot (dish) Small glass or plastic receptacle for drugs and liquids used in dentistry.

day-patient Person who spends a large part of the day in hospital for examination, observation and/or treatment but who does not remain there overnight.

DCPs (dental care professionals) Members of the dental team recognized and registered by the appropriate authority (the General Dental Council in the United Kingdom) and entitled to carry out certain dental procedures (clinically or in the laboratory): clinical dental technicians (q.v.); dental hygienists (q.v.); dental therapists (q.v.); dental nurses (q.v.); dental technicians (q.v.); orthodontic therapists (q.v.).

de- Prefix denoting loss or removal, e.g. demineralization (of teeth).

dead tooth *See* tooth.

dead tract Dark tract in dentinal tubules seen in ground section under a microscope. The tubules appear dark because they contain air and not dentinal processes.

deadman switch In radiology, a timer switch constructed so that it makes an electrical contact only when pressed and switches off when released by the operator.

deafferentation Total or partial loss of the afferent nerve supply or sensory input derived from a particular body area.

debilitate To render weak or feeble.

debilitation Effect of previous disease or malnutrition giving rise to weakness, loss of weight and a feeling of being run down.

debride To remove debris, foreign matter and dead tissue from a wound.

debridement Removal of foreign matter and dead tissue from a wound or root canal.

debris In dentistry, an accumulation of unwanted fragments such as food, pieces of tooth, drill dust and caries.

decalcification Removal of calcium or its salts from a tissue such as bone or enamel.

decalcify To remove calcium or its salts from a tissue.

decay 1. Gradual chemical decomposition of organic matter when exposed to the atmosphere. 2. In dentistry, a deprecated term for caries (q.v.). 3. Process of radio-active substance disintegration.

deciduous Shed periodically, as the leaves of trees or the primary dentition. *D. dentition. See* primary dentition.

DEF index *See* index.

defibrillation Use of a controlled electric shock to stimulate and restore normal heart rhythm in cases of cardiac arrest due to atrial or ventricular fibrillation.

defibrillator An electronic instrument used to abolish atrial or ventricular fibrillation and thus allow the resumption of normal cardiac rhythm.

deficiency disease Disease caused by a deficiency of certain substances in the diet.

definition 1. The precise limits of anything. 2. In optics and radiography, the sharpness, distinctiveness and clarity of a projected image. 3. In microscopy, the clarity with which an object is viewed.

deflashing The finishing process of removing the flash or rind produced by spaces between mould cavity edges.

deflective occlusal contact Tooth-to-tooth contact that alters the direction of mandibular movement during closure.

DEFS index *See* index.

degassing The process of releasing trapped gases from a metal casting by heating.

degeneration Breaking down and deterioration of tissues.

degloving 1. In medicine, the tearing off, by injury, of the skin of a hand or a foot in a manner comparable to the removal of a glove. 2. In dentistry, term used to describe the reflection of a mucoperiosteal flap from bone, in order to expose a larger area of bone.

deglutition The act of swallowing.

dehiscence 1. Splitting open of a surgical wound. 2. In dentistry, a vertical defect of the alveolar margin and plate of bone.

dehydration Loss or deficiency of water from the tissues of the body.

demi- Prefix denoting half.

demineralization Reduction of the mineral content of a tissue.

demulcent Substance that protects and soothes mucous membranes and relieves irritation, e.g. gum tragacanth or milk.

dendrite Protoplasmic (tree-like) process of a nerve cell (neurone) (q.v.) by which impulses are transmitted towards the cell body.

dendritic Relating to or having dendrites.

dens in dente Term meaning 'tooth within a tooth', sometimes used for a dens invaginatus (q.v.).

dens invaginatus Developmental tooth anomaly in which there is a deep invagination on the lingual or palatal surface of incisor teeth, generally maxillary laterals. The invagination may be wholly or partially lined with enamel.

density 1. The mass of a unit volume of a substance. 2. In radiology, the comparison of one tissue's image with another when exposed to X-rays. Those images appearing lighter (less dense) on a radiological film indicate that the object is more dense to X-rays than the others.

dent- (denti-, dento-) Prefix denoting the teeth.

dental Relating to a tooth or teeth. *D. arch.* Curved arrangement of the teeth in the jaws. *D. caries. See* caries. *D. engine.* Rotary electric or foot-driven machine driving rotary instruments by means of a handpiece through a pulley or cable drive, or directly. *D. floss.* Thread or tape of waxed or unwaxed silk or synthetic material passed between the teeth to remove plaque or food debris. *D. follicle.* Fibrocellular layer of tissue surrounding a developing tooth before it erupts. *D. formula.* Standard formula used to designate the number and types of teeth of a dentition. *See* charting. *D. hygienist.* Member of the dental team qualified to practise preventive and certain therapeutic aspects of dentistry, including plaque control measures, removal of deposits from the teeth, application of fissure sealants and topical fluoride, and instruction in oral hygiene measures. The treatment must be prescribed by a dentist. *D. jurisprudence. See* jurisprudence. *D. nurse.* Member of the dental team who provides close support for the dental surgeon and is responsible for the cleanliness and tidiness of surgery equipment, instruments and materials. The dental nurse should have a general understanding and working knowledge of the sterilization and disinfection of surgery instruments and equipment—and be responsible for the preparation of the dental surgery for all dental procedures. Training includes: the recording of dental charting; maintenance of dental treatment records; assisting at the chairside during all dental procedures; assisting in the care of the patient before, during and after an anaesthetic; oral hygiene instruction and advising patients on what actions to take following certain dental procedures; the taking, processing, mounting and filing of radiographs; upholding the ethical standards of the dental profession; reception and administration procedures. *D. papilla.* Tissue partially enclosed by the enamel organ, which forms the dentine of a tooth and later becomes the pulp. *D. prop.* Instrument used intra-orally to maintain the mouth in an open position, e.g. Hewitt, McKesson, Brunton and Lane (centre prop). *D. prophylaxis.* Procedure for removing dental plaque, acquired pellicle and stains from the teeth by the use of polishing paste on a rotating brush or flexible polishing cup. *D. prosthesis.* Artificial replacement for one or more teeth and their associated structures. Constructed by the dental technician using acrylic resin or a combination of metal and acrylic resin. *D. prosthetist. See* prosthodontist. *D. pulp.* Fibro-cellular, jelly-like tissue which occupies the pulp cavity of a tooth. Consists of cell bodies, odontoblasts, blood vessels, nerve fibres and lymphatics. *D. stone.* 1. General term for model and die material. 2. Rotary abrasive instrument used for grinding and polishing. *D. tape. See* d. floss. *D. technician.* Member of the dental team who constructs dentures, crowns, inlays, bridges, orthodontic appliances, splints, etc. to the prescriptions of dentists. *D. therapist.* Member of the dental team who carries out dental treatment as prescribed by the dentist. Permitted to carry out simple fillings in primary and permanent teeth, apply preventive solutions, gels and sealants to the teeth, give plaque control instruction at the chairside and provide dental health education. *D. unit.* Combination of dental equipment in one unit. Formerly fixed and now mostly mobile. Combines high- and low-speed handpiece drivers, three-in-one air/water syringes and sometimes an ultrasonic or sonic scaler. Other appliances such as a cuspidor, dental operating light, bracket table and an X-ray machine may form part of the same dental unit.

dental erosion Irreversible loss of dental hard tissue by a chemical process that does not involve bacteria. Dissolution of mineralized tooth tissue occurs upon contact with intrinsic (see GORD) or extrinsic acids. *See also* tooth surface loss.

dental public health *See* community dentistry.

dentate Having natural teeth.

denticle (pulpstone) Deposit of amorphous calcific material occurring around the pulpal vessels in an otherwise normal tooth. May be found in pulps which have been mildly irritated over a period of time.

dentiform Shaped like a tooth.

dentifrice Collective term encompassing several kinds of tooth cleansers: tooth pastes, tooth powders, tooth 'whiteners' and mouthwashes.

dentigerous Containing teeth or tooth-like structures.

dentigerous cyst *See* cyst of dental origin.

dentinal Relating to dentine. *D. process. See* odontoblast process. *D. tubule.* Microscopic tube within the dentine of a tooth which contains the odontoblast process (q.v.).

dentine Sensitive calcified tissue forming the bulk of a tooth and surrounding the pulp. The dentine itself is covered by enamel in the crown and by cementum in the root. Consists of about 70% of inorganic salts by weight, and 30% of water plus collagen fibres. Microscopically shows a vast number of S-shaped tubules, running outwards from the pulp, which house the long, slender processes of the odontoblast cells in the pulp and are responsible for the formation of dentine. When odontoblast cells have laid down the bulk of the dentine—*primary d.*—and the tooth is fully formed, they continue to lay down further regular *secondary d.* throughout the time that the tooth remains vital. In response to any stimulus such as caries or abrasion, the odontoblast cells lay down secondary dentine at a more rapid rate. This type of dentine is known as *reparative secondary d. Adventitious d. See* secondary d. *D. pin. See* pin. *D. porcelain.* Also known as *body porcelain.* The pigmented, translucent porcelain which is used to give the overall shape and shade to a jacket crown restoration or facing. *D. screw.* Threaded length of wire inserted into the dentine to provide extra retention for a restoration, e.g. dentatus screw. *Hereditary opalescent d. See* dentinogenesis. *Hypoplastic d. See* hypoplasia. *Sclerotic* or *translucent d.* Areas of dentine whose tubules have become occluded.

dentino-enamel junction *See* amelodentinal junction.

dentinogenesis The formation of dentine. *D. imperfecta.* Grey-brown discoloration of the teeth caused by a hereditary defect in the calcification of dentine, often accompanied by a similar disturbance in bone.

dentinoma A rare tumour, arising from odontogenic mesenchymal tissue composed mainly of an irregular mass of dentine-like tissue.

dentistry Profession that cares for the teeth, their supporting structures and other oral tissues. Restores to normal function carious, fractured or badly worn teeth by means of fillings, inlays, crowns or bridges. Replaces missing teeth and other tissues by bridges and prostheses and treats dental abnormalities, diseases, traumatic injuries, and also provides preventive measures for caries and periodontal disease. *See also* aesthetic d., community d., conservative d., cosmetic d., endodontics, forensic d., four-handed d., operative d., orthodontics, paedodontics, periodontics, prosthodontics, restorative d.

dentition Natural teeth in the dental arches. In humans consists of 20 primary teeth erupting from the age of 6 months onwards. Later gradually replaced and added to by 32 permanent teeth.

dento-alveolar disproportion Disproportion between the size of the teeth and the space available for them in the dental arch. May lead to either crowding or spacing between teeth.

dento-gingival junction *See* junctional epithelium.

Dentomycin® *See* sustained release device.

denture Removable artificial substitute for missing teeth and their associated structures. May be partial or complete and is generally constructed of acrylic resin alone or in conjunction with various metals. *Acrylic d.* Denture made from acrylic resin (q.v.). *Complete d.* Correct term for full denture which replaces the whole of the normal dentition in the dental arch with the exception of the third molars. *D. base.* 1. That part of the denture

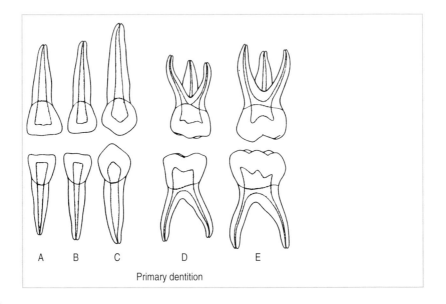

Primary dentition

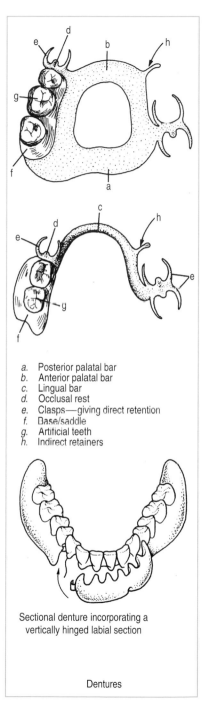

a. Posterior palatal bar
b. Anterior palatal bar
c. Lingual bar
d. Occlusal rest
e. Clasps—giving direct retention
f. Base/saddle
g. Artificial teeth
h. Indirect retainers

Sectional denture incorporating a
vertically hinged labial section

Dentures

which rests on the denture-bearing area of the oral mucosa. 2. Material, generally acrylic resin, used in the construction of dentures and other appliances by the dough moulding and curing technique. *D. bearing area.* That portion of the edentulous ridge and the surface of the teeth that is covered by a denture. *D. border.* Border of the denture base. *D. granuloma.* A deprecated term for d. hyperplasia (q.v.). *Hybrid d.* A removable dental prosthesis which is attached to a fixed substructure (such as a Dolder bar (q. v.)). *D. hyperplasia.* Area of hyperplastic fibro-epithelial tissue resulting from chronic irritation from a denture. *D. space.* Irregular space in the mouth, bounded by the cheeks, lips, tongue and floor of the mouth, and within which a denture should lie. *Duplicate d.* An exact replica of an existing denture. *Immediate replacement d.* Prosthesis constructed in advance of tooth extractions and fitted immediately after the removal of the teeth. *Implant supported d.* Prosthesis which obtains its stability and retention from a substructure lying under the soft tissues of the denture-bearing area, and which projects through the gingival tissues, e.g. asseo-integrated implant. *Interim d.* A dental prosthesis used for a short interval to check the design, the occlusion, the aesthetics or to condition the patient to accept an artificial substitute for natural teeth. The term is often used for an *immediate replacement d.* (q.v.). *Over-d.* Denture completely covering at least one tooth root or prepared tooth or asseo-integrated implant abutment. *Partial d.* Removable dental appliance which restores one or more—but less than all—of the natural teeth and associated parts, and is supported by the teeth and/or mucosa. *Sectional d.* Also known as *swing-lock d.* A denture made up of two or more separate parts connected with a mechanical device. *Skeleton d.* Prosthesis, generally of metal, designed to be as small as possible, consistent with strength, stability and retention. *Spoon d.* Small, maxillary spoon-shaped prosthesis usually replacing one or two teeth. It has no clasps, fits closely to the palatal mucosa and is not extended to the palatal necks of the maxillary teeth. *Trial d.* Denture in the process of construction when the teeth are set up in wax. It is tried in the mouth for suitability, aesthetics and stability before completion. Formerly called a '*set up*' or '*try in*'.

denturist Also called *clinical dental technician (UK)*. An accredited dental technician licensed to make and supply removable dentures to the general public.

deoxygenated Deprived of oxygen.

deoxyribonucleic acid *See* DNA.

dependence Condition of a patient who is unable to live normally without certain drugs.

depressant Agent that reduces the normal activity of any body function, e.g. anaesthetic, barbiturate.

depression 1. In anatomy, any part of the surface of an organ or structure that is lower than the general level of the surface. 2. In orthodontics, the adjustment of the vertical level of teeth that have overerupted beyond the general occlusal level of the dental arch. 3. Mental dejection; state accompanied by a loss of interest in one's immediate surroundings.

derm- (derma-, dermo-, dermat-) Prefix meaning pertaining to the skin.

dermal Relating to the skin.

dermatitis Inflammation of the skin.

dermatoid *See* dermoid.

dermatology The study of diseases of the skin.

dermis Underlayer of the skin, rich in blood vessels, nerves and lymphatics. It is covered by the epidermis.

dermoid Dermatoid. Resembling skin.

dermoid cyst *See* cyst.

desensitizing agent Preparation for topical application to sensitive areas of a tooth surface. May be in the form of a solution, gel or varnish, e.g. 2% zinc chloride solution and proprietary preparations such as Tresiolan® and Duraphat®.

desiccate To remove moisture and dry completely.

desmosomes (macula adherens) The microscopic intercellular bridges that attach adjacent epithelial cells to each other.

desquamation Process in which the outer layer of the epidermis is removed by scaling.

desquamative gingivitis Chronic, diffuse inflammation of the gingiva characterized by desquamation of the gingival epithelium.

detergent Wetting or cleansing agent which, when dissolved in water, causes dirt and grease to become detached.

detritus Debris which has disintegrated or died.

developing solution Solution which brings out the latent image on a radiographic film which has been immersed in it for a recommended period of time and temperature. It should be protected from daylight and replaced at regular intervals according to the frequency of use.

development The process of growing and differentiation. Becoming more complex.

deviation Changing from a normal course.

devitalize To kill or remove living tissue or cells. In endodontics *devitalize a pulp*, to apply a chemical agent to kill pulp tissue; *devitalize a tooth*, to remove vital pulp tissue from a tooth.

devitalizing/mummifying paste (or compound) Material, usually containing formaldehyde and various other antiseptic ingredients, which when placed in contact with an exposed pulp coagulates the protein of pulp with which it is in contact, allowing further pulp therapy at a later visit. Sometimes referred to as Easlick's Devitalising Paste. *See also* devitalizing pulp therapy.

devitalizing (mummifying) pulp treatment Method of devitalizing part of the pulp of primary teeth prior to their removal in order to preserve the remaining radicular pulp in an aseptic state until the tooth is shed normally. Rarely used in the permanent dentition.

dextran *See* Extracellular polysaccharide.

dextro- Prefix denoting the right side.

dextrose Main end-product of the breakdown of carbohydrates during digestion. Also known as *glucose*.

DF 118® *See* dihydrocodeine.

di- Prefix meaning two or double.

diabetes mellitus Condition in which lack of insulin, normally secreted by the pancreas, causes an inability to deal with sugar metabolism. Characterized by frequent passing of urine containing sugar, excessive thirst, lassitude and a lowered resistance to infection.

diabetic Person suffering from diabetes. Such people may carry a card declaring their condition and suggesting what action should be taken if they enter a state of coma. *D. coma*. Loss of consciousness due to an accumulation of ketone bodies (q.v.) in the blood.

diagnosis Identification of a disease or condition by observing the signs and symptoms and determining its nature. *Differential d.* The differentiation of two or more diseases with similar clinical signs and symptoms.

diagnostic cast *See* cast.

diagnostic injection or **analgesia** Aid to diagnosis whereby a local analgesic is injected into a specific area in order to eliminate pain, and thus prove that the pain arises from the specific site. Careful serial intraligamental injections are now used to refine this diagnostic test.

dialysis Method of separating particles of different dimensions in a liquid mixture by diffusion through a semipermeable membrane. This principle is used in haemodialysis in artificial kidney machines.

diamond Crystalline form of carbon, harder than any other naturally occurring substance. *D. instrument.* Rotary instrument, such as a bur or wheel, used as an abrasive cutting tool having commercial or synthetic diamond grit embedded in its metal surface.

diapedesis Passage of blood cells through blood vessel walls, e.g. the process in which phagocytic leucocytes (q.v.) pass through capillary walls during inflammation.

diaphragm 1. In anatomy, the thin, muscular, dome-shaped sheet separating the thoracic cavity from the abdominal cavity. Contraction causes inspiration and relaxation allows expiration. 2. In restorative dentistry, the thin veneer of metal extended from the core of a post-crown to some or all of the margins of the prepared root face. 3. In radiology, the metal plate, with central aperture, designed to limit the size of the X-ray beam.

diarrhoea Frequent bowel evacuation of abnormally soft or liquid faeces.

diastema Space occurring between two adjacent teeth.

diastole Relaxation phase of heart muscle contraction when blood enters its chambers. It is followed immediately by systole (q.v.).

diathermy Heat provided by an electric current of high frequency. Used to warm but not injure tissues. *D. apparatus.* Equipment producing high-frequency electrical currents used to cut, coagulate and fulgurate tissues. The current may pass between the two tips of the instrument (bipolar) or between the instrument and the patient, who holds an electrode (unipolar). *Short-wave d.* Used to relieve pain. *Surgical d.* Of very high frequency (VHF). May be used to dissect tissues, coagulate blood vessels and fulgurate (q.v.) tissues in periodontal procedures. Not suitable for patients with heart pacemakers.

diatomaceous (Kieselguhr) earth Form of finely divided silica used as a filler and polishing agent.

diatoric tooth *See* tooth.

diazepam Drug used in tablet form to reduce anxiety and fear, as a premedication before the use of a local anaesthetic solution or as an anaesthetic. It may be administered intravenously.

dichroic fog Chemical fog seen on radiographs and caused by exhausted fixing solutions.

diclofenac (Voltarol®) An analgesic drug that is sometimes used in the management of dental pain. The normal dose is 50 mg three times daily.

die The positive reproduction of a prepared tooth or teeth in a suitable hard material such as amalgam, stone or plaster. *D. lubricant.* A separating medium applied to the die so that the wax pattern may be withdrawn without sticking to the die.

diet A way of feeding. A prescribed course of feeding.

differential diagnosis *See* diagnosis.

differentiation 1. Distinction of one disease from another. 2. Change of function of certain cells.

diffuse Scattered over an area. Widespread.

diflunisal A drug with analgesic and anti-inflammatory properties. Trade name Dolobid®.

digastric Having two bellies, e.g. digastric muscle (q.v.). *D. muscle.* Muscle contributing to movement of the mandible and mouth during mastication. It has two bellies of muscle separated by a tendon, which runs through a pulley of fibrous tissue attached to the hyoid bone. The posterior belly is attached to the temporal bone and the anterior belly is attached at the digastric fossa near the midline, lower border of the medial surface of the mandible. Contraction of the digastric muscle, when the hyoid bone is held steady, helps to open the mouth, but during deglutition the muscle action raises the hyoid.

digestion Process performed in the alimentary tract by which food is broken down into simpler elements for tissue building and repair.

digestive system System in which food is broken down by enzymes to yield simpler substances capable of being absorbed by the body tissues. Consists of the mouth and teeth, the salivary glands, the oesophagus, stomach, small and large intestines and rectum. Digestive juices are added from the pancreas, the gall-bladder and the liver.

digit A finger or toe. *D-sucking. See* finger-sucking.

digital radiograph A computerized image obtained either directly via a charge coupled device or indirectly using a photostimulable phosphor plate and laser plate reader.

dihydrate Compound possessing two molecules of water.

dihydrocodeine Powerful analgesic prescribed in 10 and 30 mg tablets. May cause giddiness and/or nausea. Trade name DF 118®. This drug is of no use in the management of inflammatory pain of dental origin.

dilaceration Distortion occurring during the development of a tooth which disrupts the normal axial relationship between the crown and the root.

dilatation Spreading or extension in all directions. Term applied particularly

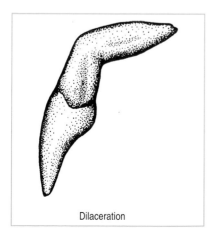

Dilaceration

to the enlargement of a cavity, blood vessel, canal or other opening.

diodontic implant Historical term used for a sterile metal rod placed in a root canal and extending through the root apex with the intention of stabilizing a tooth, especially one with a short root. Has also been referred to as *endodontic implant*.

diphtheria An infectious bacterial disease caused by *Corynebacterium diphtheriae* which multiplies in the throat, producing powerful toxins affecting the heart and nerves. The inflammatory exudate coagulates in the throat to form a characteristic false membrane. This disease is now rare owing to widespread immunization. Incubation period 2–8 days.

diplegia Paralysis of similar organs on both sides of the body.

Diprivan® *See* propofol.

direct attachment *See* direct bonding.

direct bonding Bonding of a fixed orthodontic bracket directly to a tooth surface by means of an adhesive technique, most commonly using acid etchant (q.v.) and composite adhesive.

direct fracture Fracture at the site of injury.

direct inlay technique Method of construction of an inlay or casting by using a wax pattern taken directly from a tooth preparation and not from a model. Used in the lost wax casting technique (q.v.).

direct interdental wiring *See* fixation.

direct retainer Part of a partial prosthesis designed to resist dislodgement along its path of insertion.

direct retention Retention obtained in a partial prosthesis by the use of direct retainers.

direct technique *See* direct inlay technique.

dis- Prefix denoting separation.

disaccharide Sugar which yields two monosaccharides on hydrolysis (a reaction of a substance with water), e.g. sucrose, lactose, maltose.

disarticulation Separation of the components of a joint resulting in disturbance of normal function.

disc (disk) 1. Flat, circular fibrocartilaginous structure separating the opposing surfaces of a joint, e.g. temporomandibular *articular disc*. 2. Metal, plastic or cardboard disc having one surface carrying an abrasive, glued or bonded to it. Mounted on a mandrel (q.v.), it may be used to abrade or polish restoration surfaces or to sharpen instruments. *D. guard.* Protective metal shield placed partially round a rotary disc. *Magnetic d. (disk).* A data storing device used in the operation of computers and word processors.

disclosing agent Non-toxic vegetable dye, such as erythrocin, used to reveal plaque and other deposits on a tooth surface. May be in gel, solution, capsule or tablet form.

discoid Having the shape of a hollow disc, e.g. the blade of an excavator.

disease Abnormality of structure or function, or both, as found in a part or parts of the body.

disinfect To reduce the number of pathogenic micro-organisms by physical or chemical agents to a level at which they pose little risk of causing disease.

disinfectant Agent capable of reducing the number of pathogenic micro-organisms to safe levels.

dislocation (luxation) Displacement from their natural position of the ends of bones forming a joint. Also used to describe a tooth which has been displaced from its socket. If partially displaced it is termed 'subluxation'.

disodium tetraborate *See* borax.

dispersed phase amalgam alloy *See* alloy.

displacement Malposition of a tooth or joint.

distal Situated away from the centre of the body or point of origin. *D. end cutter.* Orthodontic wire cutter with blades set at right angles to the handles and used to cut the distal ends of archwires (q.v.). *D. surface.* That surface most distant from the midline.

distortion In dental radiology, the distortion of the radiographic image from the true outline or shape of the object being radiographed. Generally due to incorrect angulation of the central beam, or to bending of the radiographic film.

distraction osteogenesis Surgical technique where a fracture is surgically created in a bone and a mechanical device is then used to slowly move the ends of the fracture apart in order to achieve bony growth in the gap, thereby achieving elongation of the bone hopefully without the need for a bone graft.

distribution Arrangement of nerves and blood vessels throughout the body.

ditch A long narrow trench.

ditching Characteristic effect seen at the periphery of an amalgam restoration at its junction with the enamel of the tooth.

divergence Spreading apart.

DMF index Index giving the total number of decayed, missing and filled permanent teeth. Used to show the

DMFS index Index giving the total number of decayed, missing and filled *surfaces* of permanent teeth. Used to show the caries incidence of an individual or an average group.

DNA (deoxyribonucleic acid) Molecules present in the nucleus of cells and which dictate hereditary traits and control all cell activity.

doctor 1. Title given to the recipient of a university degree (usually a PhD) higher than a Master's degree. 2. Courtesy title given to medical practitioners and, in some countries, to dental surgeons.

Dolder bar Metal bar of various shapes, soldered or screwed to a crown or post and core of abutment teeth or an asseo-integrated implant abutment. Provides retention for a prosthesis by means of a clip on the fitting surface of the prosthesis.

Dolobid® *See* diflunisal.

domiciliary kit Portable basic dental kit for the treatment of bedridden or disabled patients in their homes or in hospital.

-dontic Suffix meaning of the teeth, e.g. orthodontic, endodontic.

dormant In an inactive state.

dors- Prefix denoting the back.

dorsum 1. The back. 2. Refers to the superior surface of the tongue.

dosage The exact quantity of a drug that has been prescribed for a specific period of time.

dose 1. In medicine, the quantity of a drug prescribed. A general term for the prescribed quantity of medicine to be taken at any one time. 2. In radiology,

the quantity of radiation or energy absorbed by the body tissues. *D. rate.* Dose absorbed per unit time expressed in grays per second.

dosimeter Instrument used to determine the absorbed dose, exposure or similar radiation quantity.

doughing time Time elapsing after mixing a material and before it is ready for manipulation. Used in connection with denture base (q.v.) resins.

dovetail (keyway) Type of cavity retention lock which is wider at its extremity and narrower at its neck where it joins the main cavity. It provides a mechanical lock to aid retention of a restoration.

dowel crown *See* crown.

Down syndrome (mongolism) A congenital disorder characterized by varying degrees of mental retardation and developmental defects which result in the typical appearance.

doxycycline A tetracycline antibacterial drug sometimes used in the management of maxillary sinusitis.

DPF Dental Practitioners' Formulary. A publication outlining the drugs that dental practitioners can prescribe on the National Health Service.

DPT Dental pantomogram. *See also* pantogram, pantographic tracing.

drain Device such as a tube, corrugated rubber or piece of rubber dam (q.v.) used to allow drainage of fluid from an internal body or pathological cavity to the surface either passively or by use of a vacuum.

drainage Channel created in soft tissues through which accumulated exudate and gases may be released. The creation of drainage from a pulp chamber or apical soft tissue.

dressing 1. Covering which may be soothing, to protect a wound and promote healing. 2. Provisional restoration, often placed in an emergency situation. In endodontics, *see* root canal dressing.

drill Rotating cutting device for making holes in hard substances. *D. biopsy.* Biopsy of hard tissues obtained by means of a hollow drill.

droplet infection Spread of microorganisms carried in minute droplets, usually by coughing or sneezing, which may be inhaled by others, e.g. diseases of the respiratory tract such as colds and influenza.

drug Any substance used in medicine or dentistry as a medicament. *D. addiction.* The taking of certain drugs which may lead to physical and personality changes and which may prove very difficult to abandon, e.g. alcohol, morphine, heroin. The use of such drugs often follows the drugs of dependence or 'soft' drugs such as amphetamines, cannabis and LSD (lysergic acid diethylamide) and synthetic narcotics. *D. dependence.* State in which a person has a psychological longing for the effects certain drugs may produce and which may become habit forming, e.g. benzodiazipines as sleeping pills and amphetamines as 'pep' pills. *D. eruption.* Skin rash developing as a result of administration of certain drugs, e.g. penicillin rash.

dry socket *See* localized alveolar osteitis.

duct Tube or canal conveying secretions, especially those of glands, e.g. Stenson's duct from the parotid salivary gland, Wharton's duct from the submandibular salivary gland.

ductile Able to be drawn out in fine strands or wires.

ductless gland *See* endocrine gland.

duo- Prefix denoting two.

duodenum The first part of the small intestine, extending from the stomach. The bile and the pancreatic duct open into it.

duplicating material Material used in dental laboratories to produce accurate duplication of models, casts, etc.

dura mater Tough protective outer coat of the brain and spinal cord.

Duraphat® *See* desensitizing agent.

dwarfism Underdevelopment of the body. May be caused by lack of activity of the pituitary gland (q.v.).

DWSIs Dentists with Special Interests.

dwt Pennyweight.

-dynia Suffix denoting pain.

dys- Prefix denoting abnormal, impaired or difficult.

dyscrasia Developmental disorder such as may be found in blood.

dysentery Inflammation and ulceration of the large intestine lining. There are two main types, amoebic and bacillary, both giving rise to severe diarrhoea.

dysfunction State of incomplete or impaired function of a part or organ.

dysostosis Defective formation of bone. *Cleidocranial d.* Rare congenital condition characterized by abnormalities of the skull, teeth, jaws and clavicle. Orally there is usually a high arched palate, underdeveloped maxilla and sinuses, and frequently a cleft palate. The shedding of the primary teeth is retarded with consequent delay in the eruption of the permanent teeth. *Craniofacial d. (Crouzon's disease).* Congenital disease of bone characterized by bossing of the frontal region, hypoplasia of the maxilla, mandibular prognathism and often cleft palate. Other bones may be involved as well as eye changes, often resulting in blindness.

dysphagia Difficulty in swallowing.

dysphasia Difficulty in speaking and failure to arrange words in their proper order.

dysplasia Abnormal development of tissues. *Chondro-ectodermal d. See* Ellis–van Creveld syndrome. *Ectodermal d.* Hereditary condition characterized by defects in the skin, teeth, hair and other organs.

dyspnoea Difficulty in breathing.

Dysport® *See* botulinum A toxin.

dystrophy Disorder of an organ, usually of muscular tissue, due to impaired nutrition of the affected part.

E

e- Prefix denoting from, out of or without.

ear-bow An instrument, similar to a face-bow, that is centred on the external auditory meatus and records the relationship of the maxillary dental structures to the cranial structures and to the horizontal plane.

Eastman analysis An orthodontic cephalometric analysis undertaken by orthodontic tracing based on landmarks and use of A-point and B-point to define the skeletal relationship (ANB angle), measurement of maxilla plane and mandibular plane angles relative to the incisors and the angle of the maxilla and mandibular planes.

EBA cement Reinforced zinc oxide-eugenol cement (q.v.) in which some of the eugenol is replaced by 2-ethoxybenzoic acid. The zinc oxide is reinforced by the addition of inorganic fillers such as alumina and silica together with rosin.

eburnation 1. The act or process of becoming hard like ivory. 2. In medicine, the increased density of bone due to reduced vascularity or inflammation. 3. In dentistry, the change in carious dentine from a soft decalcified mass to a hard, polished, black-to-brown state.

eccentric Not having its axis placed centrally, e.g. the position of a nozzle in an intravenous syringe. *E. jaw relationship.* Any jaw relation which is lateral or protrusive to the retruded mandible relationship. *E. occlusion. See* occlusion.

ecchymosis Collection of blood under the skin causing discoloration—a bruise.

ECG (EKC) *See* electrocardiogram.

ecology The scientific study of living things in relation to each other and to their environment.

ect- (ecto-) Prefix denoting external, outer or on.

ectoderm Outer germinal layer of the three primitive germ layers of the developing embryo from which the nervous system, skin, enamel and mucous membrane of the mouth are derived.

ectodermal dysplasia *See* dysplasia.

-ectomy Suffix denoting the complete or partial removal of an organ, e.g. apicectomy.

ectopic Located away from the normal position. *E. beat.* An extra systole, i.e. a premature beat generated in the heart but outside the sino-atrial node. *E. eruption.* Eruption of a tooth in an abnormal position.

ectoplasm The cell membrane. A thin clear area at the periphery of a cell.

79

ectro- Prefix denoting absence, usually of congenital origin.

eczema Inflammation of the skin, characterized by redness, soreness and itching.

edentate Having no natural teeth.

edentulous Toothless. Without natural teeth in the mouth, as when born or following total tooth clearance.

edge 1. A margin, border or ridge. 2. Cutting aspect of a blade.

edge-to-edge bite Malocclusion in which the mandibular and maxillary incisors occlude along their incisal edges and do not overlap.

edgewise appliance *See* appliance.

edgewise bracket An orthodontic bracket used in fixed orthodontic appliances having a horizontal channel or slot, most commonly 0.018 or 0.022 inch wide. Designed to receive a rectangular, square or round wire.

EDTA (ethylenediamine tetra-acetic acid) solution Chelating solution containing ethylenediamine tetra-acetic acid used in root canal therapy to soften dentine and facilitate its removal from root canal walls by means of reamers and files.

efferent Conveying from the centre to the periphery. *E. nerves.* Motor nerves from the brain conducting impulses which cause muscles to contract and glands to secrete.

ejector That which removes or expels, e.g. saliva ejector used to remove fluids from the mouth.

elastic Capable of recovering normal shape and size after having been stretched. *E. band.* Used in orthodontics to produce tooth movement. *Intermaxillary e.* Band applied between upper and lower dental arches to exert a pulling action when the mouth is opened. *Intramaxillary e.* Band applied to orthodontic appliance in one arch only.

elastomer Polymer with rubber-like elastic properties.

elastomeric impression material Impression material (q.v.) based on a non-aqueous polymeric system and which exhibits rubber-like elastic properties, e.g. the polysulphide, polyether and silicone impression materials.

electric pulp tester Instrument used to help determine the vitality of teeth. When the patient indicates that he or she can appreciate small amounts of current applied to a tooth, then the degree of vitality is noted. Should always be used in combination with other diagnostic tests before a tooth is pronounced non-vital.

electro-anaesthesia A local analgesia or, more commonly, general anaesthesia, produced by the passing of an electric current through tissues.

electrocardiogram (ECG) Record of the electrical activities of the heart on a moving paper strip.

electrocautery Wire loop heated electrically to red heat and used to cauterize tissue. *See also* diathermy, periodontal instruments.

electrode Either of the two terminals of an electric circuit or cell.

electrolyte Solution that produces ions, i.e. particles that will conduct electricity.

electrolytic polishing Process in which a metal is placed in an electrolytic solution and an electric current passed through it. Very minute particles of the surface of the metal are removed by electrolysis, so leaving a polished surface.

electromyography A technique utilizing an electronic apparatus to detect and record skeletal muscle activity. Of use in the diagnosis of occlusal and temporomandibular joint dysfunction.

electron Unit of negative electricity revolving around the positively charged nucleus of an atom. Flow of electrons along a conductor towards a positive charge is known as a 'current'. *E. microscope.* Instrument that uses a beam of electrons as a source for viewing a specimen. Has much greater resolving power than an ordinary light microscope.

electronic apex locator *See* apex locator.

electronic pulp tester *See* pulp tester.

electronic timer *See* timer.

electroplate Archaic term. To plate by means of electrolysis. In the dental laboratory, impressions may be plated with copper or silver to provide a hard, rubproof working model.

electrosurgery Coagulation of tissues by a diathermy apparatus (q.v.) using high-frequency electric current. The current may pass between the tips of the applying instrument (bipolar) or between the instrument and an electrode held by or attached to a patient (monopolar). The apparatus may also be used to cut tissues as in gingivectomy (q.v.).

element Simplest form into which matter can be divided. Consists of atoms having the same atomic number.

elephantiasis gingivae (gingival fibromatosis, idiopathic gingival hyperplasia) *See* fibromatosis.

elevate To remove, by elevating or lifting, teeth or roots from the alveolus using an elevator.

elevator Instrument used to lever tissues from each other. *Apical e.* Set of three elevators—right, left and straight—having hollow handles, small blades and long shanks. *Boyd Gardner e.* Right and left elevators with hollow handles. *Cryer's e.* Right and left elevators with triangular sharp-pointed blades and hollow handles. *Hospital pattern (Coleman) e.* Left, right and straight serrated broad-bladed instruments with heavy serrated hollow handles. *Warwick James e.* Small-bladed, left, right and straight elevators with flat, smooth handles. *Winter e.* Set of paired levers, with corkscrew handles and various shaped blades.

All elevators must be sterile when used and their pointed blades kept sharp for each operation. Hollow-handled elevators should not be placed in a dry heat sterilizer.

Ellis–van Creveld syndrome Chondro-ectodermal dysplasia. Disease characterized by bilateral polydactylism,

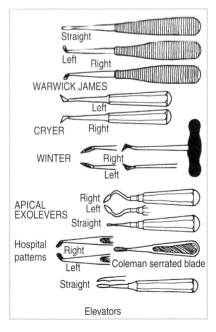

Elevators

chondroplasia of the long bones resulting in dwarfism and often in congenital heart disease. There are also disturbances in nails, hair and teeth which may be absent or defective.

elongation In radiography, a distortion of an image in which the teeth appear longer than their true size, caused by incorrect angulation of the central beam in the bisecting angle technique (q.v.).

Eludril® A mouthwash containing 0.1% chlorhexidine, 0.1% chlorbambutol and 0.5% chloroform.

Elyzol® *See* sustained release device; metronidazole.

EM Electron micrograph.

emaciation Excessive leanness due to illness or starvation.

embed In histology, the technique of fixing friable tissue in some rigid material, such as wax, so that thin sections may be prepared for microscopic examination.

emboli Plural of embolus.

embolism Sudden obstruction of a blood vessel by an embolus brought to the site by the blood circulation. May consist of a piece of tissue, fat, air bubble or a clump of bacteria.

embolus Clot or plug (usually a thrombus) in the blood circulatory system which blocks a vessel where it reduces in size. The clot then obstructs the blood circulation.

embouchure The position and use of the tongue, lips and teeth in the playing of wind instruments.

embrasure Space partially bounded by two adjacent teeth.

embryo First stages after the fertilization of a human ovum. Term usually confined to the first 8 weeks of intra-uterine life after which the embryo becomes recognizable and is described as a fetus.

embryology The study of the growth and development of the embryo.

embryonic The early stages of any process.

emery An abrasive powder, containing aluminium oxide and magnetite, used to smooth and polish metals. An impure form of corundum.

emesis Vomiting.

emetic Substance which causes vomiting, e.g. strong salt solution.

EMG Electromyogram. *See* electromyography.

emigration Passage of leucocytes through the semi-permeable single-celled epithelial lining of very small blood vessels.

eminence A projection or prominence, e.g. frontal or parietal.

emission Process of giving off or discharging.

EMLA® **(eutectic mixture of local anaesthetics)** Cream containing a 5% mixture of lignocaine and prilocaine. Used to reduce discomfort of venepuncture.

emollient 1. Soothing. 2. Agent which softens or soothes the skin.

emotive Exciting emotion.

empathy Ability to identify oneself mentally with another person's feelings.

emphysema Abnormal presence of air in the tissues or cavities of the body. Most commonly a lung disease.

empiric Treatment based on experience and not necessarily on scientific reasoning.

empirical Relating to empiric.

empyema Accumulation of pus in a cavity or hollow organ.

emulsification Splitting of a substance into minute droplets. Bile salts secreted by the liver emulsify fats during the process of digestion.

emulsion 1. Mixture in which oil or fats are suspended in a solution. 2. In radiography, coating on radiographic films composed of a gel containing silver halides. *E. speed.* Sensitivity of a radiographic film to radiation exposure.

enamel Hard outer covering of the anatomical crown of a tooth, consisting of highly calcified, acellular, generally prismatic tissue of ectodermal origin. It is the hardest tissue in the body, composed of rods and prisms, has 96% inorganic content and is not sensitive. *Decalcified e.* Enamel from which calcium has been removed. *See* white spot. *E. crystallites.* Crystals of biological apatites which occur in human enamel. *E. cuticle.* Organic film found on the surface of enamel. *E. fluid.* Aqueous solution found in the pores of the solid phase of enamel. *E. hatchet. See* hatchet. *E. lamella.* Thin sheets of imperfectly calcified organic material extending from the surface for a variable distance through the enamel. *E. matrix.* Organic base, secreted by ameloblasts, within which inorganic crystallites are laid down and grow. *E. organ.* Derived from the surrounding ectodermal tissues, the dental lamina and the tooth bud. Responsible for the formation of tooth enamel during development. *E. pearl.* Enameloma. A small bead of enamel formed apically to the cement–enamel junction and resembling a pearl. Often found in the furcation of molars. *E. porcelain.* Translucent, lightly pigmented outer covering of a porcelain jacket crown restoration used to simulate the translucency of a natural tooth. *E. prism.* Basic morphological unit of enamel running from the amelo-dentinal junction to the enamel surface. *E. protein.* Protein which forms a large part of the enamel organic material and is a product of the ameloblasts. *E. spindles.* Extensions of the dentinal tubules which can be seen under the microscope to be running across (for a short distance) the amelo-dentinal junction into the enamel. *E. striae of Retzius.* Incremental brown growth lines seen in enamel under the microscope running obliquely across the long axis of the enamel prism. *E. tuft.* Area of unmineralized enamel matrix extending from the amelo-dentinal junction a short way into the enamel. *Mottled e.* Enamel with white, yellow or brown areas—sometimes pitted—due to excessive ingestion of fluoride during enamel formation.

encapsulated Enclosed within a capsule. *E. amalgam alloy.* Preproportioned amalgam alloy and mercury supplied in a capsule which provides a standard mix.

encapsulation Enclosure within a capsule.

encephalo-trigeminal angiomatosis *See* Sturge–Weber syndrome.

endarteritis Inflammation of the lining of an artery.

endemic Referring to any disease prevalent in one particular locality.

endo- Prefix meaning within.

endocarditis Inflammation of the endocardium.

endocardium Innermost coat of the heart, lining the chambers.

endocrine gland Gland whose secretions (hormones) flow directly into the blood or lymph and greatly modify body development and metabolism. The chief endocrine glands are the pituitary, thyroid, parathyroid and suprarenal glands.

endocrine system System that consists of several ductless glands such as the pituitary, pineal, thyroid, parathyroid, thymus and adrenal, and certain cells within the pancreas and the ovaries and testes. These glands secrete hormones which pass directly into the blood circulation.

endocrinology The study of those ductless glands which secrete endocrines directly into the bloodstream or lymphatic system to affect tissues at some distance from them.

endodontic stop Device to fix the depth to which an endodontic instrument is introduced into a root canal. Usually a moveable silicone ring whose position is set with the aid of a ruler. Synonym: rubber stop.

endodontics The branch of clinical dentistry concerned with prevention, diagnosis and treatment of diseases of the dental pulp and their sequelae.

endodontology Study of the dental pulp, its form, function and behaviour in health, prevention, diagnosis and treatment of its diseases and their sequelae.

endogenous Produced from within and not from external sources.

endoscope Apparatus for viewing the interior of the body.

endosseous (endosteal) implant *See* implant.

endothelial Relating to endothelium.

endothelium Cell lining of various body cavities and of the blood vascular system.

endothermic A chemical reaction which results in the absorption of heat.

endotoxin A component, specifically lipopolysaccharide, of Gram-negative bacterial cells walls liberated after the death of the bacterial cell. Endotoxin is a powerful mediator of the inflammatory response.

endotracheal intubation Introduction of a tube into the trachea by way of the mouth or nose during an inhalation anaesthetic to maintain the airway.

energy Inhaled oxygen from the atmosphere, together with the action of enzymes in body cells, is used to oxidize glucose, converting it into carbon dioxide and water and releasing energy.

enervation 1. General weakness and loss of strength. 2. Surgical removal of a nerve.

engine mallet Dental engine-powered mallet sometimes used in the condensation of gold foil and amalgam.

enhancement In radiography, the intensification of detail, making a radiograph more easily interpreted.

enostosis Bony growth proliferating within a bone.

Entonox® A 50% mixture of nitrous oxide and oxygen that is used as a sedative.

entrance dose (skin dose) Quantity of radiation (or dose) absorbed at the site of entry of the X-ray beam.

enucleate 1. To shell out completely. 2. To remove a nucleus from a cell.

enucleation Complete removal of a cyst lining and contents, or of a tooth germ from its surrounding structures.

envelope of motion Three-dimensional space within which the mandible moves during its normal excursions.

enzyme A form of catalyst. A complex protein substance which produces fermentation and chemical change in other substances, apparently without undergoing any change itself. The substance acted upon by the enzyme is called a substrate. Enzymes are essential for many body processes such as digestion and the use of energy. There are three groups of digestive enzymes: the starch splitters or amylases (q.v.); the fat splitters or lipases (q.v.); and the protein splitters or proteases.

eosin Rose-coloured crystalline stain or dye derived from coal tar. Used to stain cells for study under the microscope.

eosinophil Leucocyte (q.v.) which readily takes up eosin dye.

eosinophilic granuloma *See* granuloma.

Epanutin® *See* phenytoin sodium.

ephedrine Drug with adrenaline-like properties used mainly in the treatment of asthma.

epidemic Disease affecting a large number of persons within a certain region.

epidemiology The scientific study of disease in order to discover means for its prevention and control.

epidermis Non-vascular outer thin layer of the skin derived from the ectoderm, consisting of layers of stratified squamous epithelium having no blood supply.

epidermoid carcinoma Malignant salivary gland carcinoma.

epidural Extradural. On or over the dura mater (q.v.). *E. analgesic.* Injection of an analgesic solution into the outer lining of the spinal cord in order to produce analgesia of part of the body. Used in patients who are not suitable for general anaesthesia.

epiglottis Cartilaginous, lid-like structure covering the opening to the larynx during the act of swallowing. Its function is to fold back over the aperture of the larynx, so preventing food from passing into the larynx, trachea or bronchi during deglutition (swallowing), directing it instead into the oesophagus.

epilepsy Disorder of the nervous system characterized by recurrent fits of convulsive muscular body movements and loss of consciousness. Severe attacks are known as *grand mal*, mild attacks as *petit mal*.

epileptic Relating to epilepsy.

epinephrine (adrenaline) *Hormone* either prepared synthetically or secreted by the medulla of the adrenal gland. Powerful stimulator of the sympathetic nervous system and a vasoconstrictor (q.v.). Increases the systolic blood pressure and tenses the body for flight or fight. Used topically (1 part per 1000 as a clear solution) to reduce haemorrhage, and in gingival retraction cords. Added to some local anaesthetic solutions (1 in 80 000 or less) to prolong analgesia by its action as a vasoconstrictor in reducing the local blood flow. Used in a concentration of 1:1000 in the emergency management of anaphylactic shock.

epistaxis Bleeding from the nose.

epithelial Referring to or composed of epithelium. *E. attachment. See* junctional epithelium. *E. cell rests of Malassez.* Cells of the epithelial root sheath of Hertwig, seen under the microscope as remains of the periodontal ligament. *E. cuff. See* junctional epithelium. *E. inlay. See* skin grafting vestibuloplasty. *E. root sheath of Hertwig.* Seen under the microscope as an extension of the enamel organ which, as it grows, forms the shape of the tooth root.

epithelialization Final stage of wound healing.

epithelioma *See* cancer.

epithelium Thin cellular layer which lines or covers internal or external surfaces of the body. It consists of cells joined together by small amounts of cementing substances. Found in many parts of the body such as the skin, where it acts as a protection against bacteria and the loss of body fluids. There are several types of epithelium. *Ciliated e.* Having mobile hair-like processes (cilia). *Columnar e.* Having cells which are taller than their width. *Crevicular e.* An extension of non-keratinized squamous cells into the crevice from the gingival crest epithelium. *Cuboidal e.* Having square-shaped cells. *Germinal e.* Covering the gonads. *Glandular e.* Having cells which secrete. *Pigmented e.* Having cells containing pigmented granules. *Sensory e.* Related to special sense organs. *Simple e.* Having a single layer of cells. *Squamous e.* Having flat, pavement-shaped cells. *Stratified e.* Consisting of several layers of different cell types.

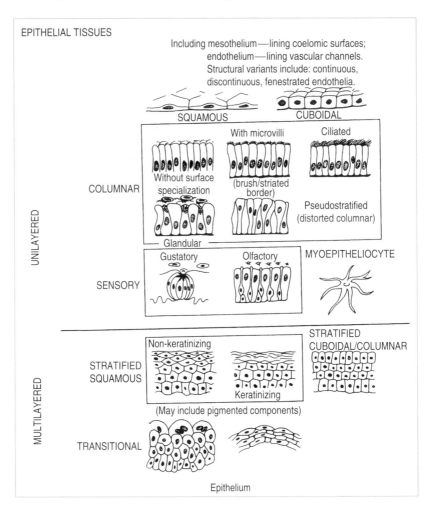

EPITHELIAL TISSUES

Including mesothelium—lining coelomic surfaces; endothelium—lining vascular channels. Structural variants include: continuous, discontinuous, fenestrated endothelia.

SQUAMOUS

CUBOIDAL

COLUMNAR

With microvilli

Ciliated

Without surface specialization

(brush/striated border)

Pseudostratified (distorted columnar)

Glandular

MYOEPITHELIOCYTE

SENSORY

Gustatory

Olfactory

UNILAYERED

MULTILAYERED

STRATIFIED SQUAMOUS

Non-keratinizing

Keratinizing

STRATIFIED CUBOIDAL/COLUMNAR

(May include pigmented components)

TRANSITIONAL

Epithelium

eponym Disease, anatomical structure or species named after the person who first described or discovered it, e.g. Ludwig's angina, Sharpey's fibres.

epoxy resin Synthetic resin used in die material and for applications using its adhesive properties.

Epstein's pearls (Bohne's nodules) Small yellowish-white nodules found on the palate and the crest of the alveolar ridges in the newborn infant. They generally disappear spontaneously after 2–3 months.

epulis Any localized enlargement of the gingiva. A benign fibroid tumour of the gingiva may be associated with pregnancy and resolves following parturition.

equilibration Maintenance or restoration of a body into a state of equilibrium. *Occlusal e.* Act of modifying the occlusal anatomy of teeth, by grinding, in order to restore a normal occlusion and thus harmonize cuspal relations in function.

equilibrium A state of balance.

ergocalciferol *See* vitamin D.

ergonomics The study of work and its environment and conditions so as to achieve maximum efficiency.

erosion 1. Wearing away of any substance. 2. A shallow ulcer. 3. Progressive loss of hard dental tissues by a chemical process without bacterial action.

erubescence Flushing or blushing—a reddening of the skin.

eructation Belching, i.e. the act of violently raising wind from the stomach.

erupt To break through.

eruption 1. A visible skin lesion. 2. In dentistry, the act of pushing or coming through the gingivae, as eruption of the teeth. *Active e.* Normal movement of a tooth into or towards the oral cavity

from its developmental position in the alveolar bone. *E. cyst. See* cyst of dental origin. *E. haematoma. See* haematoma. *E. table. See* Appendix 2.

erythema Superficial redness of the skin due to hyperaemia (q.v.)—a blush. *E. dose.* That amount of radiation which produces a temporary redness of the skin exposed to it. *E. multiforme.* Acute skin disease of unknown aetiology. Oral lesions may occur which may ulcerate, producing pain.

erythematous Characterized by erythema.

erythr- (erythro-) Prefix denoting redness.

erythritol Bulk sweetener with approx. 0.7 times the sweetness of sucrose. *See* sweetener.

erythroblast Elementary red blood cell.

erythrocyte Mature red blood cell. Non-nucleated bi-concave disc circulating in the blood. Its haemoglobin content is responsible for the transport of oxygen and the acid–base balance of the blood. The average life span of a red blood cell is 120 days and when worn out they are destroyed in the spleen and removed by the reticulo-endothelial system to the liver. They are developed in the red bone marrow of cancellous bone in such places as the ribs, sternum, vertebrae and the ends of long bones. Normally between 8 μm in diameter and 2 μm in thickness, numbering about 5 million/ml^3 in males and 0.5 million less in females. *E. sedimentation rate. See* ESR.

erythromycin Antibiotic used to treat a wide range of infections and often used in cases of sensitivity to penicillin and penicillin-resistant infections. Administered orally.

escharotic Caustic or corrosive agent often used to produce a dry scab when applied to the skin.

ESR (erythrocyte sedimentation rate) Rate at which erythrocytes (q.v.) settle out of suspension in blood plasma.

essence Solution of an essential oil dissolved in alcohol.

essential oil Volatile oil derived from an aromatic plant, e.g. oil of cloves.

Essix retainer *See* retainer.

ester Compound formed from an alcohol and an acid by the removal of water.

etching The selective dissolution of a surface by an acid or other agent. In dentistry, *acid e.* Partial demineralization of a selected area of tooth substance by the use of dilute acid in order to provide a clean and mechanically retentive surface for the retention of selected types of restorative materials such as composite and glass ionomer cements.

ethanol *See* alcohol.

ether Volatile liquid formerly used as an inhalation anaesthetic. Now largely replaced by safer and more efficient anaesthetics.

ethical 1. Relating to ethics. 2. Being in accord with professional etiquette and accepted codes of conduct.

ethics Moral principles.

ethmoid bone Perforated bone forming the roof of the nasal cavity and part of the floor of the skull.

ethoxybenzoic acid *See* EBA cement.

ethyl chloride Clear, highly volatile, colourless liquid. Used to produce surface analgesia by refrigeration or to test the vitality of pulps by their reaction to cold.

ethylenediamine tetra-acetic acid *See* EDTA solution.

ethylene oxide A chemical used in the gas sterilization process for materials that cannot be sterilized by wet or dry heat.

eu- Prefix denoting normal, easy or good.

eugenol Essential oil of oil of cloves. Liquid component of zinc oxide-eugenol cements and has sedative and obtundent properties. Classified as an antiseptic.

eukaryote An organism whose cells possess an internal membrane and associated structures including a nucleus and vesicles, including all members of the fungi plant, and animal kingdoms.

euphoria Exaggerated feeling of well-being, often not justified by circumstances. Can be induced by certain narcotic drugs.

Eustachian tube Narrow tube passing from the ear to the nasopharynx. Its function is to equalize the atmospheric pressure on each side of the ear-drum.

eutectic Describes a mixture of two or more constituents that melts and resolidifies without separation of its constituents.

evaporation Conversion of a liquid or solid into vapour.

eversion Turning inside out.

evert To turn inside out.

evulsion *See* avulsion.

ex- (exo-) Prefix denoting outside, outer, beyond or away from.

exacerbation Increase in the severity of symptoms of a disease.

examination An inspection and/or an investigation to evaluate the state of health or of a disease. In dentistry, a full examination should include a medical and dental history, a visual intra- and extra-oral inspection including palpation, auscultation, measurement of tooth mobility and gingival pocket depth, pulp tests as well as various radiographic and laboratory procedures.

excavation Process of scooping out. In dentistry, the removal of a softened dentine from a carious tooth.

excavator Hand-held cutting instrument used primarily to excavate softened dentine from a carious tooth. It has a sharp blade which may be circular, oval or spoon shaped. Usually double ended.

excipient Substance with no pharmacological action which is added to a drug to make it suitable for administration.

excise To cut out tissue in order to remove diseased from healthy matter.

excision Act of cutting out tissue.

excisional biopsy *See* biopsy.

excoriate To scratch the skin.

excrete To eliminate waste products.

excretory duct Terminal portion of the salivary duct which conveys the fully formed saliva from the striated duct into the oral cavity.

excursion Movement of the mandible laterally, protrusively or retrusively.

excursive movements Movement occurring when the mandible moves away from the intercuspal position (q.v.).

exfoliation 1. Falling away in layers, flakes or scales. 2. Natural loss of a primary tooth prior to its replacement by its permanent successor.

exit port (aperture or window) In radiography, the opening in the tube head through which X-rays leave.

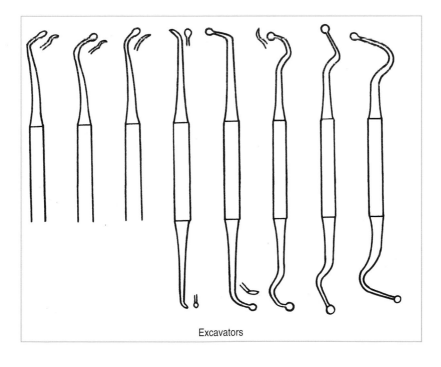

Excavators

exo- *See* ex-.

exodontics (exodontia) The subject of and the techniques used in the extraction of teeth or parts of them.

exogenous Describes a condition caused by external or environmental factors.

exolever Elevator (q.v.) for extracting whole or parts of teeth.

exostosis Developmental bony outgrowth from the surface of a bone. May be due to chronic inflammation, constant pressure on the bone or tumour formation. It may influence the positioning of a prosthesis.

exothermic 1. Heat releasing. Found in the setting process of various cements and acrylic resin as a result of chemical reactions. 2. Relating to the temperature of the external body surface.

exotic Describes a disease not found in a particular area or country; e.g. in Britain, leprosy is an exotic disease.

exotoxin A toxin made and liberated by living micro-organisms. Usually a protein, e.g. diphtheria toxin; tetanus toxin (tetanospasmin); *Staphylococcus* enterotoxin A (SEA); *Escherichia coli* enterotoxin (STa).

expansion 1. Increase in size, volume or length. 2. In dentistry, the movement of teeth by an orthodontic appliance in order to correct a malocclusion.

expectorant Drug that enhances sputum secretion thus making it easier to cough up.

expectoration Spitting out of material brought into the mouth from the air passages.

expiration 1. Exhalation: the act of breathing out. 2. The act of breathing one's last breath, i.e. dying.

expiratory Relating to expiration.

expire 1. To die. 2. To breathe out.

explorer *See* probe.

exposure 1. Act of laying open, as in a surgical exposure. 2. Subjection to infection, thermal changes, radiation, etc. 3. In radiology, a measure of the amount of exposure to radiation. 4. In dentistry, a defect in the wall of a tooth pulp cavity leading to exposure of pulp tissue. This may be the result of instrumentation (*traumatic*) or of caries (*carious*).

'extension for prevention' Extension in the course of preparation of a cavity, to include adjacent areas of sound tissue which are judged likely to become carious, i.e. pits and fissures. Now considered to be over-preparation of tooth tissue in view of current adhesive materials and concepts of caries management.

extension-cone paralleling technique (XCP) Paralleling technique (q.v.) using a long cone measuring about 40 cm (16 inches).

external On or near the outside.

external auditory meatus *See* meatus.

external bevel incision Incision designed to reduce the thickness of gingiva from the external surface.

external oblique ridge A smooth ridge on the buccal surface of the body of the mandible that extends from the anterior border of the ramus to the region of the mental foramen.

extirpation Complete removal or eradication of tissue. In endodontics, commonly used to describe the complete removal of vital dental pulp.

extra- Prefix denoting beyond or outside.

extracellular Outside the cell.

extracellular fluid Tissue fluid surrounding the cell.

extracellular polysaccharides Polysaccharides either produced outside the cell or produced inside the cell and then transported to the outside. In dentistry the term refers to a variety of polymers of glucose or fructose produced extracellularly by a mixture of different enzymes using sucrose as the substrate. Fructan and levan are polymers of fructose, glucan and dextran are polymers of glucose. EPS have a variety of functions within dental plaque and are thought to contribute to plaque pathogenicity.

extracoronal Outside the crown of a tooth. Describes a restoration which envelops the remaining natural crown. *E. attachment.* A precision attachment (q.v.) which is attached to a restoration but situated outside the coronal contours of an abutment tooth.

extract 1. Preparation containing the pharmacologically active principle of a drug. 2. In dentistry, to remove a tooth.

extraction 1. Act of drawing out or removal. 2. Process of removing teeth from the alveolus.

extraction forceps *See* forceps.

extra-oral Outside the mouth. *E.-o. anchorage.* Anchorage obtained from outside the oral cavity, usually from the head or neck. *E.-o. radiograph.* One in which the film is placed outside the mouth during exposure, e.g. panoramic radiographs, always housed in cassettes to reduce the amount of radiation used. *E.-o. tracing. See* tracing, gothic arch. *E.-o. traction (EOT).* Use of extra-oral apparatus to apply force to the teeth in orthodontic treatment.

extrusion 1. Condition of being forced or thrust out of a normal position. 2. In dentistry, the movement of a tooth to a new position beyond its normal alignment. This may be caused by trauma, as part of an orthodontic treatment plan or by the absence of an opposing occlusal force (over-eruption (q.v.)).

exuberant Prolific, copious, excessive.

exudate Fluid which passes into the adjacent tissues through vessel walls during the process of inflammation, i.e. lymph.

exudation Slow oozing of a fluid through the walls of an intact blood vessel, usually as the result of inflammation.

exude To ooze through a tissue or opening.

eye tooth Deprecated (or lay) term for the maxillary canine.

eyelet wiring *See* interdental.

face-bow 1. Instrument used in prosthetics to record the relationship of the maxilla to the transverse horizontal axis (hinge axis (q.v.)) of rotation of the

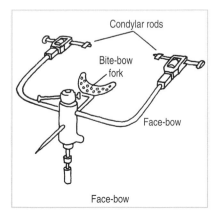

Condylar rods

Bite-bow fork

Face-bow

Face-bow

mandible. This can then be transferred to an anatomical articulator (q.v.). 2. In orthodontics, a wire frame used to transmit extra-oral forces from headgear to an orthodontic appliance.

facet 1. Face or front. 2. In dentistry, a smooth worn area on a tooth surface made by movement of another tooth upon it. 3. In anatomy, a small flat surface on a bone, especially on a surface of articulation.

facial Related to the face. *F. bones*. The group of small bones about the eyes and nose which form the architecture of the face. They include the maxilla, mandible, palatine and zygomatic bones. *F. hemiatrophy*. Wasting of the soft tissues of one half of the face and head. *F. hemihypertrophy*. Congenital condition causing enlargement of one side of the face. *F. nerve*. Seventh cranial nerve supplying efferent branches to the muscles of facial expression, the submandibular and sublingual salivary glands, and afferent branches (taste) to the anterior two-thirds of the tongue. *F. neuralgia*. Pain syndrome, generally of obscure aetiology, characterized by pain in any region of the face, teeth, tongue and often in the shoulder area. The pain is intermittent and may last for minutes or for days and is not characterized by a trigger zone. *F. palsy*. See palsy, Bell's. *F. plane*. Transverse plane through the skull represented on a lateral skull radiograph by a line joining the nasion and the pogonion. *F. seal*. In prosthetics, seal created by the contact of the lips and cheeks with the polished surface of a denture. The seal is effected by a salivary meniscus which prevents the entry of air. *F. surface*. In dental anatomy, the surface of a tooth directed towards the lips or cheeks (buccal or labial surfaces). *F. transfixation*. See fixation.

facing Veneer applied to the visible surface of a restoration to improve its appearance.

factor Substance, condition, influence or agent which contributes towards a result.

facultative A micro-organism, usually a bacterium, which has no requirement for oxygen and which can grow in its presence or absence. *f. aerobe* and *f. anaerobe* are synonymic.

Fahrenheit Temperature scale now being replaced by the Celsius or centigrade scale (q.v.). Water, at sea level, boils at 212°F and freezes at 32°F. Body temperature is normally 98.6°F.

faint 1. Weak and feeble. 2. Loss of consciousness. See syncope.

falciform Shaped like a sickle.

false pocket Deprecated term for periodontal pocket due to gingival enlargement (q.v.).

familial Describes any condition that affects a family to a greater extent than is expected by chance. *F. multicystic disease*. See cherubism.

fascia Band or sheet of fibrous connective tissue, covering the body beneath the skin and enveloping muscles and organs.

fascial Relating to the fascia.

fat 1. Adipose tissue (q.v.) of the body. 2. An oily substance. Fat consists of various combinations of oxygen, carbon and hydrogen and occurs in most foods, especially meat and dairy products.

fauces Opening from the mouth into the pharynx bounded by two folds of muscle covered by mucous membrane known as the *pillars of the fauces*. These run from the soft palate on either side of the fauces, one fold passing to the tongue and the other into the pharynx. Between them lie the tonsils.

FDI Féderation Dentaire Internationale.

febrile Describing a feverish condition. Feverish.

feedback Constant flow of sensory information to the brain.

feldspar (felspar) Crystalline mineral of aluminium silicate containing potassium, sodium, barium or calcium. An important constituent of dental porcelain.

felypressin Octapressin®. Synthetic vasoconstrictor drug used in local anaesthetic solutions containing prilocaine, e.g. Citanest®. It has little effect on blood pressure.

femur Largest long bone of the body extending between the knee and the pelvis. Its ball-shaped head articulates with the pelvic girdle.

fenestrate To pierce with one or more openings. To make a window.

fenestrated Perforated in more than one place.

fenestration 1. Act of perforating or being perforated. 2. Area of incomplete coverage of bone over a root which does not extend to the alveolar crest.

ferric oxide Impure form of naturally occurring red oxide of iron, commonly called rouge, and used as a polishing and colouring agent in synthetic teeth, ceramics and filling materials.

ferric sulphate Pulp medicament, increasingly being used in primary molar pulp therapy as an alternative to formocresol.

fetid (foetid) Foul smelling.

fetus (foetus) Developing embryo from the 8th week until birth.

fever (pyrexia) Rise in body temperature above normal ($37°C$ or $98.6°F$ taken orally). Generally accompanied by increased pulse and respiration rate, shivering, headache, and possibly nausea, constipation or diarrhoea. A rise in temperature above $40°C$ is termed *hyperpyrexia* and may lead to convulsions and delirium.

FFD (focus-to-film distance) In radiography, the distance from the focal spot to the film packet.

FGP Functionally generated path.

fibre Slender, thread-like structure. *Afferent f.* Nerve fibre conducting impulses to a nerve centre or spinal cord. *Collagen f.* White, flexible but inelastic fibre which forms the chief constituent of connective tissue. *Efferent f.* Nerve fibre conducting impulses from the brain or spinal cord. *Elastic f.* A basic constituent of loose connective tissue, elastic cartilage and skin dermis. *F. optics.* A miniaturized light source that is transmitted along flexible strands of fibre glass. In dentistry, it is commonly used as a light source attached to a handpiece. *Principal f.* The main group of collagen fibres which make up the periodontal ligament. *Sharpey's f.* Connective tissue fibre that passes from the exterior into the cortex of bone. In dentistry, the extension of collagen fibres of the periodontal ligament embedded in the alveolar bone and cementum and which contribute greatly to the anchorage of a tooth in its socket.

fibril Slender minute fibre or filament.

fibrillar Relating to one or more fibres.

fibrillation Abnormal, rapid and chaotic beating of many individual muscle fibres.

fibrin Fibrous, insoluble substance formed by the interaction between thrombin and fibrinogen during the process of clotting. It enmeshes the red blood corpuscles.

fibro- Prefix denoting fibres or fibrous tissue.

fibroblast Immature cell found in developing connective tissue which may become a chondroblast, a collagenoblast or an osteoblast, such differentiation leading to the formation of cartilage, collagen or bone.

fibroblastoma Tumour arising from a fibroblast.

fibrocartilage Form of cartilage containing collagen fibres.

fibrocyte Inactive cell present in connective tissue derived from a fibroblast.

fibro-epithelial polyp Tissue enlargement due to an overgrowth of epithelium and connective tissue.

fibroma Benign neoplasm arising from epithelial fibrous tissue.

fibromatosis A proliferation of fibrous tissue *F. gingivae* (gingival hyperplasia, idiopathic f., idiopathic gingival hyperplasia, elephantiasis gingivae). A rare condition which may be associated with either the primary or the secondary dentition. The gingival enlargement may cover the teeth and may be hereditary, idiopathic or drug induced.

fibrosarcoma Malignant neoplasm arising from fibrous connective tissue.

fibrosis Formation and ingrowth of fibrous connective tissue following chronic inflammation.

fibrositis Inflammation of fibrous tissue causing pain and difficulty of movement.

fibrous Characterized by the presence of fibres. *F. dysplasia.* Disease of bone in which bone and bone marrow are replaced by fibrous tissue and poorquality bone. *F. tissue.* Type of connective tissue having a mass of fibres present. Found in all ligaments, including the periodontal ligament. *F. union.* Union of fracture segments by connective tissue instead of bone.

field size Area of the X-ray beam at the site of entry.

filament Delicate thread or fibre.

filamentous Composed of long threadlike structures.

filariform Hair-like, thread shaped.

file 1. Means of storing information or records. 2. Metal hand instrument used in a rubbing action to reduce and smooth a surface, e.g. bone file. *See also* root canal file.

filled resin *See* composite resin.

filler In dentistry, substance or material used to fill a gap or to increase the strength of a substance.

filling 1. Lay term for a dental restoration. 2. Material placed in a preparation or cavity in order to fill it. *F. material.* Suitable material inserted into a tooth preparation or cavity in an attempt to restore form or function, e.g. amalgam or composite. *Retrograde f.* Filling placed in the apical area of a root following the surgical removal of a root apex. *Root canal f. See* root. *Temporary f.* Filling, usually of temporary cement, which is intended to remain in place for a short time only. *See* provisional restoration.

film 1. Thin layer or coating. 2. Thin sheet of material such as cellulose acetate which has been treated for use in photography or radiography. *F. badge.* Radiation dose meter containing a radiation-sensitive film, worn by dental and medical staff to detect exposure to radiation.

F. development. Chemical reaction in reducing the latent image in the emulsion of an exposed photographic or radiographic film in order to produce a stable image composed of minute grains of metallic silver. *F. fixation*. Chemical removal of metallic salts from the emulsion of an exposed film to produce a stable, permanent image. *F. hanger*. Device to hold radiographic films during processing. *F. holder*. Device to hold and stabilize a radiographic film in the mouth. *F. packet*. Lightproof and moisture-resistant sealed packet or envelope containing one or more radiographic films for use in intra-oral radiography. *F. processing*. Chemical transformation of a latent image, produced by exposure to either light or radiation, on the film emulsion, into a stable permanent image. *F. sensitivity* or *speed*. Amount of light or radiation required to produce a given image density. This property is largely related to the grain size of the emulsion. *Non-screen f.* or *direct action f.* Film whose emulsion is more sensitive to radiation than to light. *Screen f.* Film whose emulsion is more sensitive to light than to radiation and often used in cassettes (q.v.) fitted with intensifying screens (q.v.).

filter 1. Device consisting of a membrane or other permeable material (e.g. filter paper) which prevents the passage of some of the components of a mixture. 2. In radiography, device placed in the path of an X-ray beam to reduce selectively the intensity of certain undesirable wavelength components. 3. In photography, a transparent coloured material placed in front of a lens to remove or reduce the intensity of certain colours. 4. In sound physics, a device to reduce the intensity of undesirable frequencies.

filtration 1. Process of passing liquids through a material so as to suspend impurities. The liquid, once filtered, is known as the *filtrate*. 2. In radiology, process in which a material is placed in the path of an X-ray to remove its undesired longer wavelengths of radiation.

final impression Also called *master, working* or *second impression*. The impression used to construct the master cast. *See* impression.

fineness (of alloy) A method of rating the gold content of a gold alloy. The fineness of gold is the parts per thousand of pure gold, e.g. pure gold is 1000 fine. A gold alloy containing 800 parts gold and 200 parts of other metals is 800 fine. The relationship between carat and fineness is given by the equation:

$$\frac{Carat}{24} = \frac{Fineness}{1000}$$

finger spring Palatal spring or retractor. A cantilever spring attached to the fitting surface of a removable orthodontic appliance.

finger-sucking Common habit in young children which, if it persists, can lead to various occlusal discrepancies such as anterior open bite, proclination of maxillary incisors and retroclination of mandibular incisors.

finishing In denture construction, the term is used to describe the final stages of denture construction. After the denture has been processed, the flask is opened and the denture cut out of the plaster. It is then cleaned of plaster, trimmed and polished, and thus made ready for insertion in the mouth. *F. bur. See* bur. *F. line. See* line. *F. strip. See* strip.

Fish gingivectomy knife *See* periodontal instruments.

fission Act of splitting.

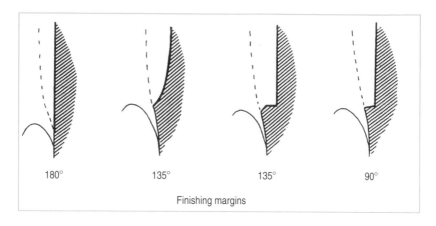

180°   135°   135°   90°

Finishing margins

fissural (inclusion) cyst Cyst arising in the lines of junction of the embryonic processes forming the jaws.

fissure 1. A groove, cleft or furrow. 2. In dentistry, a small groove or trough in the enamel of a tooth. An unfolding of the enamel between cusps and ridges. Fissure burs (q.v.) are designed to cut along the fissure. *F. sealant.* Hard insoluble substance (usually unfilled composite resin) used in liquid form to seal the vulnerable pits and fissures in teeth against bacterial plaque and food debris. May be self-processing or require a curing light to activate setting (polymerization).

fissured tongue *See* tongue.

fistula Abnormal epithelialized connection between two hollow organs or from a cavity to the external body surface, e.g. oro-antral fistula.

fitted labial bow Wire closely adapted to the labial surfaces of a number of anterior teeth in orthodontic treatment. Usually has one or two small loops to allow for adjustment.

fitting (tissue) surface *See* tissue surface.

fixation 1. Retention. The means by which a prosthesis or orthodontic appliance is kept in position. 2. Maintenance,

in correct position, of the displaced fragments of a fractured bone. *Arch bar f. See* arch (archaic). *Cap splint f.* (archaic) Splint used in oral surgery to immobilize fractured bone ends. May be cast in silver alloy or other metals, to be a close fit over the crowns of the existing teeth, extending to the gingival margins. It is cemented in place and usually retained for at least 8 weeks. *Craniomandibular f.* (archaic) The fixation of the mandible to the cranium with rods connected either to bone pins or to a head frame and denture splints. The fixed mandible is then used to reposition and stabilize the fractured maxilla. *Cranio-maxillary f.* (archaic) External metal rods or wires, running from a cast maxillary splint to a plaster of Paris head cap or metal halo, used to immobilize fragments of a fractured maxilla. *Direct interdental wiring f.* Method of wiring the teeth together, generally in fracture cases, in which wires are passed round the necks of the teeth in both dental arches and their ends twisted together. Such ends are then themselves twisted together. *Facial transf.* (archaic) Method of immobilizing maxillary fractures by passing pins, e.g. Steinmann pin (q.v.), or wires, e.g. Kirschner wire (q.v.), through the face and bone fragments, and the non-fractured zygomatic arch bones. *Gunning type f.* Used in edentulous fracture cases where existing dentures, or an acrylic resin splint, are wired circumferentially to the maxilla and the mandible and then wired together. *Intermaxillary f.* Fixation of the lower to the upper jaw by means of splints or wiring. *Internal skeletal f.* Stabilization of a fractured bone by internal or direct wiring, by bone plate and screws, or by transfixation by medullary pins. *Intramedullary f.* Surgical technique in which a metal pin is inserted into the interior of the bone (in the medulla) across the line of fracture. *Open reduction internal f. (ORIF).* Fracture is surgically exposed and reduced under direct vision using fixation appropriate to the bone involved, e.g. mini titanium plates and screws for a mandible or maxilla. *Pin f.* (archaic) Immobilization of bone fragments in fracture cases by the use of steel pins inserted from the external surface of the face. The protruding pins are connected together by a system of rigid bars and universal joints. *See also* internal wire suspension, per-alveolar wiring.

fixed appliance Orthodontic appliance involving the use of attachments, either bands or bonds to one or more teeth. It cannot be removed by the patient and at the completion of the treatment is removed by the operator. Unlike removable appliances, its action is constant and can achieve all orthodontic tooth movements, including moving teeth bodily and not just by tilting. Plaque control is rendered more difficult by these appliances.

fixed-fixed bridge *See* bridge.

fixed-movable bridge *See* bridge.

fixing solution Acid solution into which are placed photographic or radiographic films that have previously been placed in a developing solution and then washed in running water. Further development of the film is arrested by it and the film can then be inspected before being replaced in the solution for some 10 minutes when all emulsion has been dissolved and the film is clear.

Flagyl® *See* metronidazole.

flange 1. Projecting flat rim. Some saliva ejector attachments have flanges to control and protect the tongue, and reflect light during dental procedures. 2. That part of a denture base that lies in a sulcus.

flap Flat portion of tissue, either skin, mucosa or mucoperiosteum, utilized for access to underlying structures or repair of a surgical defect. They may be partially severed from their bed or deeper surroundings. The blood supply can be preserved by keeping intact one of the margins, usually referred to as the base of the flap, or in the case of free tissue transfer reconstruction, may be dissected free from the donor site and re-anastomosed at the recipient site, e.g. radial forearm free flap.

flask 1. Sectional metal case containing and supporting the mould in which dentures are formed. 2. Also used to describe the action of investing a pattern (q.v.) in the flask.

flasking Investing a wax denture or pattern in a flask.

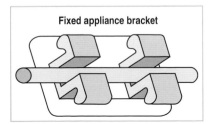
Fixed appliance bracket

97

flocculent Resembling tufts of wool. A fluid containing fluffy particles.

floss Waxed or unwaxed thread or cord used to remove plaque from the interproximal surfaces of the teeth. *F. silk. See* dental f.

flow 1. To circulate freely. To glide along. 2. Plastic deformation, under load, exhibited by some dental materials under certain conditions, e.g. amalgam, impression material, wax.

fluconazole An antifungal drug used to treat oral fungal infections.

fluctuation A variation, a rise and fall.

flumazenil (Anexate®) A benzodiazepine drug that acts as an antagonist to other benzodiazepines such as diazepam and midazolam. It is used as a reversal agent during benzodiazepine intravenous sedation. It is supplied in vials containing 500 μg in a 5 ml solution.

fluorescence Property of some substances which can emit surface reflections of light that differ in colour from the light absorbed.

fluorescent agent (or pigment) Material used in the fabrication of artificial teeth, crown and bridge porcelain and filling materials to impart fluorescence and thus simulate the fluorescence of natural teeth.

fluoridation Adjustment of the amount of soluble fluoride in water supplies in order to reduce the incidence of dental caries. In temperate climates, the optimum level of the fluoride ion in the water supply is between 0.7-1.0 part per million (or 0.7 -1.0 mg/litre). This has been found to reduce dental decay by as much as 40–50%. Naturally fluoridated water may contain a much higher fluoride ion concentration, especially in parts of Africa and Asia. Milk, salt and fruit juices may be artificially fluoridated for use in communities where water fluoridation is not possible.

Excessive exposure to ingested fluoride may produce fluorosis (q.v.) of teeth.

fluoride Naturally occurring inorganic ion of fluorine which when used topically or systemically renders teeth less susceptible to caries.

fluorine Non-metallic gaseous element.

fluorosis Mottled discoloration of the teeth due to a excessive ingestion of fluoride when the teeth are forming.

flux Material used to prevent oxidation and facilitate the flow of solder.

FMPA Frankfort mandibular plane angle. *See* Appendix 10.

focal infection The mechanism in which micro-organisms from one site of the body are disseminated into other areas of the body and set up secondary areas of infection.

focal plane (plane of cut) In tomography, the selected plane that provides a clear image.

focal spot (source) That portion of the target on the anode of the X-ray tube which is bombarded by the electron stream.

focal trough (image layer) In dental panoramic tomography, the depth of focus in which the selected layer provides a clear and distinct image.

foci Plural of focus.

focus Point at which reflected or refracted rays meet. The centre of activity, the centre. *F.-to-film distance. See* FFD. *F.-to-skin distance. See* FSD.

foetid *See* fetid.

foetus *See* fetus.

fog In radiography, the partial or complete darkening of a developed photographic or radiographic film due to sources other than the primary beam or to light exposure.

foil Very thin sheet of metal such as tin, platinum or gold. *Cohesive gold f.* 24 carat or 1000 fine pure gold, whose surface is completely pure so that it will cohere or weld at room temperature. *Gold f.* Pure gold rolled into extremely thin sheets and historically used in the restoration of teeth. *Platinum f.* A precious metal foil with a high fusing point. In dentistry, it is most often used as the internal matrix onto which porcelain restorations are built up, prior to firing (q.v.).

folic acid Vitamin B_{12}. *See* vitamin.

follicle 1. Small cavity or recess with an excretory or secretory function. *Dental f. See* dental.

follicular Relating to a follicle. *F. cyst.* Cyst arising from the dental follicle (q.v.). Follicular cysts include the dentigerous and eruption cysts. *See* cyst of dental origin.

food impaction Forceful wedging of food interdentally

foramen Opening or hole in a bone which allows the passage of blood vessels, nerves and lymphatics. *Apical f.* Opening at or near the apex of a tooth root through which nerve, blood and lymphatics enter and leave. *F. magnum.* Large foramen in the occipital bone of the skull through which the brainstem joins the spinal cord. *F. ovale.* Opening in the greater wing of the sphenoid bone which conducts the mandibular division of the trigeminal nerve and the small meningeal artery. *F. rotundum.* Foramen in the greater wing of the sphenoid bone through which passes the maxillary division of the trigeminal nerve. *Greater palatine f.* Conducts the greater palatine nerve and blood vessels to and from the mucous membrane of the palate. Situated close to the posterior border of the hard palate in the region of the palatal root of the upper third molar on each side of the midline. *Incisive f. (nasopalatine f.).* Connects the nasal cavity to the oral mucosa. Lying in the midline internal to the upper central incisors, beneath the central papilla of the rugae. It has four openings, two for the nasopalatine nerves and two for the nasopalatine blood vessels. *Infra-orbital f.* Situated on the facial aspect of the maxilla below the orbital cavity. The infraorbital artery exits from it and the afferent maxillary division of the trigeminal nerve enters it from the tissues around the nose, face and upper lip. *Lesser palatine f.* Situated close and posteriorly to the greater palatine foramen at the posterior border of the hard palate. Conducts the afferent lesser palatine nerve and blood vessels from the soft palate to the sphenopalatine ganglion. *Mandibular f.* Situated on the internal aspect of the ascending ramus of the mandible, halfway between the sigmoid notch and the lower border of the body of the mandible, at the upper end of a narrow groove against which the mylohyoid nerve and blood vessels run to the floor of the mouth. The mandibular artery and vein and the afferent inferior dental nerve from all lower teeth are protected by a triangular spur of bone known as the lingula. This is the area sought when giving an inferior dental block injection. *Mental f.* Opening on the buccal aspect of the body of the mandible usually in the region below and between the premolar teeth. Afferent nerves from the lower lips and labial incisal gingivae pass through it, together with blood vessels, to join the incisive branch of the inferior dental nerve within the bone. *Nasopalatine f. See* incisive f. *Palatal f. See* incisive f. *Posterior palatal f. See* greater palatine f. *Supra-orbital f.* Groove in the supra-orbital margin of the frontal bone conducting the supra-orbital nerve and vessels.

foramina Plural of foramen.

forceps Instrument having two beaks and handles, used for grasping instruments, dressings, needles, etc. and for the extraction of teeth. *Artery f.* Metal forceps with serrated, sometimes curved beaks and scissor-like handles with a ratchet device to maintain the grip until released. *Spencer Wells artery f.* Original pattern of forceps used to clamp arteries. *Mosquito artery f.* Similar to Spencer Wells artery forceps but with fine beaks. *Bone-cutting f.* Two-handled instrument with knife- or chisel-shaped blades, also known as *bone shears. Bone-nibbling f.* (*rongeurs*). Two-handled, pincer-like instrument used to cut away small portions of bone by means of cup-shaped beaks. *Dissecting f.* Tweezer-like instrument with curved, straight, serrated or rat-toothed jaws. Some are insulated for electro-surgery. *Extraction f.* Pincer-like instruments for tooth extraction. Consist of handles, joints and beaks or blades, made in various shapes and widths. Classified by numbers stamped on the inner side of the handle by the makers, according to the shape of the beaks or handles or to their special uses. *Lower molar f.* Forceps with both beaks set at right angles to the handles and arrow shaped to fit the bifurcation of the two roots of lower molars. *Lower root f.* Straight-handled forceps with hollowed-out beaks in various widths, set at right angles to the handles. Used to extract lower incisors, canines, premolars and roots.. *Upper anterior f.*

(*straight*). Forceps with hollowed-out straight blades of various widths in line with the handles. *Upper molar f.* Right and left instruments having one hollowed-out beak to fit the palatal root of upper molars and a pointed, spade-shaped beak to accommodate the bifurcation of the buccal roots. There are several other patterns including a range of smaller children's extraction forceps. *Upper root f.* Forceps with curved, hollowed-out beaks of various widths and curved handles (*Read's pattern*), one to fit into the palm of the hand and the other to provide a comfortable grip for the fingers. *Upper root bayonet pattern f.* Having straight beaks set at an angle to the handles which may be curved (*Read's pattern*) or straight. Used for extraction of upper teeth and roots in the posterior part of the mouth. *Maxillary disimpaction f.* Instrument in which one blade passes into the nasal cavity and the other fits against the palate so that the displaced maxilla may be grasped, disimpacted and repositioned. *Needle-holding f.* Instrument with scissor-type handles and often a ratchet device, to hold needles during suturing. *Cow's horn f.* Forceps with cutting blades bearing resemblance to cow's horns in shape used to split and separate the roots of multi-rooted teeth. *Rubber dam clamp f.* (*cervical clamp f.*). See rubber dam. *Tissue f.* Fine-bladed forceps with scissor handles and with or without ratchet device to hold their jaws together once closed.

Fordyce's spots (or disease) Developmental anomaly consisting of enlarged sebaceous glands of the oral mucosa and genitals. Clinically it appears as a collection of small yellowish spots.

forensic Pertaining to courts of law. *F. dentistry. See* jurisprudence and odontology, forensic.

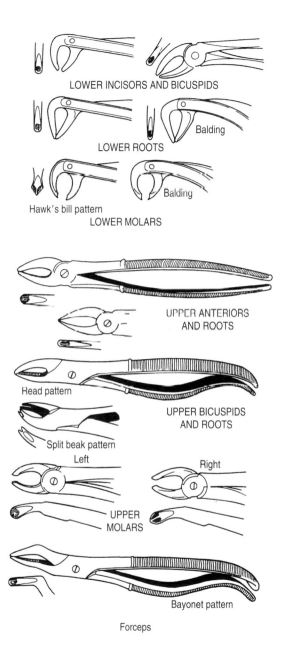

LOWER INCISORS AND BICUSPIDS

Balding

LOWER ROOTS

Balding

Hawk's bill pattern

LOWER MOLARS

UPPER ANTERIORS
AND ROOTS

Head pattern

UPPER BICUSPIDS
AND ROOTS

Split beak pattern

Left

Right

UPPER
MOLARS

Bayonet pattern

Forceps

foreshortening In radiography, the decrease in length of the radiographic image of the tooth due to incorrect technique.

formaldehyde Gas with a strong pungent odour used in solution as a disinfectant and in some cases mixed with cresol as a root canal medication.

formalin A 37% aqueous solution of the gas formaldehyde used to fix tissues for histological examination.

formants Two major resonating frequencies determining the sound of a vowel.

formocresol A pulp medicament, usually used in a 1:6 dilution (Buckley's formocresol). Used in primary molar pulp therapy to mummify or 'fix' pulpal tissue.

fossa A depression in bone or on the surface of a tooth, e.g. glenoid fossa.

four-handed dentistry Dental surgeon and surgery assistant working together as a team on operative procedures.

foveae palati Two pits situated near the junction of the hard and soft palate, one on either side of the midline.

fracture A breakage. Bone fractures may be simple, compound or comminuted. Jaw fractures are treated by reducing the fracture so that the bone ends are in approximation. The fractured bone is then immobilized by means of splints, pins or wires for a period of weeks to allow the bone ends to unite, after which the splints, etc. are removed. *Closed f. See* simple f. *Comminuted f.* Bone fracture in which the bone is fragmented into several pieces. *Compound f.* Bone fracture in which the bone fragments are exposed externally to communicate with the surface. *Greenstick f.* Incomplete fracture. *Impacted f.* Condition in which one portion of a fractured bone is driven into the other portion. *Indirect f.* Fracture at any distance from a point of impact or trauma, e.g. a blow on the chin may cause a fracture of one or both condyles of the mandible *(guardsman's f.)*. *Le Fort f. classification. See* Le Fort classification. *Linear f.* Fracture running along the long axis of a bone. *Middle third f.* Fracture of the bony complex that comprises the middle third of the facial skeleton. *Simple f.* Bony fracture in which the bone ends do not appear through the skin.

fraena Plural of fraenum.

fraenal Relating to the fraenum.

fraenectomy Excision of a fraenum. The operation, sometimes carried out for orthodontic reasons, includes the removal of interdental fibrous tissue.

Fraenkel A German orthodontist known for his devlopemnt of myofunctional appliances. Fraenkel 1 is used to correct Class II Division I malocclusions; Fraenkel 2 to correct Class II Division II malocclusions; Fraenkel 3 to correct Class III malocclusions.

fraenoplasty Repositioning of attached fraenum.

fraenotomy Cutting of a fraenum.

fraenum (frenum, frenulum) Fold of mucous membrane extending from the inner surface of the lip, cheek or tongue, to the alveolar process. *Abnormal f.* Abnormal fold of mucous membrane which may obstruct the seating of a denture, or influence the periodontal attachment. *Labial f.* Fold of mucous membrane in the midline, anterior to the upper central incisors, extending from the inner surface of the upper lip to the alveolar process. Its surgical removal is known as a *fraenectomy* (q.v.). *Lingual f.* Midline fold of mucous membrane extending from the inferior surface of the tongue to the floor of the mouth.

fragmentation Breaking up into small parts.

Frahm's carver *See* carver.

framework The skeletal metal part of a partial denture to which the remaining denture components are attached.

Frankfort mandibular plane angle The angle formed by the Frankfort horizontal plane and the mandibular plane. (*See* Appendix 10).

Frankfort plane Plane passing through the lowest point in the floor of the left orbit (the orbitale) and the highest point of each external auditory meatus of the skull (the porion). It is horizontal when the head is in the normal upright position. *See* Appendix 10.

free articulation *See* articulation.

free cleansing Improving the shape of a tooth surface or space between two teeth. This makes it easier to keep clean, by opening up the contact area, ensuring smooth margins on restorations or recontouring the tooth surface to discourage plaque build-up.

free end saddle Partial denture whose distal extension base terminates without support from a natural tooth or an implant.

free graft *See* graft.

free radicals Any species capable of independent existence, which contains one or more unpaired electrons occupying an atomic or molecular orbital by itself. Thought to contribute to cell and tissue damage in many disease states including, for example, periodontal diseases.

freeway space *See* interocclusal clearance.

freeze drying Technique in which tissues for pathological examination, or dental materials such as the glass ionomer and carboxylate cements, are subjected to freezing and then dehydration in a high vacuum.

frenulum *See* fraenum.

frenum *See* fraenum.

Frey's syndrome Condition sometimes occurring as a sequel to operations involving the parotid gland. Characterized by sweating and redness of the cheeks in the area of distribution of the auriculotemporal nerve on mastication.

frit The material from which dental porcelain is made. It consists of partially or completely fused hot porcelain which is plunged into cold water. The mass cracks and fractures and is then pulverized into the correct grade of particle and packaged as dental porcelain (q.v.).

frontal bone Skull bone forming the forehead and protecting the frontal lobes of the brain.

frontal plane *See* coronal plane.

frontal sinus One of a pair of air-containing cavities situated above the eyes in the frontal bone.

fructan *See* Extracellular polysaccharide.

fructose A fruit sugar. A monosaccharide found in honey and fruits.

FSD (focus-to-skin distance) In radiography, the distance from the focal stop to the point where the X ray beam enters the skin.

fulgurate To flash as lightning. To destroy tissue by high-frequency electrical currents.

fulguration Destruction of tissues by electrical means.

full denture *See* denture, complete.

Fuller's earth *See* kaolin.

full-mouth disinfection Treatment method for periodontal diseases that involves the conventional removal of tooth surface deposits by scaling and root planing over two visits, usually within 24 hours. Various chlorhexidine preparations are also used to help eliminate oral pathogens from periodontal pockets and other 'infected' sites in the mouth such as the tonsils and surface of the tongue. The aim is to reduce the likelihood of re-infection.

full-mouth radiological survey Complete radiographic examination of the teeth and surrounding bone, in which the film is positioned periapically in each tooth area. Normally consists of 10 films. Now superseded by panoramic techniques which subject the patient to less radiation and are usually extra-oral.

full-mouth rehabilitation or full-mouth reconstruction Treatment intended to restore the integrity of the dental arches by the use of directly applied composite restorations, inlays, crowns, bridges, precision-attached prostheses, implants or partial prostheses.

full-thickness flap Flap of mucosal tissue, including the periosteum, reflected from bone.

full-thickness graft (Wolfe graft) Free graft of the full thickness of skin removed from one part of the body and sutured in another part to repair a defect.

full-veneer crown Restoration that replaces the entire surface of the clinical crown.

functional appliance See myofunctional appliance.

functional articulation See articulation.

functional impression See impression.

functional impression material See impression material.

functional record See record.

functionally generated occlusal path Movement made by opposing cusp or cusps from centric occlusion to a number of eccentric positions.

fungal Referring to a fungus or fungi.

fungi Plural of fungus.

fungicidal Relating to fungicide.

fungicide Agent destructive to fungi.

fungiform Shaped like a fungus or mushroom.

Fungilin® See amphotericin.

fungoid Having the characteristics of a fungus.

fungus Eukaryotic organisms belonging to the kingdom Fungi, including mushrooms, toadstools, moulds, rusts, yeasts which are characterized by a lack chlorophyll and vascular tissue and by the presence of a rigid *cell wall* composed of *chitin*, *mannans* and sometimes *cellulose*. Fungi range in form from a single cell to a body mass of branched filamentous hyphae that often produce specialized fruiting bodies.

furcation Anatomical area where the root of a multirooted tooth divides. Known as a *bifurcation* in two-rooted teeth and *trifurcation* in three-rooted teeth. *F. involvement*. Pathological condition involving the alveolar bone in the furcation of a multirooted tooth. *F. tunnel procedure*. A periodontal procedure where a mandibular molar, with bifurcation involvement and a wide U-shaped arch between the roots, is treated surgically by osteoplasty (q.v.) and odontoplasty (q.v.) in order to allow cleaning of the postsurgical site with an interdental brush. The horizontal furcation involvement may be classified as *Grade I*, where there is incipient involvement in which the opening of the furcation is exposed with horizontal involvement of less than 1/3 the width of the tooth; *Grade II*, where the involvement extends beyond 1/3 the width of the tooth; and *Grade III*, where there is a through-and-through involvement.

furnace A high temperature oven used in dentistry for firing ceramics, and in the preparation of an inlay pattern for casting. **glaze** 1. To produce a smooth, shiny surface on porcelain or composite filling materials. 2. Resinous material applied to the surface of a composite resin filling, to enhance its surface finish.

fusible Able to be melted. *F. alloy. See* low-fusing alloy.

fusiform Spindle shaped. Tapering towards each end.

fusion Blending or uniting of substances into a whole.

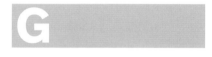

GA General anaesthesia. *See* anaesthesia.

GABA (gamma amino butyric acid) An inhibitory neurotransmitter. A number of sedative agents such as benzodiazepines achieve their effect by enhancing GABA activity.

gabapentin. An analogue of the inhibitory neurotransmitter GABA (gamma amino butyric acid) that is used in the management of trigeminal neuralgia.

gag 1. To retch without actually vomiting. 2. Instrument used during an anaesthetic to prise and hold open the jaws. *See* mouth gag.

gallipot Small receptacle for drugs, solutions and lotions.

galvanic 1. Pertaining to production of direct electric current by chemical means. 2. Similar in effect to an electric shock.

galvanism In dentistry, the electrical effect produced when two dissimilar metals contact one another in the mouth. Most noticeable when a newly completed amalgam restoration contacts a gold restoration.

Gamgee tissue Absorbent cotton wool covered by gauze, as used in a throat pack.

gamma rays Form of electromagnetic radiation similar to X-rays but shorter in wavelength. Emitted from radioactive substances and used commercially to sterilize such items as sutures, injection needles, scalpel blades and local analgesic cartridges.

ganglia Plural of ganglion.

ganglion In anatomy, a mass of nerve cells found in the course of certain nerves. In surgery, a swelling containing fluid or a jelly-like substance, on the sheath of a tendon. *Gasserian* or *trigeminal g.* Situated on the sensory root of the fifth cranial nerve close to the brain on the anterior aspect of the petrous portion of the temporal bone. In severe facial neuralgia, the sensory nerve is

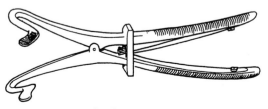

Gag (Ferguson)

sometimes cut at this point or the ganglion destroyed by injected drugs to obtain relief. Also called the *semi-lunar g. Otic g.* Parasympathetic ganglion arising on the glossopharyngeal nerve. Its nerve fibres supply the parotid salivary gland, its sensory and sympathetic fibres passing through the gland. *Sphenopalatine g. (Meckel's g.).* Parasympathetic ganglion derived from the facial nerve. Its postganglionic fibres supply the palatal glands, and the sensory and sympathetic fibres pass through the ganglion. *Submandibular g.* One of the four associated with the cranial nerves and located close to the submandibular gland. Its preganglionic fibres are derived from the seventh (facial) nerve and its postganglionic nerve fibres supply the submandibular and sublingual salivary glands.

gangrene Breakdown or necrosis of tissue owing to lack of blood supply.

gangrenous The state of a tissue affected by gangrene.

Gardner's syndrome Familial disease characterized by multiple polyposis of the colon, osteomas of bone, sebaceous cysts and multiple impacted supernumerary or permanent teeth.

gargoylism *See* Hurler's syndrome.

garnet Abrasive powder composed of a crystalline silicate mineral. Used as a polishing material when embedded on rotary, plastic and cardboard discs.

Garré's osteomyelitis Chronic, non-suppurative, low-grade sclerosing osteitis or osteomyelitis due to infection by pyogenic cocci.

gas Completely elastic substance which, whatever its quantity, can distribute itself evenly over the whole volume of its container. *Nitrous oxide g.* Supplied in French blue cylinders and used in dentistry—together with more than 22%

oxygen—as an anaesthetic. *Oxygen g.* Supplied in black cylinders with white tops. *See* Appendix 9.

gastr- (gastro-) Prefix denoting stomach.

gastric Concerning the stomach.

gastritis Inflammation of the stomach lining.

gastroenteritis Inflammation of the stomach and intestines as a result of food poisoning or poor hygiene. A serious complaint for infants.

Gastro-oesophageal reflux disorder (GORD) Increased frequency and duration of gastric reflux following relaxation of the lower oesophageal sphincter. Reflux of acidic stomach contents into the mouth can cause dental erosion, particularly of the palatal aspects of the upper teeth.

gauge Instrument for measuring physical properties such as length, volume or pressure.

gauze Thin fabric of cotton, silk or metal. May be impregnated with a medicament such as iodoform for use as a dressing. *Tulle gras* is a gauze soaked with soft paraffin containing 1% Peru balsam used in dressing wounds. *Metal g.* May be used as a strengthener in the construction of prostheses.

GDC General Dental Council.

GDP General dental practitioner.

Geiger counter Device to monitor radiation.

gel Semisolid or gelatinous colloidal suspension that has set to form a jelly. Gel-containing fluoride is used to harden and protect teeth.

gelatin Protein obtained from the collagen of bones, cartilage and connective tissue. *G. sponge.* Absorbable sponge made of gelatin which may be placed in a tooth socket to reduce bleeding and promote clotting.

gelation Process wherein a colloid changes from a sol to a gel.

gemination Condition in which twin tooth forms develop from a single bud or follicle. They are rare, have only one pulp chamber and a dividing groove down their centre.

gene One of thousands of biological units present in the chromosomes of the early germinal cells. They determine the inherited characteristics of an individual. Low doses of ionizing radiation may cause changes in them.

general anaesthetic *See* anaesthetic.

generic Relating to a genus. Of a general nature and not specific. A family name.

genetic dose The dose (q.v.) or quantity of radiation received by the germ cells of an individual at risk during his or her lifetime.

genetic effect Effect of radiation on the genes.

genetics The study of heredity.

geni (genio-) Prefix denoting the chin.

genial Relating to the chin. *G. tubercle.* One of two raised nodules of bone, one above the other, on each half of the lower border of the mandible near to the symphysis menti (q.v.) to which muscles are attached.

-genic Suffix meaning 'producing' or 'produced by'.

genioglossus muscle A tongue muscle and the main protruder of the tongue. It arises from the inner surface of the mandible near the symphysis and is inserted in the body of the hyoid bone.

geniohyoid muscle Muscle arising from the inner surface of the mandible near the symphysis and inserted into the anterior surface of the hyoid bone.

genioplasty Reconstruction of the chin by either an enlarging or reducing procedure.

genus Category made up of several closely related species, in the classification of animals and plants.

geographic tongue A condition in which smooth, red depapillated patches on the superior aspect of the tongue are said to resemble a map.

ger- (gero-, geront-) Prefix denoting old age.

Gerber attachment *See* precision attachment.

geriatric Pertaining to geriatrics or old age.

germ A trivial term for a microorganism, especially one causing disease.

German measles (rubella) Mild but highly contagious virus disease producing a red rash and widespread enlargement of glands. It has an incubation period of 2–3 weeks and is a dangerous contact for women during the first 3 months of pregnancy as the child may suffer from heart disease, blindness and deafness.

germicidal Referring to the power to destroy germs.

germicide Agent that kills germs.

germinal Relating to the primary cells of a fetus at their earliest stage of development.

gerodontics The treatment of dental problems and diseases peculiar to ageing persons.

gerontology The study and treatment of diseases of old age.

GI Gingival index. *See* index.

giant cell granuloma (lesion) *See* granuloma.

Gigli's wire saw Flexible toothed wire used to transect bone.

Gillies' approach Surgical approach to the zygomatic arch area through an incision in the temporal region, above the hairline.

gingiv- (gingivo-) Prefix denoting the gingivae or gums (lay term).

gingiva Fibrous connective tissue, covered by epithelium, that surrounds and is attached to the tooth and alveolar bone and extends to the mucogingival junction. On the palatal aspect it is a rim of tissue that merges with the masticatory mucosa of the hard palate. Referred to in lay terms as *the gum. Attached g.* In health, salmon- or coral-pink-coloured tissue, stippled like orange peel, situated between the gingival crest and the mucogingival junction. It is attached to the underlying cementum and bone.

gingival Relating to the gingiva. *G. cleft.* Narrow, V-shaped split in the marginal gingiva. *G. col.* Depression or valley in the interdental papilla. *G. corium.* Lamina propria of the gingiva. *G. crater.* Concave shape of the gingival papilla resulting from necrosis. *G. crest.* The coronal border of the gingiva. *G. crevice. See* g. sulcus. *G. fibres.* Network of fibres that produce close apposition of the marginal gingiva to the tooth. *G. fibromatosis.* Dense overgrowth of gingival tissue. *G. crevicular fluid.* Transudate of blood plasma found in the gingival sulcus due to leakage of plasma from blood capillaries in the free gingiva. *G. graft.* Gingival tissue that has been completely detached and replaced on a different site. *G. groove.* Shallow, V-shaped groove sometimes seen on the outer aspect of the marginal gingiva.

G. margin. That part of the gingiva surrounding the tooth and nearest to its crown. The crest of the free gingiva. *G. margin trimmer.* Hand instrument similar to a hatchet chisel but having its sharp blade curved in its length. Used to trim the cervical margin of a tooth preparation. *G. morphology.* Shape, contour and profile of the gingiva. *G. papilla.* That part of the gingiva which occupies the interproximal space between the teeth. *G. recession.* Loss of gingiva over the root of a tooth on the vestibular or oral aspect. *G. retraction.* Process of temporarily expanding the gingival sulcus by displacing the gingival tissues to allow visualization of the margins of a restoration, e.g. crown preparation. May be undertaken with the use of gingival retraction cord soaked in an astringent solution. More recently, expandable 'putty' materials have been brought to market that are injected into the gingival sulcus. *G. stippling.* Minute depressions on the attached gingival surface. *G. sulcus.* Shallow sulcus lying between the gingival crest and the neck of a tooth, extending from the margin of the free gingiva to the junctional epithelium. This may deepen, due to pathological processes, to produce a periodontal pocket. In health the sulcus may be up to 2 mm in depth. Previously known as the *gingival crevice. See also* index, gingival, and index, bone count.

gingival contouring The carving on the base material of a denture to simulate the natural curved gum outline about the necks of the teeth.

gingivectomy Excision of excess gingival tissue to reduce pocket depths. Indicated, for example, in cases of drug-induced gingival overgrowth. *G. knife. See* periodontal instruments.

gingivitis Inflammation of the gingivae. Signs and symptoms are: local and generalized redness of the gingivae, bleeding of the gingivae on brushing or spontaneously in severe cases, and swollen gingivae. *Necrotizing ulcerative g.* (NUG). Previously called *Vincent's angina, trench mouth, acute ulcerative necrotizing gingivitis (AUNG) and acute ulcerative gingivitis (AUG)*. Acute inflammation of the gingivae associated with spontaneous bleeding, pain, the presence of a grey slough called a pseudomembrane, and a characteristic halitosis. Usually occurs in young adults. Of unknown cause but associated with poor oral hygiene and the presence of a fusiform bacillus/spirochaete complex. Treatment is by prophylactic measures and, in severe cases, administration of metronidazole. *Pregnancy g.* Transient gingivitis occurring during pregnancy and which may be avoided by strict bacterial plaque control.

gingivoplasty Periodontal procedure by which gingival deformities, not accompanied by pocketing, are reshaped to create a correct anatomical form.

gingivostomatitis Inflammation of both oral mucosa and the gingivae.

glabella Smooth bony surface connecting the two superciliary arches of the frontal bone.

gland Organ consisting of specialized cells secreting substances necessary for special functions as a response to a stimulus. Glands usually discharge through ducts, except for the endocrine ductless glands, into or outside the body. *Adenoid g.* Lymphatic glandular growth situated on the posterior wall of the throat in the nasopharynx. *Ductless g.* ADRENAL G. *(SUPRARENAL G.)*. One of a pair of glands situated close to and above the kidneys. They secrete adrenalin into the bloodstream. PITUITARY G. Situated at the base of the brain. The master endocrine gland whose secretions regulate the function of the other ductless glands. THYROID G. Situated in the lower part of the neck in front of the trachea. Controlled by the pituitary gland and secreting iodine-containing hormones such as thyroxin, which influences the metabolism of the body tissues and is distributed in the bloodstream. *Lymphatic g.* Found throughout the body in connection with the lymphatic system. Acts as filter of the lymphatic fluid. *Mammary g.* In the female, one of a pair of glands situated in the skin over the anterior aspect of the chest which secrete milk for a time after giving birth. *Mucous g.* Mucus-secreting gland situated beneath the surface of mucous membrane. *Salivary g.* PAROTID G. One of a pair of glands on each side of the head, below and in front of the ear, and wrapped round the posterior border of the ramus of the mandible. Stensen's duct runs forward from it, across the masseter muscle to pass through the buccinator muscle and open into the mouth opposite the second upper molar. The gland secretes serous saliva and is supplied by the facial nerve and a branch of the external carotid artery. SUBLINGUAL G. The smallest of the salivary glands situated in the floor of the mouth against the deep surface of the mandible, above the mylohyoid line and close to the midline. One of a pair of almond-shaped glands with 8–20 small ducts opening on the crest of the sublingual fold of mucous membrane beneath the tongue. Supplied by the lingual nerve and artery. SUBMANDIBULAR G. One of a pair of glands, about half the size of the parotid gland, situated partly under cover of the mandible, below the mylohyoid line in the region of the angle. Its duct passes forwards and upwards to open on the floor of the mouth, beneath the tongue at a small papilla on the crest of a fold of mucous membrane. Supplied by the lingual nerve. *Sebaceous g.* Widely distributed over the skin surface and which secretes an oily substance. *Sweat g.* Gland secreting sweat as a part of the body temperature control system.

glandular Relating to a gland. *G. fever.* Infectious disease affecting the lymph nodes of the neck, armpits and groin. Thought to be caused by the Epstein–Barr virus.

glass bead sterilizer *See* sterilizer.

glass ionomer cement Semitranslucent, tooth-coloured, fluoride-releasing cement used to restore anterior teeth, especially labial cavities, pits and fissures. Also used to lute, line tooth preparations and act as a fissure sealant. Must be used in dry conditions and be protected by varnish after being placed. By virtue of its molecular make-up, it has the unique ability of forming adhesive bonds with enamel and dentine. *Resin modified g.i.* contain resin monomers, setting by acid base reaction and resin polymerization. Properties generally considered superior to conventional g.i.c.

glazing porcelain *See* porcelain.

glenoid fossa Depression in the temporal bone in which the condylar process of the mandible rests and which forms part of the temporomandibular joint (q.v.).

globulo-maxillary cyst Developmental cyst (q.v.) seen in the maxillary lateral incisor and canine regions.

gloss- (glosso-) Prefix denoting the tongue.

glossectomy Partial or complete removal of the tongue.

glossitis Inflammation of the tongue. *Median rhomboid g.* A condition of the tongue, in the region of the foramen caecum, which is reddened and lacks papillae.

glossodynia Painful or burning tongue.

glossopharyngeal Relating to that part of the throat formed by the tongue and the pharynx.

glossoptosis Abnormal downward displacement of the tongue.

glossopyrosis A painful burning sensation of the tongue.

glottis Opening between the vocal cords in the larynx protected by the epiglottis. Produces sound later modified as speech.

glucan *See* extracellular polysaccharide.

glucogenic Producing glucose.

glucose Colourless, crystalline, water-soluble sugar in a form which is absorbed and circulated in the bloodstream and to which all forms of sugar and starches are converted in the small intestine. Present in fruit and honey.

glucose oxidase Enzyme capable of breaking down glucose to form gluconate and water.

glycerin Clear, colourless, syrupy liquid obtained as a by-product of soap manufacture and sugar fermentation. It is tasteless and hygroscopic.

glycerin thymol compound Mouthwash containing borax, sodium carbonate, sodium benzoate, sodium salicylate, menthol, thymol, cineole, methyl salicylate, pumilio pine oil and glycerol 10% v/v.

glyceryl trinitrate (nitroglycerin) Drug that dilates blood vessels and is used to prevent and treat angina pectoris (q.v.).

glycogen Produced by the breakdown of carbohydrates and stored in the body, especially the liver, until required for use. It is then further broken down by the liver to form glucose.

gnath- (gnatho-) Prefix denoting the jaw.

gnathic Relating to the jaw or teeth. *G. index.* Classification of skulls founded on measurements of the jaw and skull.

gnathion A craniometric point. The most anterior and inferior point of the body outline of the chin, equidistant from the pogonion and menton.

gnathodynamometer Instrument used to record and measure the forces exerted by the muscles in closing the jaws.

gnathology That branch of dental science that deals with the physiology of the masticatory mechanism.

gnathosonics The study of the sounds made by the occlusion of teeth during mastication or during voluntary tooth tapping.

gnathostat Mechanical appliance used to mount and orientate plaster casts so that the Frankfort, orbital and mid palatal planes are constantly related.

goitre Swelling of the thyroid gland.

gold Heavy, soft, yellow, ductile and malleable precious metal found in its natural state and which is not dissolved by most acids. Pure gold is described as being 24 carat. Other metals may be added to it to harden it and also to change its melting point, thus reducing its carat measure or fineness. Used in dentistry, because of its favourable properties, in the construction of inlays, crowns, bridges, precision attachments and other prostheses. *Casting g.* Alloy, mainly of gold, with small quantities of silver, copper and platinum. It is heated to the required temperature to become molten and then cast into a mould. Variations of the ingredients produce castings of different strength and

hardness. *G. foil.* Thin gold sheet historically condensed directly into cavity as a restorative material. *G. solder.* Alloy consisting of gold, silver, copper, tin and zinc, whose melting point has been adjusted to occur some 50–100°C below the melting point of the gold alloy to be soldered. *White g.* Gold alloy with a high platinum content. *See also* carat and fineness (of gold).

gomphosis Articulation of a fibrous type such as a tooth in its socket.

gonad Male or female reproductive organ, i.e. ovary, testis.

goni- (gonio-) Prefix denoting an anatomical corner or angle.

gonion A cephalometric landmark defined as the most posterior, inferior point of the angle of the mandible. It is constructed in orthodontic tracings by bisecting the angle formed by the tangents of the posterior and inferior borders of the mandible. *See* Appendix 10.

Gothic arch tracing (arrow point tracing) *See* tracing.

gouge Bone chisel of curved cross-section, used to cut and remove bone.

GPT General professional training (trainee).

graft Portion of tissue removed from one site and transplanted in another, either in the same or in another individual, in order to repair a defect caused by disease, accident or by a developmental anomaly. *Allog.* Graft obtained from a donor of the same, but genetically dissimilar, species as the recipient. *Allelog.* Graft material not obtained from any human or animal source, used to restore tissues or organs, e.g. acrylic, polyethylene, titanium, tantalum, chrome cobalt and stainless steel alloys. *Autogenous g. (autog).* A graft removed from one site and transplanted to another in the same individual. *Free g.* Tissue completely removed from one site and transplanted to another. *Onlay g.* Graft applied directly onto the surface of a bone. *Osseous g.* A portion of bone taken from the patient, or a synthetic bone substitute, and used to repair or replace alveolar bone. *Pedicle g.* Full-thickness skin graft used to transplant tissue from one area of the body to another in the form of a tube, which is always connected at one end to an established blood supply. In the first operation the skin is raised and sutured into a tube-like structure, both ends being left attached. Later one end is severed and moved to another site. This can be repeated at intervals. *Split skin g.* Very thin shaving of skin containing epidermis and a portion of dermis used as a graft leaving exposed tissues from which regeneration of the epithelium may occur. *Xenog.* Graft taken from a donor of different species from that of the recipient.

gram (g) Unit of mass defined as 1000th part of a kilogram.

-gram Suffix denoting a tracing or record.

Gram negative Type of bacteria which does not retain Gram's stain.

Gram positive Type of bacteria which retains Gram's stain.

Gram stain Method of staining microorganisms in order to aid their identification. Gram-positive organisms stain blue-black, whilst Gram-negative organisms stain pink.

grand mal *See* epilepsy.

granular Containing grains or granules. *G. cell myeloblastoma.* Tumour of unknown aetiology seen primarily in the tongue. Clinically, it may protrude above the surface of the tongue and histologically is made up of large cells that exhibit a granular eosinophilic cytoplasm.

granular layer of Tomes Granular layer found in the dentine immediately below the cemento-dentinal junction. It is not fully mineralized. Possibly a consequence of the unique arrangement of matrix proteins or the terminal loops of the dentinal tubules at the dentino-cementum interface.

granulation 1. Subdivision of a solid into a small particle. 2. Formation of small rounded masses in tissues. 3. Process of healing by the development of young connective tissue and blood vessels on the surface of a wound. *G. tissue.* Consists of new tissue by which wounds heal. Contains new capillary vessels and fibroblasts to fill in the space and later become fibrous tissue. A scar tissue. A barrier of this tissue forms the walls of an abscess cavity and the floor of an ulcer. It is localized by the process of inflammation.

granulocyte One of the two main types of white blood cells (q.v.) having a granular cytoplasm. There are three main subclasses: polymorphonuclear leucocytes, eosinophil leucocytes and basophil leucocytes.

granuloma Spherical mass of tissue, mainly consisting of histiocytes, which occurs in reaction to chronic inflammation. *Apical* or *dental g.* Mass of granulation tissue associated with the apex of a tooth and formed as a sequel to infection of the root canal. *Eosinophilic g.* Composed of eosinophils and histiocytes occurring in bone or soft tissue. *Giant cell g.* or *lesion.* Of unknown aetiology but thought to be associated with an exaggerated inflammatory response. Consists of a vascular connective tissue with many giant cells. The lesion may grow to a large size and show aggressive neoplastic behaviour.

granulomatous Having the appearance of a granuloma.

granulosis Formation of a mass of granules.

-graph Suffix denoting a recording instrument.

graphite Black lead, plumbago. One of the allotropic forms of carbon, the other being diamond. A soft, dark grey-to-black crystalline substance used as a lubricant and for the fabrication of lead pencils, furnace crucibles and as a conductor of electric currents.

grave Critical, as of the symptoms of a serious condition.

Graves' disease Exophthalmic goitre.

gray (Gy) SI unit of absorbed dose of ionizing radiation (q.v.).

green rouge Very fine polishing powder containing green chromium oxide. Used in the technician's laboratory to polish chrome metal prostheses.

green stick Specific type of thermoplastic impression material (q.v.).

greenstick fracture See fracture.

grey matter Tissue found in the brain and spinal cord, composed of collections of intricately connected nerve cells with a rich blood supply.

grid 1. Series of horizontal and vertical lines forming squares of uniform size, used as a reference for the plotting of curves. 2. In radiography, a device used to prevent scatter radiation from reaching the film during exposure. Consists of alternate strips of lead and radiolucent material placed in apposition to the film.

grind 1. To sharpen or smooth by friction. 2. To crush food with the posterior teeth. 3. Elimination of high spots on tooth contours by the use of abrasive tools.

grinding-in Fine adjustment to the occlusion of artificial teeth by selective grinding.

groove A long narrow depression.

group function The simultaneous contact of a group of mandibular and maxillary teeth in lateral movements on the working side thus distributing occlusal forces.

growth 1. Process of development. An increase in size. 2. Swelling or tumour which may be benign or malignant. Benign growths do not necessarily affect or endanger the general health or recur elsewhere in the body as secondary growths. Malignant growths may be fatal.

GTR Guided tissue regeneration (q.v.).

guard wire The baseplate of an orthodontic appliance may have a guard wire attached to its fitting surface, to limit any distortion of small springs while in use and under pressure.

guardsman's fracture See fracture.

gubernacular Relating to a gubernaculum. *G. canal*. Canal in the alveolar bone through which the dental follicle and unerupted teeth are connected to the oral mucosa by a cord of connective tissue known as the gubernaculum.

gubernaculum A guiding pathway. *Dental g.* Leads from the developing tooth follicle to the surface of the gingiva.

Guérin fracture See Le Fort I fracture.

guidance A method of controlling the direction or regulation of movements. *Anterior g.* 1. The moving anterior tooth contacts that guide mandibular movements. 2. That part of an articulator on which the guide pin (q.v.) slides and thus mechanically reproduces mandibular movements. *Canine g. See* canine protected articulation.

guide pin A metal rod attached to one part of an articulator and contacting the anterior guide table on the opposing portion of the articulator.

guide plane The two or more prepared parallel surfaces of abutment teeth used to limit and guide the path of insertion (q.v.) of a removable prosthesis.

guide table That part of an articulator on which the anterior guide pin (q.v.) rests and thus maintains the established vertical dimension.

guided tissue regeneration (GTR) A technique used in surgical periodontics in which membranes are used to guide the path of epithelial cell regeneration and thus permit unhindered regeneration of connective tissues.

gum 1. Colloquial term for gingiva. 2. Adhesive material prepared from the dried viscous sap exuded by certain trees and plants. *G. benzoin.* Balsam resin employed in Whitehead's varnish. *G. boil.* Commonly used to refer to a sinus leading from a subperiosteal abscess. *G. dammar.* Natural resin used in the manufacture of waxes, baseplate materials and impression compounds. *G. scissors. See* scissors. *G. tragacanth.* Dried gummy exudate obtained from the incised stems of certain trees. Used in dentistry as a denture fixative.

gumma Rubbery localized lesion that occurs irregularly during the third stage of syphilis.

Gunning type fixation *See* fixation.

gustation The act of tasting. Substances must be in solution in order to be tasted.

gustatory Pertaining to the sense of taste. *G. stimulus.* Substance which stimulates the taste receptor nerve endings in the mouth and causes a flow of saliva.

Recognized as sweet, sour, salt and bitter. *G. sweating. See* Frey's syndrome.

gustatory sweating *See* Frey's Syndrome

gutta percha Substance obtained from the sap of trees. Available in sheets, points and sticks, it softens when warmed and may be used as a temporary dressing or in root canal treatment to obliterate the pulp canal and seal the apical foramen. *G. p. point.* Slender cone of gutta percha used in endodontic treatment to obturate the entire root canal.

gypsum Naturally occurring calcium sulphate ($CaSO_4 2H_2O$) that is calcined to provide plaster of Paris—calcium hemihydrate ($CaSO_4 \frac{1}{2}H_2O$).

H

habit 1. Settled, fixed way of behaving. 2. In orthodontics, a persistent tendency to repeat the practice of thumb, finger, lip or tongue sucking which sometimes displaces the teeth.

habit posture Instinctively and reflexively produced and maintained posture in which the muscles are in active contraction.

habitual posture of the mandible *See* rest position of the mandible.

haem- (haema-, haemo-, haemat (o)-) Prefix meaning 'of the blood'.

haemangioblast Embryonic cell that develops into the cells of the blood vessels, endothelium, reticulo-endothelial elements and their cells.

haemangioma Benign tumour involving newly formed blood vessels that appear as a network beneath the skin. May be aneurysmal, capillary, congenital or cavernous.

haematemesis Act of vomiting blood.

haematologist Scientist who makes a special study of blood physiology and disorders.

haematology The study of blood, blood-forming tissues and associated disorders.

haematoma Collection of blood in the tissues that causes a swelling, generally following an injury. *Eruption h.* Eruption or dentigerous cyst (q.v.) associated with erupting deciduous or permanent teeth. A dilatation of the normal follicular space around the crown of the tooth caused by the accumulation of blood or tissue fluid.

haematuria Presence of blood in the urine.

haemoglobin Pigmented principal protein of red blood cells giving blood its bright red colour when carrying oxygen in the form of oxyhaemoglobin. Otherwise of a darker colour.

haemolysis Rupture of the red blood cell walls releasing haemoglobin into the blood plasma. Caused by a surrounding hypertonic fluid.

haemolytic Causing a breakdown of red blood cells.

haemophilia Blood disease inherited by males and transmitted by females. Gives rise to prolonged bleeding, even from very minor injuries. Special centres exist for the medical treatment of haemophiliacs.

haemophiliac Person afflicted by haemophilia.

haemoptysis Expectoration or coughing up of blood.

haemorrhage Internal or external bleeding due to injury to blood vessels, allowing the escape of blood. May be trivial, severe or fatal, and may be *primary*, as at the time of injury to blood vessels, *secondary* or *reactionary*, due to infection. Haemorrhage from an artery tends to be bright red in colour, while darker from a vein. Bleeding from the nose is known as *epistaxis* and from the respiratory tract and lungs as *haemoptysis*.

haemostasis Arrest of bleeding either physiologically, surgically or mechanically.

hairy tongue (black hairy tongue) *See* tongue.

halitosis Foul-smelling breath. May be temporary, e.g. after eating strongly flavoured food or taking drugs such as paraldehyde, or long lasting, due to disease of the gingivae, teeth, throat, nasal sinuses, lungs and stomach or liver.

hallucinatory drug Drug that produces an idea of imaginary objects or events.

halo head frame Metal band of varying design attached to the head by screws that are inserted through incisions until they contact the outside of the skull. Used for the attachment of various immobilizing devices in the treatment of fractures of the facial skeleton.

halothane Volatile, non-explosive, non-inflammable, clear liquid, the vapour of which is a powerful anaesthetic. Used as an additive to inhalation techniques giving rapid induction and muscular relaxation. Pregnant women should not be exposed to its vapour, owing to the possibility of miscarriage.

hamartoma Tumour-like overgrowth of mature tissue whose elements show disordered arrangement but are normal to the site.

hand mallet Instrument used in oral surgery. Usually metal with a cylindrical head and obtainable in various weights.

handpiece Hand-held connecting device placed between the driving force and rotary cutting and polishing instruments such as burs and discs. May be *straight, contra-angled* or *miniature* to hold smaller burs. Driven by the rotating shaft of an electric motor, or by compressed air. *Reciprocating h.* Handpiece that changes the rotating movement to a reciprocating one of an alternating quarter-turn movement, e.g. the *Giromatic h.* used in endodontic therapy. *Turbine-driven h.* Handpiece driven by compressed air, with friction grip chucks. The air pressure causes the small turbine or rotor in the head of the handpiece to rotate at very high speed. The rotor may be mounted on bearings or be air-borne.

Hand–Schüller–Christian disease Variant of the reticulo-endothelioses (histiocytosis X) characterized by defects in the facial bones and skull, exophthalmos, often dwarfism and a brown colour of the skin.

hanger Device to which radiographs are clipped in a known order during the processes of developing, fixing and drying.

haplodont Possessing peg-like molar teeth.

hard palate Anterior bony part of the palate formed by the fusion of the two maxillae in the midline, supported by the palatine processes of the maxilla and the palatine bone. Presents three foramina through which nerve and blood vessels pass carrying sensation and nutrients to and from the mucosa of the palate.

hard radiation In radiography, 'hardness' indicates in a general sense the quality of the radiation as a function of the wavelength, i.e. the shorter the wavelength, the 'harder' the radiation.

hardness scale Scale of the ability of a material to resist indentation,

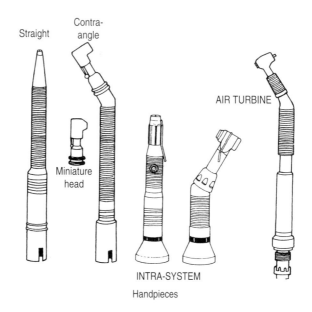

Straight

Contra-angle

Miniature head

AIR TURBINE

INTRA-SYSTEM

Handpieces

scratching, abrasion or attrition. Commonly used scales are: *Brinell h.s.* or *number (BHN)*. Scale in which a hardened steel sphere is pressed into the surface of the material being tested under a specified load. The hardness number is calculated by dividing the load by the area of indentation after removal of the load. *Knoop h.s.* or *number (KHN)*. A rhomboidal pyramid of diamond is pressed into the material being tested and the degree of hardness is calculated by measuring the length of the long axis of indentation produced. *Mohs h.s.* or *number (MHN)*. Scale for measuring the hardness of minerals by scratching one mineral against another of lower value. Diamond has an MHN of 10, quartz 7 and gypsum 2. *Rockwell h.s.* or *number (RHN)*. The hardness of the material being tested is measured by the difference in indentation produced by a hardened steel ball or diamond conical point under two different loads. *Vickers h.s.* or *number (VHN)*. Hardness is measured by indenting a material with a pyramidal diamond that has a square base.

harelip *See* cleft lip.

hatchet Hand-held cutting chisel with bevelled blade used to trim hard tooth tissue.

haversian canal *See* bone.

Hawley bow Variant of the short labial bow with adjustment loop in the canine region.

Hawley retainer *See* retainer.

hay fever (allergic rhinitis) Allergic reaction to some pollens and dusts, characterized by inflammation of the membrane lining the nasal passages and sometimes the conjunctiva.

HBIG Hepatitis B immunoglobulin. *See* hepatitis.

HBV Hepatitis B virus. *See* hepatitis.

head 1. That part of the body that contains the brain, the special sense organs and the mouth. 2. Rounded portion of a bone which fits into the hollow or groove of another bone to form a movable joint.

headcap 1. Rigid cap made of plaster of Paris and gauze strips, incorporating anchorage wires. Used in the treatment of jaw and facial fractures. 2. Removable head harness applied to the head and neck to provide for the transmission of extra-oral forces to an orthodontic appliance.

headgear Apparatus applied to the head and neck for the transmission of extra-oral forces to an orthodontic appliance.

heart Hollow muscular organ lying in the chest cavity which, by rhythmic contractions and relaxations, pumps blood round the circulatory system of the body. The human heart consists of four chambers—the left and right auricles (LA and RA) and ventricles (LV and RV)—each separated from the next by a valve which prevents backflow. Normal rate of contraction is 72 times per minute. Blood to the heart muscle itself is supplied by the coronary arteries.

heat-cured polymer Mixture of powder (polymer) and liquid (monomer) which can be hardened or cured by heat.

Hedström file Tapered, flexible, endodontic file consisting of a series of sharp, milled, conical-shaped blades and used with an outward rasping motion to plane canal walls and remove materials from root canals.

Heerfordt's syndrome *See* uveoparotid fever.

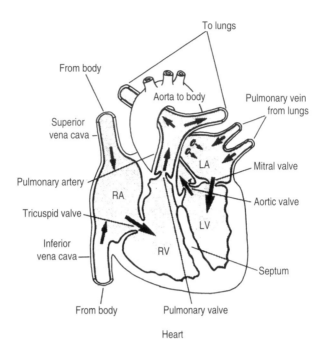

Heart

hemi- Prefix denoting half.

hemidesmosome (half-desmosome) A similar structure to a desmosome (q.v.) but with a plate of one cell only and without a companion cell butting up against it.

hemiglossectomy Surgical removal of half of the tongue.

hemihydrate Hydrate containing one molecule of water for every two molecules of other substance in the compound. *See also* plaster of Paris.

hemimandibulectomy Surgical removal of one half of the mandible.

hemimaxillectomy Surgical removal of one half of the maxilla.

hemiplegia Paralysis limited to one side of the body.

hemisection 1. Removal of one half of an organ or anatomical structure.

2. In dentistry, the division of a tooth in half and the removal of the unwanted diseased portion together with its root or roots.

hemiseptum That portion of bone remaining between two adjacent teeth, when an infrabony lesion is present in the approximal aspect of the other tooth.

heparin Anticoagulant present in the tissues, especially the liver. Used in the treatment of thrombosis.

hepat- (hepato-) Prefix denoting the liver.

hepatitis Inflammation of the liver. Characterized by nausea, vomiting, loss of appetite, weight loss and giving rise to a condition known as jaundice (q.v.). *Hepatitis A.* Less serious illness thought to be spread by droplet infection. *Hepatitis B.* Serious illness with a high death rate. The virus is blood-borne and can be transmitted from an infected person by means of contaminated needles and instruments. Extra care is required in treating such patients and sterilizing methods must be strictly observed. Some patients, known as carriers, may carry the disease without knowing it or showing any symptoms. *Hepatitis C.* Blood-borne infection acquired through contact with infected blood thus transmitted through contact with contaminated needles and instruments. Up to 30% of affected individuals may be unaware that they carry the virus.

Herbst appliance *See* appliance.

hereditary Relating to characteristics transmitted from one generation to another. Such characteristics concern the various peculiarities of body form, structure and function. Human germinal cells repeatedly divide into two after fertilization. Each half contains a number of rod-like chromosomes which decide the character of an individual. These carry the genes or hereditary factors. *H. haemorrhagic telangiectasia (Rendu–Osler–Weber disease)*. Hereditary disease characterized by numerous angiomatous and telangiectatic areas on the oral mucosa and the skin, that tend to undergo haemorrhage. *H. gingival fibromatosis. See* gingival fibromatosis. *H. intestinal polyposis. See* Peutz–Jegher's syndrome. *H. opalescent dentine. See* dentinogenesis imperfecta.

herpes *Orig.* one of a number of diseases of the skin characterized by eruptions of an acute nature. *Mod.* Infection with one of a number of herpesviruses which characteristically can remain dormant in the body for long periods, e.g. herpes simplex virus 1 (HSV-1), the aetiological agent of herpetic stomatitis (cold sores); HSV-2, genital herpes; varicella-zoster virus (VZV), varicella (chickenpox) and zoster (shingles) when sensory ganglia become infected; Epstein-Barr virus (EBV), infectious mononucleosis (glandular fever); cytomegalovirus (CMV), frequently asymptomatic and seldom recognized clinically, a mild mononucleosis syndrome is seen occasionally in young adults; human herpesvirus 6, 7 and 8 have been described recently. HHV8 is also referred to as Kaposi's sarcoma-associated herpesvirus (KSHV).

herpetic Relating to herpes.

herring-bone pattern Effect produced when radiographic film has been exposed with the incorrect side towards the central ray. The lead backing within the film produces the pattern on the developed film.

heter- (hetero-) Prefix denoting difference or dissimilarity.

heterodont Possessing teeth of several shapes, such as incisors, canines, premolars and molars.

heterogeneous graft (xenograft) *See* graft.

heterograft Obsolescent term for xenograft. *See* graft.

Hewitt's prop *See* mouth prop.

hiatus A gap or opening.

Higginson syringe *See* syringe.

high copper amalgam alloy *See* alloy.

high labial bow Thick stainless steel wire bent to conform to the buccal aspect of the upper dental arch above the teeth. It can carry thinner wires wound on to it in the form of T-springs or apron springs to retract the upper incisor teeth. The ends of the bow are anchored in the acrylic baseplate as a removable orthodontic appliance.

high-level fracture *See* Le Fort III fracture.

high lip line *See* lip.

hind-brain *See* cerebellum.

hinge axis *See* transverse horizontal axis.

hinge axis locating face-bow (hinge bow, kinematic face-bow) *See* adjustable axis face-bow.

hinge movement Joint movement comparable to that of a hinge but allowing more laxity than a straight hinge. The temporomandibular joint allows forward (incisive), lateral and rotational as well as retrusive movements.

hist- (histio-, histo-) Prefix denoting tissue.

histamine Substance occurring naturally in an inactive form in most body tissues. It is released in response to injury, irritant chemicals, animal stings, antibodies and allergies. It affects the gastric secretions, muscles and blood vessels which dilate, so causing a drop in blood pressure. Unwanted effects are swelling, circulatory collapse and bronchospasm. The most effective antidote is adrenalin. Antihistamines may also be employed, especially in allergic reactions.

histiocyte A fixed macrophage, i.e. one that is stationary within connective tissue.

histiocytosis-X Complex group of diseases in which there are abnormalities of certain large phagocytic cells (histiocytes). The group includes eosinophilic granuloma (q.v.), Hand–Schüller–Christian disease (q.v.) and Letterer–Siwe disease. *See* Langerhans cell histiocytosis.

histogram Bar chart. Graph in which values are plotted in the form of rectangles.

histology Study of the microscopic structure of body tissues by means of special staining techniques.

histopathology Microscopic study of the diseases of tissues.

HIV *See* human immunodeficiency virus.

Hodgkin's disease A form of lymphoma. Painless, progressive and often fatal enlargement of the lymphatic glands of the whole body. It may continue over a period of years, causing the patient to become anaemic and weak.

hoe Chisel-like instrument used to remove hard tooth tissue by trimming and chipping. *See also* periodontal instruments.

holder Device for holding nerve canal broaches, napkins, needles, radiographic films and rubber dam.

homeo- (homo-, homoeo-) Prefix denoting alike or similar.

homeopathy System of medicine based on the theory that diseases are curable by those drugs which produce similar symptoms to those caused by the disease. The drugs are administered in minute doses, obtained by extreme dilution.

homogeneous Having a uniform structure or quality throughout. *H. graft (allograft). See* graft.

homograft Obsolescent term for allograft. *See* graft.

homologous Alike. Having the same relation or value.

hook Surgical instrument with a fine bent or curved tip used to retract and hold tissue at operation. *Poswillo h.* Hook used percutaneously to elevate the zygoma.

horizontal overlap *See* overjet.

horizontal reference plane *See* plane.

hormone Substance secreted by the ductless glands and carried in the bloodstream to stimulate other organs. Hormones act as chemical messengers to the organs, stimulating or retarding certain activities such as growth, reproduction and mental processes.

Horner's syndrome Unilateral disturbance of the cervical sympathetic nerves characterized by pupil constriction, ptosis of the upper eye-lid and skin dryness due to an absence of sweating in the affected part.

host Organism on or in which another organism can live as a parasite or commensal.

Howe's pliers See pliers.

Howship's lacunae (resorption lacunae) Depressions in the surface of mineralized tissue undergoing resorption.

human immunodeficiency virus A retrovirus that causes immune system failure and debilitation. The infectious and aetiological agent of acquired immune deficiency syndrome.

humerus Upper-arm bone extending from the shoulder to the elbow.

Hurler's syndrome (gargoylism) Inborn defect of metabolism leading to mental retardation, flattening of the nasal ridge and other bone deformities, sometimes deafness and cardiac anomalies.

Hutchinson's teeth See tooth.

hyal- (hyalo) Prefix denoting transparent or glassy.

hyaline Nearly or completely transparent. Glass-like. *H. cartilage.* Homogeneous cartilage of glassy appearance.

hybrid Union of two different varieties. *H. denture. See* denture.

hybrid layer Dentine layer which has been infiltrated with resin-based adhesive.

hydro- (hydro-) Prefix denoting water.

hydrocolloid Substance which when combined with water initially forms a sol and then a gel. May be reversible, changing its state by heat (agar), or irreversible (alginate). Used for dental impressions. *H. impression material.* General term to describe agar and alginate impression materials (q.v.).

hydrocortisone Product of the human adrenal cortex, or a synthetic anti-inflammatory drug classed as a steroid. Used in dentistry as a topical medication on ulcers and inflamed pulps. *H. lozenge.* Topical application of corticosteroids for mouth ulcers. Should be allowed to dissolve slowly and is most effective when applied at the onset of an ulcer. Reduces the painful symptoms of ulcers but does not cure them.

hydrogen peroxide Colourless, odourless liquid capable of oxidation and having antiseptic and deodorating properties. Commonly made up in water to the strength of 10 volumes which means that any quantity of that strength will give off 10 times its volume of oxygen gas. Sometimes used to irrigate root canals and in diluted form as a mouthwash to destroy anaerobic micro-organisms.

hydrolysis The splitting of a compound by the addition of water.

hydroquinone Inhibitor used in minute amounts to prevent premature polymerization of methyl methacrylate.

hydrous Containing water.

hydroxyapatite Form of basic calcium phosphate from which bone salts are derived.

hygienist See dental hygienist.

hygr- (hygro-) Prefix denoting moisture.

hygroscopic Tending to absorb moisture from the atmosphere. *H. expansion.* Phenomenon of increased expansion, exhibited by gypsum products, after the initial set, when exposed to excess water.

hyoid U-shaped. *H. bone.* U-shaped bone situated between the thyroid cartilage and the base of the tongue.

hyoscine (scopolamine) Drug that prevents muscle spasm.

hyp- (hypo-) Prefix denoting small, lack of, deficiency, below or beneath.

hyper- Prefix denoting over, beyond the normal, excessive or above.

hyperaemia Presence of an excessive amount of blood in any tissue. Condition found in early stages of inflammation.

hyperaesthesia Greatly increased sensitivity to painful stimulation.

hypercementosis Excess deposition of cementum around a tooth root.

hyperdontia Term used to describe greater than normal number of teeth in cases of supplemental and supernumerary teeth.

hyperkeratosis Excess of keratin on an epithelial surface.

hyperparathyroidism Disease due to overactivity of the parathyroid glands which results in bone resorption and replacement by fibrous tissue and/or giant cell granuloma (q.v.).

hyperplasia Overdevelopment of a tissue due to an increase in the production of its cells. *Gingival h. See* gingival.

hyperplastic Relating to hyperplasia.

hyperpnoea Increased rate of breathing proportional to an increase in metabolism, for example during exercise. *See also* hyperventilation.

hypersensitive tooth Tooth reacting more than normally to a stimulus such as heat, cold, sweetness and pressure.

hypersensitivity A more than normal reaction to a stimulus.

hypertension Abnormally high blood pressure.

hyperthyroidism Excessive activity of the thyroid gland as found in exophthalmic goitre.

hypertonic Term used to describe a solution whose acid/alkali level of pH value is above that of normal blood levels. Hypertonic saline into which blood cells are placed will cause the cells to give up their fluid content and become shrivelled or crenulated. This applies to local analgesic solutions which must be isotonic (q.v.) in order not to affect the fluid balance of the tissues.

hypertrophy State of an organ, or part of an organ, that has become enlarged symmetrically, without pathological involvement. Often due to an increased work demand of its existing cells. For example, if one kidney is removed then the other will become enlarged. The opposite state of shrinkage is known as atrophy (q.v.).

hyperventilation Forced breathing at an abnormally high rate while at rest. This lowers the carbon dioxide concentration and may lead to unconsciousness.

hypnotic Any drug which induces sleep.

hypnotism The practice of inducing hypnosis.

Hypnovel® *See* midazolam.

hypo- *See* hyp-.

hypoaesthesia Decreased sensitivity to painful stimulation.

hypocalcification Lack of calcium salts in a calcified tissue. In teeth, a deficiency in the normal content of enamel due to a disturbance during the maturation period of the tooth.

hypodermic Under the skin. *H. syringe. See* syringe.

hypodontia Developmental absence of up to 6teeth. *See* oligodontia.

hypoglossal Situated beneath the tongue.

hypoplasia Underdevelopment of an organ or tissue. *Dental h.* Defective formation of dentine due to illnesses such as measles or due to starvation.

hypoplastic Relating to hypoplasia.

hypothyroidism Condition due to lack of thyroid hormone which causes a low rate of metabolism, dry skin, hair loss and retarded mentality. Causes cretinism at birth.

hypotonic Describes a solution whose pH, or acid/alkali balance, is below that of normal blood levels and may cause haemolysis (q.v.) of blood cells.

hypoxia (hypoxaemia) State of reduced oxygen content of the blood.

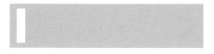

-ia, -ics, -logy Suffix meaning the 'practice of'.

-iasis Suffix denoting a diseased condition.

iatro- Prefix denoting medicine or doctor.

iatrogenic Brought about by surgical or medical treatment.

ibuprofen (Nurofen®) A non-steroidal anti-inflammatory drug that is useful in the management of dental pain. The normal dose is 400 mg three times a day.

ICON Index of Complexity of Orthodontic Need. An orthodontic index aimed to combine both treatment need and the complexity of treatment that would be required to correct a malocclusion.

ICP Intercuspal position.

icterus *See* jaundice.

ideal occlusion Occlusion based on the morphology of unworn teeth.

identification dot Mark embossed on the corner of a radiographic film to indicate which side was facing the source of X-rays on exposure. Consists of a raised pimple which should face the tube head during exposure.

ideo- Prefix denoting mental activity or ideas.

idio- Prefix denoting peculiar to an individual.

idiopathic Self-originated. Applied to a condition, the cause of which is not known or which arises spontaneously.

idiosyncrasy Unexpected or unusual reaction or sensitivity exhibited by an individual to a particular food or drug.

i/m Abbreviation for intramuscular (q.v.).

image Shadow of a structure cast by X-rays on to a radiographic film. *I. intensification.* Method of producing a brighter radiographic image than that obtained by the unaided action of the X-ray beam. The technique utilizes accelerated electrons focused on a fluorescent screen. *I. layer. See* focal trough.

imbricated Overlapped like tiles.

imbrication Overlapping of adjacent incisor teeth.

immature Not fully developed.

immediate replacement denture *See* denture.

immiscible Unable to be mixed, e.g. oil and water.

immobilization Fixation (q.v.) of fractured bone ends to prevent movement until they are firmly joined together by new bone. May be effected by wiring, splinting, plating and bone grafting.

immobilize To render fixed.

immune Protected against a disease either by natural means or by inoculation.

immunity Inbuilt protection of the body against infection by any particular pathological micro-organisms and their toxins. Immunity may be natural (racial, familial or inborn) or acquired. *Acquired i.* May result from a previous attack of a disease or from artificial means such as the effects of repeated small injections of toxins, antitetanus sera or vaccines which produce antibodies.

immunization Process of rendering a person immune, so protecting them against certain diseases.

immunology The science dealing with the various phenomena of allergy, induced sensitivity and immunity.

impaction State of being firmly lodged or wedged. *Food i.* Accumulation of food, generally interproximally, because of an open contact, a 'plunger' cusp or uneven marginal ridge height. *Tooth i.* Situation in which a tooth is so placed that it is unable to erupt normally. May be due to a wedging against another tooth or teeth or to the abnormal development or siting of the tooth.

impermeable Impenetrable. Refers to a substance or tissue that does not permit the passage of fluids through it.

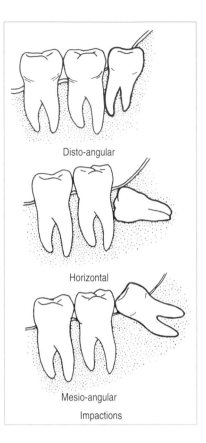

Disto-angular

Horizontal

Mesio-angular

Impactions

impervious Unable to be penetrated. Not affording a passage.

impetigo Superficial infection of the skin caused by Group A streptococci or *Staphylococcus aureus*. Highly contagious, common in babies and children, and occurring mainly on the face and limbs. *I.* is not a serious disease and complications are rare.

implant 1. To insert or fix. 2. Portion of tissue used in a graft. 3. Tooth that has been reimplanted. 4. Metal screw, pin, blade or casting inserted into or placed on the alveolar bone in order to provide anchorage or stabilization either to teeth or to a prosthesis. An implant may consist of three parts. a. The

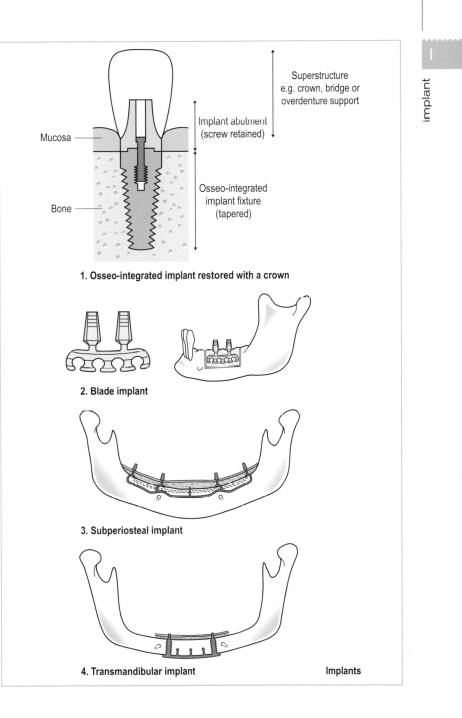

Superstructure
e.g. crown, bridge or
overdenture support

Implant abutment
(screw retained)

Mucosa

Osseo-integrated
implant fixture
(tapered)

Bone

1. Osseo-integrated implant restored with a crown

2. Blade implant

3. Subperiosteal implant

4. Transmandibular implant

Implants

FIXTURE (previously BODY) which is placed in the bone. b. The ABUTMENT, which connects to the fixture and is visible in the mouth and supports and/or retains the prosthesis (or superstructure) and c. The SUPER-STRUCTURE which may be an integral part of the final restoration (a bridge) or supports the final restoration (an overdenture). *I. denture. See* denture. *Endosseous (Endosteal) i.* Implant, usually of metal, introduced into bone; in dentistry this will usually be the maxilla or mandible. *Asseo-integrated i.* An implant which is placed within bone; and has a direct interface between its surface and the host's bone. *See also* diodontic implant and mandibular staple implant. *Subperiosteal i.* An implant that is introduced between the bone surface and overlying periosteum with a part of it protruding through the mucosa into the mouth.

impression Imprint, mould or negative form from which a model or positive reproduction may be obtained by casting. *Final, master, major, second or working i.* Impression used to make the master cast. *Functional i.* Impression which, during its formation, is modified by masticatory loads and adjacent muscular activity and is mucodisplacive. *Mucostatic i.* Impression made with the intention of minimizing the displacement of soft tissues. Formerly termed *functional i. Primary i.* An impression made for construction of a model or to construct a custom or special tray. *Sectional i.* Impression built up in the mouth from two or more parts that are removed separately and reassembled out of the mouth for casting.

impression material Material used to take an impression. *Compound i.m.* (compound, thermoplastic impression material, composition). Thermoplastic material consisting of natural and synthetic resins, fillers and plasticizers. Used mainly for edentulous mouth impressions. Softened by placing in hot water at 60°C or by holding over a flame. Obtainable in sticks, sheets or cones. Not sufficiently elastic to reproduce undercut areas accurately. *Elastomeric i.m.* Very accurate impression material used in inlay, crown, bridge and precision attachment work. Especially useful for multi-unit preparations. May exhibit a rubber-like behaviour. Must be mixed and used strictly in accordance with the manufacturer's instructions. Usually presented in tubes or cartridges with mixing tips and used on preparations which must be dry. There are three main types: SILICONE I.M. Addition or condensation curing polymeric materials. Highly elastic but hydrophobic materials. Usually presented in 4 viscosities (light, medium, heavy, putty) which are used in combination. POLYETHER I.M. Clean to use, based on an organic polymer having an ether linkage. Marketed in tubes of pastes and accelerator. POLYSULPHIDE I.M. Material with a characteristic odour, based on an organic polymer linked with disulphide groups. Sometimes referred to as *rubber base, thiokol* or *mercaptam.* A two-part mixture of light body, intermediate or regular, or heavy body, with a catalyst—all in tubes. *Green stick i.m. (tracing stick).* Thermoplastic impression material in stick form. Used to build up the margins of impression trays or in copper rings. May not be green colour. *Inlay wax i.m.* Wax used for obtaining patterns for castings. Blue inlay wax is harder than the green variety, the working properties being varied by their ingredients. A mixture of waxes such as paraffin wax, beeswax, ceresin, carnauba and candelilla wax. Obtainable in sticks, sheets and prefabricated shapes used for clasps and bars. *Irreversible hydrocolloid (alginate) i.m.* Powder containing soluble alginates and additives mixed in correct proportion with water (at room temperature) to form a gel on setting. Cannot be re-used. Mixing instructions must be followed exactly to obtain accurate and standard results. The set material dehydrates if left exposed to air for any length of time, causing shrinkage. *Plaster of Paris i.m.* Finely ground plaster of Paris containing such substances as potassium sulphate and borax to reduce setting time and expansion. The powder is mixed with water and spatulated in a flexible bowl. Used mostly for edentulous cases but seldom as a routine. *Reversible hydrocolloid (agar) i.m.* Agar aqueous gel that liquefies when heated and gels on cooling. Provides very accurate impressions and is used on wet preparations. Marketed in tubes or cartridges. Heated before use in electrically controlled water baths at various temperatures. The material is contained in water-cooled impression trays held in the mouth. *Zinc oxide-eugenol i.m.* Paste used for rebasing or relining a complete denture, and in some cases as a wash covering an existing impression. Obtained by mixing pastes from two tubes, one containing zinc oxide, an oil and accelerator, and the other a resin dissolved in eugenol or other substance.

impression tray Metal or plastic tray used to carry, control and support an impression material. May be perforated to improve the adherence of the material to the tray, so reducing the possibility of distortions. *Anatomical i.t.* Used for edentulous cases and shaped to accommodate and follow the contours of the denture-bearing area. *Box i.t.* Stock impression tray of metal or plastic used for impressions of partially dentate arches. *Special i.t.* Tray made from an individual patient's models to control the impression material accurately. *Stock i.t.* Metal or plastic tray used to obtain a first impression model on which a special tray may be constructed.

in- (im-) Prefix denoting not, in, within or into.

incidence The number of occurrences of something (e.g. a disease) in a population over time.

incipient In medicine, the initial stages or onset of a disease.

incisal Cutting edge of an incisor tooth. *I. angle.* Angle formed with the horizontal plane by drawing a line in the sagittal plane between the incisal edges of the mandibular and maxillary central incisors when the teeth are in intercuspal occlusion. *I. edge.* Cutting surfaces of the incisor and canine teeth. This edge is bounded by the labial and lingual or palatal surfaces. *I. guide* or *table.* Anterior guide of an articulator which maintains the incisal angle. *I. guidance.* Guidance provided by the palatal surface of the maxillary incisors during the lateral movement of the mandible. *I. rest. See* rest.

incision In surgery, a cut made in body tissues. *See also* external bevel incision, inverse bevel incision.

incisional biopsy *See* biopsy.

incisive canal Bony canal running from the incisive foramen in the anterior inferior aspect of the maxilla behind the central incisors, to the floor of the nasal cavity. Conveys the long sphenopalatine nerve, blood vessels and lymphatics. *I.c. cyst. See* nasopalatine cyst.

incisive papilla Raised portion of soft tissue covering the incisive foramen in the hard palate.

incisor Single-rooted tooth with a cutting or shearing edge. The four most anterior maxillary and mandibular teeth. Classified as *central* and *lateral* incisors. The upper incisors develop and erupt in the premaxilla and the lower incisors gain contact with them when the mouth is closed. The lateral incisors are situated on each side of the central incisors and are bounded by the canines.

incisor relation In orthodontics, classification based on the anteroposterior relationship of the incisors. *Class I.* When the incisal edges of the lower incisors occlude with the central portion or cingulum of the upper central incisors. *Class II.* When the incisal edges of the lower incisors lie posteriorly to the upper central incisor cingulum. DIVISION 1. Proclined upper central incisors with an increased overjet. DIVISION 2. Retroclined upper central incisors. *Class III.* The lower incisor edges lie anteriorly to the upper incisor edges. There is a reduced or reversed overjet.

inclusion cyst *See* fissural cyst.

incompatible Mutually repellent.

incompetent lips Condition where the lips remain apart when the muscles of facial expression are relaxed and the mandible is in the rest position. Leads to mouth breathing and to orthodontic and periodontal problems.

incomplete lip seal *See* incompetent lips.

incomplete overbite Seen when the posterior teeth are in occlusion but the lower incisors do not occlude with the upper incisors or with the mucosa of the palate.

increment An increase, an added amount.

incremental Variable increase in quantity. Additional small dose of a drug given at intervals.

incremental growth lines of dentine Lines seen under the microscope to be running across the long axis of the dentinal tubules representing the rhythmic deposition of dentine matrix (q.v.).

incremental growth lines of Von Ebner Microscopic lines seen in dentine, 20 μm apart, that represent 4-5 day increments in rhythmic growth of the tissue.

incubation 1. Process of egg development. 2. Development of a bacterial culture. *I. period.* Period between exposure to an infection and the appearance of symptoms.

indentation State of being notched. A pit or depression.

index 1. Method of recording the progress of a disease or condition by using established criteria. 2. Fore- or pointing finger. 3. Value expressing the ratio of one measurement to another. *Bleeding on Probing I. (BoP).* Usually 4 or 6 surfaces (periodontal pockets) around each tooth are tested by gentle probing and the results recorded as a percentage. *Calculus I. See* oral hygiene i. *Community Periodontal Index of Treatment Needs (CPITN).* WHO designated index in which a special ball-ended probe is used to determine the severity of periodontal involvement and treatment need, usually in each of the sextants of the dentition. Identifies bleeding on probing, subgingival calculus, deficient restoration margins, extent of probing depth, furcation involvement and recession. Now also referred to as the Basic Periodontal Index (BPE). *Cumulated I. Medicus (CIM). See* Index Medicus. *DDE*

I. Developmental defects of enamel index. *Dean's I.* Used to measure dental fluorosis. *DEF I.* A method of measuring caries experience. It is obtained by counting the Decayed, Extracted or Filled teeth in the primary dentition. Missing teeth are not counted as it may be difficult to determine if they were exfoliated normally or extracted. *DEFS.* Similar to DEF but filled *surfaces* rather than filled teeth are counted and added to the decayed and extracted score. *DMF.* An index giving the total number of Decayed, Missing and Filled permanent teeth. *dmft/dmfs index* the decayed missing and filled components of primary teeth and primary teeth surfaces, used in dental epidemiology to measure caries prevalence and incidence. *Gingival (Loe and Silness) I. (GI).* The scoring depends on the severity of the condition and ranges from 0 for normal gingiva to 3 for gingiva showing severe inflammation with marked oedema, redness and ulceration. *I. Medicus (IM).* A monthly bibliography of the principal worldwide biomedical literature produced by the MEDLINE system from the MEDLARS data base. It is cumulated annually into the Cumulated I. Medicus (CIM). *Index of Tooth Mobility (ITM).* Tooth mobility is scored in four stages. 0, where there is no detectable mobility; 1, where there is barely discernable mobility; 2, where there is crown movement in any direction and 3, where there is crown movement in any direction including rotation and depression. *Oral Hygiene I. (OHI).* A quantitative index for determining oral hygiene in population groups and individuals. Measurements are taken to determine the extent of debris, calculus (q.v.) and plaque (q.v.). *Papillary Bleeding I. (PBI).* An index based on the bleeding resulting from the gentle probing of the interdental papilla. *Periodontal Disease (Ramfjord) I.*

(PDI). A quantitative index (now seldom used) of the periodontal state of individuals or groups. It is assessed by examining six teeth only and scoring the teeth into six grades ranging from health (0) to severe gingivitis with over 6 mm of crevice formation (6). *Periodontal (Russell) I. (PI).* An index (now seldom used) for assessing gingival and periodontal disease. The scoring is in six steps and ranges from 0 where there is no inflammation or loss of function and with normal radiographic appearance to 8 where there is advanced destruction of the supporting tissues, loss of masticatory function, drifting and looseness of the tooth and where there is radiographic evidence of bone loss in more than one-half of the length of the tooth root. *Plaque (Silness and Loe) I.* There are 4 criteria for scoring ranging from 0 (no plaque) to 3 where the interdental region is filled with debris and there is heavy accumulation of soft material filling the niche between the gingival margin and the tooth surface. *Plaque score I.* 4 or 6 surfaces of each tooth are examined for the presence or absence of plaque and the total score of surfaces expressed as a percentage. *PMA (Schour and Massler) I.* This was probably the first numerical system for recording and evaluating the progress of periodontal disease. The abbreviation letters refer to the examination carried out of the Papillary, Marginal and Attached gingivae. *Retention (Loe) I.* This index evaluates the degree of plaque retention resulting from defective margins of restorations and from carious cavities. It is scored in 4 stages, 0 (no caries, calculus or imperfect restorations in a gingival location) to 3 (large cavity, abundant calculus and/or grossly infected margin). *Thylstrup Fejerskov I.* Used to measure dental fluorosis.

indication In medicine, a belief that a particular course of action or treatment plan is desirable. *See also* contra-indication.

indices (indexes) Plural of index.

indigenous Occurring naturally in one area. Native.

indirect Acting through an intermediate agent. *I. fracture. See* fracture. *I. pulp capping. See* pulp capping. *I. retention. See* retention. *I. technique.* Method of making a gold casting in which a wax pattern is obtained from a model of the tooth preparation and not directly from the preparation in the mouth.

induction Activation by indirect stimulus. *I. of anaesthesia.* The initial stages in the administration of a general anaesthetic so that the patient passes smoothly from consciousness to unconsciousness. *Root end closure i. See* apexification.

indurated Hardened.

induration Abnormal hardening of an organ or tissue.

inert Lifeless. Having no chemical reactions.

infantile cortical hyperostosis *See* Caffey's disease.

infarct Area of dead tissue within an organ where the blood supply has been cut off, as may occur by the impaction of an embolus.

infect To contaminate with harmful micro-organisms.

infection Successful invasion of the body by a harmful micro-organism. *Cross-i.* Transfer of an infection esp. to a patient in a surgery, waiting room or during treatment due to inadequate procedures or use of inadequately sterilized equipment, materials or instruments. *See* Droplet i.

infectious (contagious or communicable) disease Any disease caused by a micro-organism that can be transmitted from one person to another by direct or indirect contact. *See* Appendix 1.

infective endocarditis *See* bacterial endocarditis.

infective mononucleosis *See* glandular fever.

infectivity The degree of infectiousness.

inferior In anatomy, below, or lower in the body in relation to another structure.

inferior vena cava Major vein into which veins from the lower aspect of the body and trunk carry deoxygenated blood to enter the right atrium of the heart.

infiltration Spreading of a substance not normally present in a tissue.

infiltration analgesia *See* analgesia.

inflammation Reaction of the body tissues to invasion by pathogenic microorganisms, or to trauma by wounds, burns or chemicals. May be acute or chronic and is characterized by five cardinal signs: redness, swelling, pain, a rise in temperature and loss of function. *Acute i.* Inflammation of rapid onset, severe symptoms and, generally, of brief duration. *Chronic i.* (frustrated healing). Longstanding, less painful condition that may lead to drainage through a sinus.

inflammatory exudate Fluid liberated at the site of an acute inflammation which dilutes toxins and any irritants present and allows phagocytosis (q.v.) to take place. Also causes swelling.

influenza An acute, highly contagious disease, commonly of epidemic proportion, caused by the influenza virus and characterized by inflammation of the respiratory tract, fever, chills, muscular pain. Pneumonia is a rare complication except for those at risk, e.g. the elderly and immunocompromised.

infra- Prefix denoting below.

infrabony pocket Periodontal pocket, the base of which lies below the margin of the surrounding alveolar bone. It is described according to whether it has one, two or three bony walls.

infrabulge *See* undercut (preferred term).

infradentale Most anterior point of the mandibular alveolar crest, situated between the lower central incisor teeth.

infra-occlusion Where a tooth is below the level of the occlusal plane either due to supereruption of the adjacent teeth or due to ankylosis or other pathology preventing eruption of the tooth. *See* submerging teeth.

infra-orbital Below the orbit. *I.-o. canal.* Bony canal running through the maxilla below the orbit. Conveying the infra-orbital artery and the maxillary division of the trigeminal nerve carrying afferent nerve impulses from all of the upper teeth. *I.-o. pointer* or *indicator.* Part of a face-bow that records the infra-orbital notch, thus aligning it with the Frankfort plane (q.v.).

ingestion Method of taking food into the body. Process by which a cell takes in foreign matter.

inhalation (inspiration) 1. Act of drawing air into the lungs through the mouth and nose. 2. Gas, vapour or aerosol breathed in for the treatment of upper respiratory tract infections. *I. anaesthetic. See* anaesthetic. *I. sedation See* sedation.

inherent filtration Unavoidable filtration due to the components of an X-ray tube, e.g. the glass of the tube.

inhibitor Any substance that prevents or slows down the occurrence of a given process or chemical reaction, e.g. the

metabolic process or the growth of bacteria.

initial Of, or belonging to, the beginning. *I. contact. See* premature contact.

initiator Any substance that activates a given process or chemical reaction.

injection Forcing of a liquid into a substance, usually by means of a syringe. Common routes for injection are into the skin (*intracutaneous* or *intradermal i.*), into the periodontal ligament, which produces instant analgesia (*intraligamentary i.*), into muscle (*intramuscular i.*), into cancellous bone (*intra-osseous i.*) or directly into a vein (*intravenous i.*). *I. moulding.* A manufacturing process whereby a plastic material is forced into a mould cavity under pressure. *I. needle.* Hollow needle with a bevelled sharp end used to introduce fluid into the body. *Submucosal i.* An injection of a solution beneath the mucosa.

inlay Restoration of composite, ceramic or gold which is made to have a precise fit into a tooth preparation, retained by being cemented in place. Inlays can be prepared in two ways. By the *direct method* where the inlay pattern is prepared in the mouth using wax or by optical scanning of the preparation in the patient's tooth and by the *indirect technique* where an accurate impression of the prepared teeth is made, a model is poured and the restoration constructed in the laboratory on the prepared model. *I. wax. See* impression material, wax.

innervation Nerve system serving an area of the body.

inoculation 1. Introduction of dead or attenuated micro-organism, toxins or prepared antigens into the body with the aim of stimulating an immune response and preventing disease, e.g. mumps, hepatitis and tetanus. 2. In microbiology, the deliberate introduction of a small number of micro-organisms into a growth medium for cultivation.

inorganic Not derived from plant or animal life and having no ordered structure. In chemistry, refers to those substances that do not contain carbon.

inpatient Person admitted to a hospital and remaining there overnight so that examination, observation and/or treatment may be carried out. *See also* day-patient, outpatient.

INR International Normalized Ratio. A measure of prothrombin time, useful in monitoring warfarin therapy and detecting abnormalities of the extrinsic clotting pathway.

insertion 1. In dentistry, the placing of an inlay into a tooth preparation or a prosthesis into the mouth. 2. The site of attachment of the distal portion of a muscle into bone.

in situ In position.

insoluble Not able to be dissolved.

inspiration Act of breathing in.

insulin Endocrine secretion of the pancreas that regulates the metabolism of carbohydrates by controlling blood sugar levels and ensures complete fat combustion. It is excreted directly into the bloodstream. Used in the treatment of diabetes.

integral The greater part or the whole of an object. *I. absorbed dose. See* i. dose. *I. dose.* Total energy absorbed by an object during exposure to radiation.

intensifying screen Sheet of plastic coated with calcium tungstate crystals or rare earth material, positioned in contact with an unwrapped radiographic film in a cassette. X-rays striking the screen during exposure cause it to fluoresce and enhance the image on the film.

intensity In radiography, the degree of density and contrast of an image on a radiographic film.

intention The process of healing. Healing by *first i.* is the natural healing of a wound or surgical incision across the exposed edges of the wound. Healing by *second i.* occurs when an open wound granulates from its base and gradually fills the deficiency.

inter- Prefix denoting between, and, among others.

interalveolar distance (inter-ridge distance) Vertical distance between fixed points in the maxillary and the mandibular alveolar ridges at the vertical dimension of occlusion.

interarticular Within a joint, e.g. the intercondylar disc of the cartilage interposed between the glenoid fossa and the mandibular condyle in the temporomandibular joint.

intercellular Between the cells of a structure. May be applied to the connective tissue or fluid bathing the cells.

interceptive orthodontics Method used in orthodontics to prevent malocclusion of the permanent dentition. Generally applied during the mixed dentition period.

intercondylar axis *See* axis.

intercondylar disc Oval disc of fibrocartilage whose edges are fused with the capsular ligament of the temporomandibular joint, dividing the joint into an upper and a lower compartment.

intercuspal contact The contact between cusps of teeth in opposing jaws.

intercuspal (centric) occlusion *See* occlusion.

intercuspal position Position of the mandible when the teeth are in intercuspal occlusion.

intercuspation Condition in which the cusps of the teeth of both arches meet together.

interdental Situated between the approximal surfaces of adjacent teeth. *I. brush.* Brush designed to remove plaque from the interdental spaces. Shaped somewhat like a small bottle brush and passed between the teeth. *I. eyelet wiring.* Method of immobilizing the jaws by applying preformed eyelet wires to both the maxillary and the mandibular teeth. Intermaxillary tie wires are then passed through one eyelet in the maxilla and one in the mandible and the ends twisted tightly together, thus immobilizing the mandible against the maxilla. *I. papilla.* Papilla of the gingiva situated in the interdental space. *I. stick. See* i. wood point. *I. wood point.* Hard- or softwood piece of stick used to displace food debris and plaque from the interdental spaces.

interior Situated inside a part.

intermaxillary fixation *See* fixation.

intermaxillary space Space between the upper and lower jaws when the latter is in the rest position. Normally contains the teeth and the alveolar processes.

intermaxillary traction In orthodontics, treatment to produce movement of either or both dental arches, generally by means of elastic bands applied between brackets fixed to the teeth of opposing arches. Divided into three classes: *Class 1.* Where a force is applied within the same arch to produce movement. *Class 2.* Where a force is applied from the posterior part of the mandibular arch to the anterior area of the maxillary arch to produce movement in one or both arches. *Class 3.* Where a force is applied from the anterior part of the mandibular arch to the posterior part of the maxillary arch.

intermediate In a middle position.

intermittent Occurring at intervals. Not continuous.

internal Placed or existing inside, inner. *Open reduction i. fixation (ORIF). See* fixation. *I. wire suspension.* Method of immobilizing the fractured facial skeleton by means of wires passing above the fractured area and threaded through the soft tissue into the mouth where they are connected to arch bars or splints.

international unit system System of units used in international scientific work based on the metric system of SI units.

interocclusal Situated between opposing occlusal surfaces. *I. record.* Record made of any occlusion position in order to transfer it to an articulator. May be retrusive, protrusive, lateral, intercuspal or initial cuspal contact. Generally obtained by using a warmed or softened occlusal wax wafer or a registration paste/material. *I. clearance* (freeway space). Space existing between the occlusal surfaces of the maxillary and mandibular teeth when the mandible is in the resting position.

interproximal Between adjoining spaces such as those between teeth. *I. attrition.* Rubbing or wearing away of the proximal surfaces of adjacent teeth. *I. cavity.* Cavity involving the mesial or distal surface of a tooth. Also called *interstitial cavity. I. clearance.* Space between the proximal surfaces of two adjacent teeth. *I. or bite-wing projection.* Radiographic technique that demonstrates the crowns and the adjacent alveolar crests of maxillary and mandibular teeth. Primarily used in the diagnosis of interproximal caries. *I. space.* The triangular space between two adjacent teeth. *I. stripping.* An orthodontic technique to remove enamel from between adjacent teeth in order to provide space to allow alignment. Enamel removal is limited to the thickness of the enamel present which limits the amount of space that can be achieved. *I. surface. See* approximal surface.

interproximal stripping *See* interproximal.

inter-radicular Area between the roots of multirooted teeth.

inter-ridge distance *See* interalveolar distance.

interstitial Small space between two objects. 1. Between the specialized tissues such as the connective tissues. Interstitial fluid bathes the body cells. 2. Refers to the space separating the clinical crowns of adjacent and contiguous teeth. *I. cavity.* Cavity involving the mesial or distal surface of a tooth. *I. surface. See* approximal surface.

intestine That part of the alimentary canal extending from the stomach to the anus. The small intestine is about 6 m long and the large intestine about 2 m in length. The intestines complete the processes of digestion and elimination of waste products.

intima 1. Innermost thin layer of cells lining arteries and veins. Composed of endothelium that lines the lumen (interior) of the vessels. 2. Innermost layer of various other organs or parts.

intra- Prefix meaning within, inside.

intra-articular Located within the cavity of a joint.

intracanal medicament *See* root canal dressing.

intracapsular Located within a capsule.

intracellular Within a cell.

intracoronal Within the crown of a tooth. *I. attachment.* Precision attachment, one part of which (usually the female part) is embedded in a restoration.

I. restoration. Restoration lying within the confines of the crown of a restored tooth.

intractable Not manageable; resisting relief, cure or control.

intraligamentary injection *See* injection.

intramaxillary traction Traction applied between groups of teeth situated in one dental arch only.

intramedullary fixation *See* fixation.

intramuscular (i/m) Within the muscle substance. *I. injection. See* injection.

intranasal Within the nose.

intra-oral anchorage Anchorage provided from within the mouth, i.e. by the teeth or other oral structures.

intra-oral cassette Small cassette used with occlusal radiographic films, generally placed in the mouth. Used to reduce exposure time to X-rays by the presence of its intensifying screens.

intra-oral radiograph Radiograph of the teeth and surrounding tissues obtained by placing a film inside the mouth during exposure.

intra-oral tracing *See* tracing.

intra-oral tube Small X-ray tube placed inside the patient's mouth when taking a panoramic dental radiograph.

intra-osseous injection *See* injection.

intratracheal Within the trachea. *I. intubation. See* endotracheal intubation.

intravascular Within the blood or lymphatic vessels.

intravenous (i/v) Within a vein. *I. anaesthetic. See* anaesthetic. *I. injection. See* injection.

intrinsic Situated within or relating entirely to one part.

intro- Prefix denoting into, inward.

intubation Passing of a tube into the air passages to act as an airway or conduct the vapour of an inhalation anaesthetic into the lungs.

invagination Insertion or folding one part of a tissue into another portion of the tissue so that the former is ensheathed by the latter.

invasion Encroachment. The spread of a tumour by invading nearby tissues.

invasive Having a tendency to spread and invade nearby tissues.

inverse bevel incision Incision made in periodontal procedures to raise a flap of gingiva from the underlying alveolus.

inverse square law In radiology, the principle which states that the intensity of radiation from a point source varies inversely as the square of the distance from the point source provided there is no absorption or scattering by the X-ray apparatus.

inverted L osteotomy Surgical operation to correct prognathism (q.v.) or retrognathism.

invest 1. To wrap around or envelop. 2. To embed in an investment material.

investing In dentistry, the process of investing an object such as a wax inlay pattern in a refractory investment material prior to casting. Prostheses in the wax stage are invested in plaster of Paris in metal flasks. *Vacuum i.* Technique in which investment material is subjected to a vacuum before, and in some cases during, the time that it is being poured into a casting ring, so removing air bubbles from the mixture.

investment cast *See* cast.

in vitro Literally 'under glass'. Describes experimentation outside the living body.

in vivo Describes experimentation in, or observation of, bodies of living organisms.

involucrum Growth of new bone surrounding the necrotic bone in an area of osteomyelitis (q.v.).

involuntary muscle One of the three main types of muscle which cannot be controlled by will. It is plain or unstriped when examined under the microscope. Found in the digestive system, blood vessels and glands.

iodine Used in tincture form as a locally applied antiseptic, germicide and disclosing solution.

iodoform (tri-iodomethane) Yellow, crystalline antiseptic powder containing iodine and having a characteristic pungent odour. It has weak antiseptic powers but is no longer used because of its toxicity on absorption.

ionizing radiation Radiation that produces ions in the tissues exposed to it.

IOTN Index of Orthodontic Treatment Need. Orthodontic criteria for defining the need for treatment based on dental health and functional benefit. Categorized from 1-5 where 1 is minimum need and 5 is the greatest need.

ipsilateral (homolateral) On the same side of the body. *I. side. See* working side.

irradiation Exposure of a person or object to radiation such as X-rays.

irreversible Unable to be reversed. *I. hydrocolloid impression material. See* impression material.

irrigant Solution for rinsing or washing. In endodontics, agent for flushing root canals, ideally combining antimicrobial activity and the ability to dissolve necrotic pulp tissue (e.g. sodium hypochlorite solution).

irrigation Act of washing out a wound or hollow organ with water or an antiseptic solution to remove debris, thereby helping reduce inflammation. A disposable plastic syringe with or without a curved plastic tip may be used to irrigate sockets and cyst cavities, a three-in-one syringe to wash out debris from a cavity preparation and a hypodermic syringe to irrigate a pulp cavity during endodontic procedures. *See also* syringe.

irritant Any substance that irritates body tissues.

ischaemia Localized lack of blood in a tissue, produced by a reduction in the blood supply. The effect of vasoconstrictor (q.v.) drugs in local analgesic solutions can be observed when the tissues become blanched or ischaemic following an injection.

ischaemic Relating to ischaemia. An area of the body that is receiving an inadequate supply of blood.

ISO International Organization for Standardization.

iso- Prefix meaning equal, uniform or similar.

isograft Graft taken from one twin and transplanted to the other twin.

isotonic Describes a solution that has the same power of diffusion as another one. An isotonic or normal solution can be mixed with body fluids without causing them any disturbance. Hypotonic (q.v.) solutions will cause haemolysis or bursting of blood cells, while hypertonic (q.v.) solutions will cause shrinkage or crenulation of the cells.

isotope Chemical element that has the same atomic number but a different atomic mass as another. Radio-active isotopes may be used to act as tracers in the body.

isthmus In anatomy, a narrow connecting band of tissue, or a narrow passage connecting two cavities.

-itis Suffix denoting inflammation.

ITM Index of tooth mobility. *See* index.

i/v Abbreviation for intravenous (q.v.).

ivory Dentine. The term is generally restricted to the teeth and tusks of elephants and other large mammals.

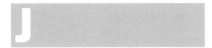

Jhook Part of an external oral traction orthodontic appliance used to transmit extra-oral forces from a headgear to the appliance.

jacket An outer covering. *J. crown. See* crown.

Jacquette scaler *See* periodontal instruments.

jaundice (icterus) Yellow discoloration of the skin and eyeballs due to the presence of excess bilirubin (a bile pigment) in the blood.

jaw Tooth-bearing bones of the face. The upper jaw comprises the two maxillae and the premaxilla and the lower jaw, the mandible. *J. augmentation procedure.* Surgical technique in which various materials, usually autogenous bone or cartilage, are grafted onto the jaws. *J. bone.* Either the maxilla or, more commonly, the mandible. *J. chattering.* Clonic spasm of the jaw muscles that may occur with rigor or as a habit spasm. *J.-closing reflex.* Reflex, by mandibular elevation, following certain oral or facial stimuli. *J.-jerk.* Reflex jaw closure occurring on stretching the jaw-closing muscles. *J. movement profile.*

1. Plot of the mandibular position against time. 2. Projection of the envelope of motion (q.v.) on the coronal or sagittal plane. *J. reflex*. Reflex action produced on the muscles moving the jaws following stimulation of the oral cavity or orofacial region. *J. relation*. Any relationship of the mandible to the maxilla. *Lock* or *locked j*. *See* trismus. *Lumpy j*. *See* actinomycosis. *Phossy j*. *See* phosphonecrosis. *Wooden J*. *See* actinomycosis.

jet injection Spring-loaded instrument, with no needle, used to rapidly inject a small amount of a solution directly into the tissues.

jeweller's rouge *See* rouge.

Jiffy tube Small celluloid or plastic tube with an extended end of reduced dimension. Used to introduce lubricant gels, dressings, cements and root-filling materials into a root canal.

joint Articulation or junction of two or more bones, e.g. the temporomandibular joint.

jugular Relating to the neck or supplying the neck or throat. *J. vein*. Any one of several veins on either side of the neck which carry venous blood from the head and brain down to the superior vena cava.

junction A joining or meeting place; an interface. *See also* amelo-dentinal junction, cemento-enamel junction, dentino-enamel junction, dentino-gingival junction.

junctional epithelium (dento-gingival junction, epithelial cuff) Epithelium at the base of the gingival sulcus which attaches the gingiva to the enamel or cementum. The term *epithelial attachment* is deprecated.

jurisprudence The philosophy of law. *Dental j*. (forensic dentistry). The science

that deals with the application of dental science to the civil and criminal law.

juxta- Prefix denoting close to.

juxtapose To position objects side by side.

juxtaposition Act of placing objects side by side.

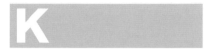

kaolin (Fuller's earth, terra alba) Purified china clay (q.v.) used in ceramics, as a demulcent and as an absorbent.

Kaposi's sarcoma Neoplastic disease of the vascular system associated with multiple red or dark brown neoplastic nodules which have a tendency to ulcerate. Primary involvement of the oral cavity is rare but secondary lesions may occur in the buccal mucosa, the lower lip and the tongue. The condition is thought to be associated with human herpesvirus 8 (q.v.).

keloid (cheloid) Overgrowth of hard fibrous tissue in a scar at the site of skin injury.

Kelvin (K) SI unit of thermodynamic temperature defined as the fraction 1/273.16 of the temperature of the triple point of water. The temperature in Kelvin is equal to a Celsius temperature plus 273.15°C.

Kennedy bar (continuous bar connector (deprecated term)) That part of a partial prosthesis consisting of a narrow bar lying in contact with the lingual surfaces of mandibular incisors, which connects the saddles and may provide indirect retention.

Kennedy bar (continuous bar connector (deprecated term))

Kennedy classification A method of classifying partially edentulous mouths and the partial dentures required to restore these edentulous areas. It is based on the location of the edentulous area relative to the remaining teeth.

kerat- (kerato-) Prefix denoting: 1. horny skin or tissue. 2. the cornea.

keratin Insoluble protein present in the epidermis, horny tissues and the organic matrix of tooth enamel.

keratinized That part of the surface tissue which has become hardened or horny by the formation of keratin.

keratoconjunctivitis Inflammation of the conjunctiva and cornea. *See* Sjögren's syndrome.

keratogenesis Formation of keratinized tissues.

kerma (*kinetic energy released in material*) Quantity representing the kinetic energy transferred to charged particles per unit mass of an unirradiated medium.

ketone bodies Compounds of acetoacetic and β-hydroxybutyric acids and acetone which are formed in the liver and are released into the blood and

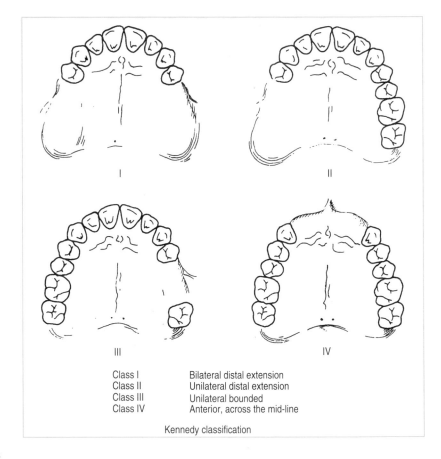

Class I	Bilateral distal extension
Class II	Unilateral distal extension
Class III	Unilateral bounded
Class IV	Anterior, across the mid-line

Kennedy classification

urine during excessive fat use, which occurs in diabetes or starvation.

keyway *See* dovetail.

K-file Tapered, flexible endodontic file, traditionally created by twisting lengths of square or triangular cross-section wire. Used in rotational or rasping motions to negotiate and enlarge root canals.

kidney One of two glandular urine-secreting organs situated in the small of the back in the lumbar region. *K. dish.* Semilunar shaped bowl for the reception of soiled swabs and instruments. Also held under the chin during mouth irrigation.

Kieselguhr *See* diatomaceous earth.

kilo- Prefix signifying one thousand (10^3).

kilogram (kg) (1000 g) The kilogram is the unit of mass and is equal to the mass of the international prototype of the kilogram. It is equivalent to about 2.2 pounds avoirdupois.

kilovolt (kV) Potential difference of 1000 V. The kilovoltage determines the quality of radiation produced by the X-ray tube and thus the qualities of the final radiograph.

kin- (kine-, kineto-) Prefix denoting movement.

kinematic face-bow Face-bow used in conjunction with an articulator in the construction of prostheses. The ends can be adjusted to permit location of the axis of rotation of the mandible.

kinematics The study of motion and the forces required to produce it.

-kinesis Suffix denoting movement.

Kirschner wire (archaic) Stout wire used to immobilize fractured bone by intramedullary fixation.

kiss of life Mouth-to-mouth emergency artificial respiration. Air is blown into the victim's lungs in order to inflate them. Exhalation is allowed to occur automatically and the process is repeated.

Koplik's spots Small red spots with a bluish centre occurring on the buccal and lingual mucosa of the mouth as an early sign of measles, often on the 2nd day of the onset prior to the appearance of a general rash.

kryo- *See* cryo-.

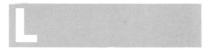

LA Local anaesthesia.

labial Pertaining to the lips. *L. bar.* Major connector of a mandibular partial denture which is placed between the reflection of the labial sulcus and the gingival margin. *L. bow. See* bow. *L. fraenum. See* fraenum. *L. surface.* A surface in contact with the lip.

labially Towards the lips.

labio- Prefix denoting lip or lips.

labioplasty *See* cheiloplasty.

laboratory putty A multipurpose vinyl polysiloxane material consisting of a base and a catalyst, which is mixed together by hand, used for a wide variety of applications in the dental laboratory such as matrices.

labrale inferius Lowest point in the midline on the vermillion margin of the lower lip.

labrale superius Uppermost point in the midline of the vermillion margin of the upper lip.

laceration Wound with torn ragged edges, not cut cleanly.

lactase Enzyme that converts lactose to glucose and galactose.

lactic acid Acid that attacks the surface enamel of teeth. A product of the conversion of carbohydrates.

lactitol Bulk sweetener with approx. 0.4 times the sweetness of sucrose. Used in sugar-free foods and confectionery. *See* sweetener.

lactobacillus Rod-shaped, Gram-positive bacteria belonging to the genus *Lactobacillus* which ferment carbohydrates with lactic acid as a by-product. *L.* grow best in slightly acid conditions, are common in the mouth and gut and are associated with dental caries. Commonly used in the food industry to produce fermented dairy products, e.g. yoghurt.

lactose Disaccharide, found in milk, which yields glucose when hydrolysed.

lacuna Hollow cavity or small pit.

lamina A thin layer. *L. dura*. Hard bony plate which appears on a radiograph as a whitish radio-opaque line situated close to and surrounding the tooth root and its periodontal ligament image.

laminated Composed of layers.

lance To cut into, and thus obtain drainage of, a fluctuant swelling.

lancinating Describes a sharp stabbing pain.

Lane centre prop *See* mouth prop.

Langerhans cell histiocytosis *See* histiocytosis X.

laryngeal Relating to the larynx. *L. reflex*. Reflex cough caused by irritation of the larynx. *L. spasm*. Spasm of the larynx.

laryngitis Inflammation of the larynx.

laryngoscope Instrument used to examine the larynx or to aid the insertion of an endotracheal tube for anaesthetic purposes.

larynx The voice organ. Situated at the upper end of the trachea having the vocal cords of elastic tissue stretched across it. The passage of air causes the cords to vibrate and produce sounds.

laser (light amplification of stimulated emission radiation) Device that concentrates energy into an intense and extremely concentrated beam of light—a laser beam. Used in surgical and diagnostic procedures.

lassitude State of weakness or weariness.

latent Existing but not yet active or developed. Hidden.

lateral 1. Related to or situated at the side of an organ. 2. In anatomy, relating to a structure or part of the body furthest from the median plane. *L. canals*. *See* accessory canal. *L. excursion*. Movement of the mandible in a lateral direction with the opposing teeth in contact. *L. interocclusal records*. *See* interocclusal record. *L. middle third fracture*. *See* fracture. *L. periodontal cyst*. Developmental or inflammatory cyst situated by the side of a tooth. *L. spreader*. *See* root canal spreader. *L. transcranial projection*. *See* transcranial projection. *L. transpharyngeal projection*. *See* transpharyngeal projection.

lathe Machine for holding and turning materials against a cutting tool, to shape and polish them. Dental laboratory lathes are electrically driven, double ended and have metal chucks pushed onto their rotating shafts. Chucks hold burs, stones, polishing brushes (bristle, felt and linen), felt cones and abrasive wheels. *L. cut amalgam alloy*. *See* alloy.

laudable pus Formerly used to describe the abundant and thick pus discharged from a wound and which was considered a sign of wound healing.

laughing gas *See* nitrous oxide.

lavage Act of washing out a cavity.

law In medicine and dentistry, a principle, rule or formula stating a fact based on experience.

laxative Agent stimulating bowel evacuation.

Le Cron's carver *See* carver.

Le Fort classification Classification describing fractures of the middle third of the facial skeleton. *Le Fort I fracture (Guérin type fracture)*. Where the maxilla is fractured transversely just above the apices of the teeth and the palatal vault, thus separating this segment from the rest of the maxilla. *Le Fort II fracture (pyramidal fracture)*. Where the fracture occurs in the central region of the middle third of the facial skeleton and passes through the bridge of the nose and backwards below the zygomatic bones. *Le Fort III fracture (high level or craniofacial dysjunction fracture)*. Where there is a transverse craniofacial bone fracture occurring above the zygomatic bones.

lead Heavy, grey, soft metal relatively impermeable to radiation. The element forms several poisonous compounds. *L. apron.* Protective apron placed on patients to protect the spinal column and reproductive organs from excess radiation during the taking of radiographs. *L. poisoning.* May result from absorption of lead salts. Seen (rarely) in the mouth as a bluish-black line at margins of the gingivae.

leakage radiation Radiation escaping from the X-ray tube head rather than through the tube aperture.

lentulo filler *See* root canal paste carrier.

lesion Broad term used to describe a zone of tissue with impaired function due to disease or trauma. The term may be applied to *primary l.*, e.g. abscesses, ulcers or tumours, or to *secondary l.*, e.g. scars or crusts, which are derived from primary lesions.

LET *See* linear energy transfer.

lethal Causing death.

letter of referral A letter from a dentist or other health professional referring a patient to another dentist, to a consultant or specialist or to another health professional. The purpose of the letter being to introduce the patient, describe the clinical history and seek advice and/or treatment on behalf of the patient.

Letterer–Siwe disease Variant of histiocytosis-X (q.v.).

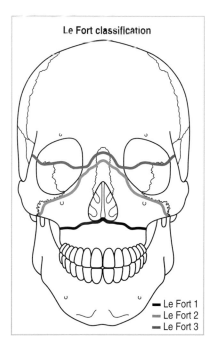

Le Fort classification

■ Le Fort 1
■ Le Fort 2
■ Le Fort 3

leuc- (leuco-, leuk-, leuko-) Prefix meaning white or lack of colour.

leucoblast Immature white blood cell.

leucocyte Colourless white blood cell of which there are two main types. *Granular l.* Consists of polymorphonuclear leucocytes, eosinophils and basophils. *Non-granular l.* Consists of monocytes and leucocytes.

leucocytosis Transient increased number of leucocytes present in the blood.

leucopenia Decreased number of leucocytes in the blood.

leukaemia Progressive malignant disease of the blood-forming system characterized by an increase in the number of white blood cells and a decrease in the number of red cells and platelets. The gingivae may become dark red in colour and subject to continuous haemorrhages.

leukoplakia White thickening of the mucous membrane in some areas of the mouth which cannot be diagnosed either histologically or clinically as any other recognizable disease. May be precancerous.

levan *See* extracellular polysaccharides.

levobupivacaine (Chirocaine®) An amide local anaesthetic agent. It is a single isomer (levo) of the long-acting agent bupivacaine.

lichen planus Group of inflammatory maculo-papular reactions of the skin and/or mucous membranes of unknown aetiology.

lichenoid Lichen planus-like lesion often of hypersensitivity origin.

lidocaine (lignocaine) A dental local anaesthetic agent. A 2% solution marketed as Lignospan®, Lignostab®,

Rexocaine®, Xylocaine® and Xylotox®, with or without epinephrine (adrenaline). Also used as a topical anaesthetic in the form of paste, gel, ointment, spray, mouthwash and lollipops. *See* Oraqix®

ligament Tough, flexible, fibrous tissue, containing both elastic and non-elastic fibres, connecting bones and cartilages and supporting joints. *Capsular l.* Ligament that completely encircles a joint.

ligamentous Relating to a ligament.

ligamentous position *See* retruded contact position.

ligate To tie with a ligature.

ligation Application of a ligature.

ligature 1. Material used to tie off blood vessels or stitch tissues together. When used externally it may be of any durable material, e.g. silk, cotton, and is removed when sufficient healing has taken place. When used internally it is usually of resorbable material, e.g. vicryl, and later becomes absorbed. 2. In orthodontics, a length of soft wire or elastic material used to retain an archwire in a bracket. *L. and pin cutting pliers. See* pliers. *L. locking pliers. See* pliers. *L. wire.* Soft, corrosion-resistant wire used in jaw fixation and splinting natural teeth. *See also* interdental eyelet wiring.

light fog Clouding or darkening on a radiographic film that has been exposed unintentionally to light, either before or during processing.

lightning strip *See* strip.

light wire pliers *See* pliers, bird beak.

lime (quicklime, unslaked lime) Calcium oxide. A constituent of silicate powder and some root-filling pastes.

line 1. Thin continuous mark, ridge or strip. 2. In anatomy and radiography, an imaginary line connecting certain landmarks on the body or passing through them. 3. A boundary. *Cervical l. See* cervical. *Finishing l.* In cavity preparation, the line of demarcation between prepared tooth substance and tooth substance untouched by instruments. *L. angle. See* angle. *See also* neonatal line, survey line.

linear energy transfer (LET) Average energy transfer imparted to a medium by a charged particle of specified energy per unit distance traversed by the particle.

liner 1. Substance applied to the walls of a cavity preparation to protect the pulp from irritation by restorative materials. *See also* cavity liner. 2. Insulating substance placed inside a casting ring.

lingual 1. Adjacent to or relating to the tongue. 2. Resembling the tongue. *L. arch.* In orthodontics, the heavy-gauge archwire that is attached to bands on the posterior teeth and which lies on the palatal or lingual aspect of the standing teeth. *L. bar.* Major connector of a mandibular partial denture and which is normally placed between the floor of the mouth and the gingival margin. *L. button (cleat or lug).* Orthodontic attachment situated on the lingual aspect of a tooth and to which a wire or elastic may be secured. *L. cleat. See* l. button. *L. fraenum. See* fraenum. *L. lug. See* l. button. *L. rest.* Occlusal rest placed on the lingual surface of a tooth. *L. surface.* Any surface of an organ adjacent to the tongue. *L. thyroid.* Rare developmental condition in which the thyroid tissue is found in the posterior superior surface of the tongue.

lingually Towards the tongue.

lingula Small, tongue-like projection of bone. The mandibular foramen is protected by a lingula of bone.

lingular Relating to a lingula.

linguo-occlusion Displacement of a tooth or teeth towards the tongue.

linguo-version Unusual position of a tooth that is inclined lingually.

lining Covering for a surface such as the inner walls of a cavity preparation. Often contains calcium hydroxide. Applied to seal the dentinal tubules and protect the dental pulp as well as to promote the growth of reparative dentine. *Resilient/ soft l.* A form of relining which provides a soft or resilient tissue-bearing surface for a removable prosthesis. *See also* zinc oxide-eugenol and zinc phosphate cements.

lip 1. Fleshy fold bordering the external entrance to the cavity of the mouth. 2. Prefix denoting fat. *Cleft l. See* cleft. *Hare l. See* cleft. *Hapsburg l.* Overdeveloped thick lower lip said to be similar to that which characterized the jaws of the Hapsburg monarchs. *High l. line.* In the upper lip, the greatest height to which the *inferior* border of the upper lip can be raised by muscle power. In the lower lip, the greatest height to which the *superior* border of the lower lip can be raised by muscle function. *Incomplete l. seal. See* incompetent lips. *L. bumper.* Orthodontic appliance that affects the dentition in one arch only. It is connected to the teeth and utilizes the resistance of the lips to that part of the appliance designed to displace the lips from their resting posture. *L. reading.* Ability of deaf persons to understand the spoken word by observing the movement of the lips and associated facial muscles. *L. seal.* The ability of the lips to come together and thus seal the oral cavity. *Low l. line.* 1. The lowest position of the *inferior* border of the upper lip at rest. 2. In the lower lip, the lowest position of the *superior* border during smiling or voluntary retraction.

lipase Constituent of the pancreatic juice that digests fats to form fatty acids and glycerol.

lipo- Prefix denoting fat.

lipoma Benign tumour of fatty tissue arising anywhere in the body.

litmus Blue pigment, either in solution or on absorbent paper, used to detect acidity or alkalinity of fluids. Blue litmus turns red in acids and remains unchanged in alkalines.

litre (l) Measure of volume equivalent to a cubic decimetre or 1000 millilitres.

liver Large, dark-red gland situated in the upper right area of the abdomen, just below the diaphragm. Its chief functions are: (1) secretion of bile (a greenish liquid aiding the breakdown of fats and the digestion); (2) maintenance of the blood composition; (3) regulation of the body metabolism; (4) storage and filtration of blood.

LJP Localized juvenile periodontitis. *See* periodontitis.

local Confined to one part or spot. Not spread. *L. analgesic cartridge.* Glass vial containing a sterile analgesic solution for use in a cartridge syringe. *L. analgesic solution.* Solution used to block the conduction of pain impulses from pain receptor nerve endings before they reach the brain. Consists of Ringer's solution (q.v.) containing 2 or 3% lignocaine, procaine or prilocaine, plus very small amounts of a bacteriostatic, and buffer salts. It may be plain or contain minute quantities of a vasoconstrictor.

local anaesthesia/analgesia Chemically induced numbness of body tissues in order to allow painful procedures to be carried out. The terms 'analgesia' and 'anaesthesia' are often used interchangeably, which is not correct. *Local* *anaesthesia.* Complete local absence of sensation and feeling including pain, pressure, temperature and touch. *Local analgesia.* Local absence of pain sensation only.

localized Bounded. Kept within a limited area. *L. alveolar osteitis* (dry or septic socket). Extremely painful inflammation of a tooth socket following extraction.

locator Device to determine the true location of an object, e.g. a needle broken in the tissues.

lock That part of a tooth preparation used to increase the retention of a restoration.

lockjaw *See* tetanus and trismus.

locomotor Concerning motion. *L. system.* System composed of bones and joints, together with the skeletal muscles, and concerned with movement.

loculated Divided or containing a number of loculi.

loculi Plural of loculus.

loculus In anatomy, a small cavity or space.

-logy (-ology) Suffix denoting field of study or science of a subject.

long cone technique *See* paralleling technique.

longitudinal axis *See* axis.

'lost wax' casting technique A casting process where a pattern, usually of plastic or wax, is embedded in investment material and later removed by heating in order to form a mould in which molten metal may be cast.

lotion Medicated solution used for washing or bathing external parts of the body.

low silver amalgam alloy *See* alloy.

lozenge Medicated tablet that has a sugar base. Also known as a *troche*.

lubb-dubb Description of the normal heart sound heard through a stethoscope. The 'lubb' coincides with the closure of the mitral and tricuspid valves and the 'dubb' with the closure of the aortic and pulmonary valves.

Luborant® *See* artificial saliva.

lubricant Any substance or secretion that acts as a surface coating and reduces friction, heat or wear and tear. In dentistry, liquid or gel agent to ease the passage or use of an implement or instrument (e.g. negotiation and enlargement of root canals).

Ludwig's angina *See* cellulitis.

Luer fitting Fitting for needles of most medical syringes, consisting of a conical projection from the syringe barrel onto which the needle hub is pushed.

lug Projecting part of an object or prosthesis.

lumen 1. The bore of a tube. In anatomy, the bore of a tube such as a duct or artery. 2. SI unit of luminous flux and equal to 1 candela.

luminescence Phenomenon in which the absorption of primary radiation by a substance gives rise to the emission of light characteristic of the substance.

'lumpy' jaw *See* actinomycosis.

lung One of a pair of conical organs consisting of air tubes ending in alveoli and filling almost the whole of the chest cavity. They are open to the atmosphere via the bronchi, trachea, nasopharynx, nose and mouth.

luting Use of a cement-like substance to seal the junction of two substances such as a crown on a tooth. *L. agent.* Fine-grained, thinly mixed cement used for the cementation of inlays, crowns, bridges and orthodontic bands.

lux SI unit of intensity of illumination.

luxation *See* dislocation.

luxator Thin, sharpened instrument used to cut periodontal ligament of a tooth to be extracted. Produces some luxation of the tooth but if used as an elevator is liable to fracture. Main indication for usage is preservation of bony structure, for example prior to implant placement.

lymph Transparent opalescent fluid that circulates in the lymphatic system. *L. gland* or *node.* Organs found throughout the body and containing lymphoid tissue, the cells of which act as filters to remove bacteria and other foreign bodies by phagocytosis (q.v.). They produce lymphocytes and are concerned with chronic inflammatory conditions, providing immunity against some diseases, fat storage and the destruction of worn-out red blood cells.

lymphadenitis Inflammation of the lymph nodes.

lymphadenoma *See* Hodgkin's disease.

lymphadenopathy Abnormal texture or enlargement of lymph nodes.

lymphangioma Tumour of lymphoid tissue.

lymphatic system Consists of lymph glands containing lymphoid tissue and lymphatic vessels. The tissue spaces contain tissue fluid carrying nutrients to the tissue cells. The fluid is returned either directly into the blood supply or to the blood via the lymphatic system through the main lymph vessels or ducts, which act as filters to remove bacterial and tumour cells.

lympho- Prefix denoting lymph or lymphatic system.

lymphocyte Mononuclear white blood cell with a clear, non-granular cytoplasm.

Formed in lymphoid tissue throughout the body. They are concerned with immunity to certain diseases. They amount to about 30% of all leucocytes, are usually about the same size as erythrocytes (7–8 μm in diameter) and are the smallest of the leucocytes. A roughly spherical nucleus occupies most of the cell.

lymphoid tissue Tissue found in lymph glands which produces lymphocytes.

lymphoma General term for a group of neoplasms derived from the basic cells of lymphoid tissue.

lys- (lysi-, lyso-) Prefix denoting destruction or dissolution.

lysis The dissolution of cellular material by chemical or physical agents, enzymes, etc.

lytic Relating to lysis.

M

maceration Term describing the softening due to excessive moisture, e.g. skin under a wet dressing.

macro- Prefix denoting large.

macrocheilia Hypertrophy of the lips, usually of congenital origin.

macrodontia Condition of having abnormally large teeth.

macroglossia Abnormal enlargement of the tongue.

macrognathia Overgrowth of the maxilla and/or the mandible.

macrophage Large mononuclear phagocytic mobile cell of the reticuloendothelial system which, together with polymorphonuclear leucocytes, appears in increasing numbers at the site of any inflammation. *M. system. See* reticuloendothelial system.

macroscopic Capable of being seen by the naked eye.

macrostomia Uni- or bilateral increased width of the mouth.

macula adherens *See* desmosomes.

macules Spot, blotch or rash not raised above the surface of the skin.

magnetic disc *See* disc, magnetic.

magnification The apparent enlargement of an image in relation to an object when viewed through an arrangement of lenses, as in a microscope.

major connector *See* connector.

mal- Prefix meaning sickness or disease.

malaise Feeling of general discomfort and illness.

malalignment Displacement of an object, such as a tooth, from its normal position.

malar bone Cheek bone, forming part of the zygomatic arch.

malformation A fault in development. A deformity.

malignant Refers to the uncontrollable growth and dissemination exhibited by some tumours.

malleable Capable of being hammered into a thin sheet, e.g. gold.

mallet Tool for hammering, having a head made of metal, wood, plastic, leather or horn. *See also* automatic mallet.

malnutrition Lack of sufficient nutrition.

malocclusion Abnormal occlusion characterized by an incorrect relationship between the arches in any spatial

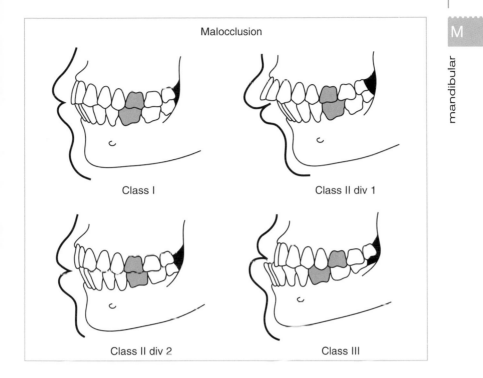

Malocclusion

Class I

Class II div 1

Class II div 2

Class III

plane or by abnormal anomalies in tooth position. *See* Angle's classification.

malposition Abnormal position of any part.

maltase Digestive enzyme converting maltose into glucose.

maltitol Bulk sweetener with approx. 0.8 times the sweetness of sucrose. *See* sweetener.

maltose A sugar (disaccharide) formed when starches are broken down by amylase.

malunion Union of the fragments of a fractured bone in an incorrect position.

mandible The lower jaw, slung below the base of the skull by two temporomandibular joints. The tooth-bearing area is known as '*the body*' and each of the two upright ends is called '*the ramus*'. The

junction of these is known as '*the angle of the mandible*'. Each ramus has an anterior process called '*the coronoid process*' and a posterior one called '*the condyle*'. The alveolar process, or tooth-supporting part, lies on the superior surface of the body. The mandible forms the shape of the lower face, the floor of the mouth and supports the lower teeth and tongue. Its movement assists in mastication and speech. *Condyle of the m. See* condyle.

mandibular Relating to the mandible. *M. canal.* Bony canal commencing at the mandibular foramen on the inner aspect of each ramus, where it is protected by the lingula. It runs through the body of the mandible, conveying the mandibular nerve, which receives afferent nerve branches from all the lower teeth. *M. condyle. See* condyle of the mandible. *M. displacement.* Deviation from a centric occlusal relationship as a result of deflection from an initial tooth contact. *M. joint. See* temporomandibular joint. *M. notch (sigmoid notch).* Separates the condyles and coronoid process of the mandible. *M. plane.* In orthodontics, a line joining the gnathion (q.v.) and gonion (q.v.) and representing the lower border of the ramus of the mandible. *M. protrusion.* An abnormal protrusion of the mandible. A Class III malocclusion (q.v.). *M. staple implant.* Modified endosseous implant (q.v.) in which the metal appliance passes through the entire height of the mandible in the anterior region where posts pierce the oral mucosa in order to give fixation points to a suitable superstructure.

mandibulofacial dysostosis *See* Treacher–Collins syndrome.

mandrel Rotary metal shank to fit a mechanical handpiece having a screw (Huey's) or split stud (Moore's) at one end to secure a disc or wheel.

manikin *See* phantom head.

manipulation time That part of the working time (q.v.) during which it is possible to manipulate a material without adversely affecting its properties.

mannitol Bulk sweetener with approx. 0.7 times the sweetness of sucrose. *See* sweetener.

mantle dentine First-formed dentine layer at the periphery of the dental pulp.

MAOI *See* monoamine oxidase inhibitors.

marble bone disease *See* osteopetrosis.

Marcain® *See* bupivacaine.

margin The edge or border of a surface. *Cervical m. See* cervical.

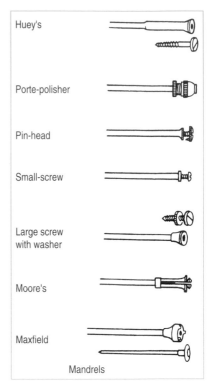

Huey's

Porte-polisher

Pin-head

Small-screw

Large screw with washer

Moore's

Maxfield

Mandrels

marginal Relating to a margin. *M. bone. See* alveolar margin.

marrow The soft centre of bone cavities.

marsupialization Surgical method of opening a cyst cavity by removing one wall to convert it into a pouch.

Maryland bridge *See* bridge.

masking 1. Covering up or concealing 2. Opaque material used to cover metallic or dark areas of restorations or prostheses.

masseter muscle Powerful, thick, square-shaped muscle of mastication attached to the lower border of the zygomatic arch and to the outer surface of the ramus of the mandible. It closes the jaw and can be palpated when the teeth are clenched. The nerve supply is from a branch of the mandibular nerve and the blood supply from the external carotid artery.

master cast *See* cast.

master impression *See* impression, final.

mastication Act of chewing when the molar teeth are used for grinding and the incisors for cutting food.

masticatory system The oral structures involved in mastication, including the muscles of mastication, the facial muscles, tongue and teeth.

mastoid process Bony prominence behind and below each external auditory meatus and containing a hollow air sinus.

materia alba Soft, white deposit consisting of food debris, dead epithelial cells and leucocytes. Found around the necks of teeth and the gingival margin, it serves as a medium for bacterial growth and is generally associated with poor oral hygiene.

materia medica Study of drugs used in medicine and dentistry.

material Any substance from which something is or can be made.

matrices Plural of matrix.

matrix 1. The ground substance of a cell. 2. Pattern or mould used in a casting. 3. Thin mould, band or strip used to contain and contour filling materials in their plastic state, during insertion and setting. 4. The female component of a precision attachment.

matrix band Stainless steel band or strip of polymeric material, which is wrapped around and held against multi-surface tooth preparations to provide a temporary wall against which the restorative material can be packed, and to impart a smooth surface and contour to the completed restoration. *M. b. retainer.* Screw, spring or clip metal device used to retain a matrix band in position. There are two main types: (1) those for use in cases of mesial occlusal or distal occlusal cavities in molars and premolars, and (2) the annular type which may also be used for mesial occlusal distal cavities. 1. IVORY NO. 1 M. B. RETAINER. For use with two surfaced cavities only. The perforated ended stainless steel bands are made in various widths and thicknesses—shorter ones being available for premolar application. They are easier to remove without disturbing the completed restoration than the annular types. The perforations allow for tension adjustment. 2. ANNULAR TYPE M. B. RETAINER. For use with two or three surfaced preparations. *a. Ivory 8 m.b. retainer.* Similar to the Siqveland but the band can be released before the holder is removed separately. *b. Siqveland m.b. holder.* A portion of ribbon band is cut and folded onto the retainer to form a ring shape which can be tightened by rotating a knurled knob. On completion of the filling the band and holder are removed together. *c. Tofflemire m.b. holder.* One of several shaped bands is selected and placed in the holder and held by screw tension. A knurled nut is rotated to tighten the annular band round the tooth. The band can be released before the holder is removed separately.

matrix metalloproteinases A family of zinc-containing enzymes, including collagenase, that are produced as part of the host immune and inflammatory response in a number of inflammatory, degenerative diseases and malignancies.

maturation 1. Process in which enamel that has just been laid down

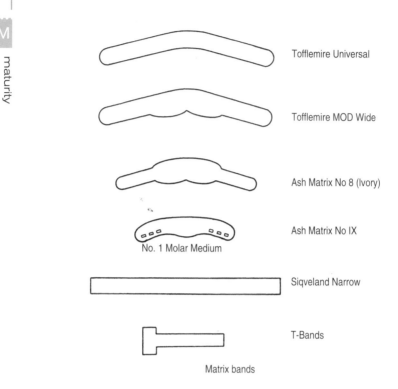

Tofflemire Universal

Tofflemire MOD Wide

Ash Matrix No 8 (Ivory)

Ash Matrix No IX

No. 1 Molar Medium

Siqveland Narrow

T-Bands

Matrix bands

becomes mineralized by the withdrawal of organic matter and water, and the deposition of apatite (q.v.). 2. The process of maturing.

maturity State of maximum development.

maxilla The upper jaw, consisting of two fused maxillae which support the upper teeth and are fixed to the skull. It separates the roof of the mouth from the floor of the nasal cavity and the floor of the orbit.

maxillae Plural of maxilla.

maxillary Relating to the upper jaw. *M. antrum* or *sinus.* Airspace within the maxilla, also known as the *antrum of Highmore,* having a lining of ciliated epithelium and draining into the nasal cavity. The roots of the upper molar

teeth and sometimes the premolars lie just below the floor of the sinus. *M. disimpaction forceps. See* forceps. *M. osteotomy.* Surgical repositioning of the maxilla. *M. plane.* Transverse plane through the skull represented on a lateral skull radiograph tracing by the line joining the anterior and posterior nasal spines. *M. resection.* The surgical removal of all or part of the maxilla and the related soft tissues. *M. tuberosity reduction.* Surgical removal of excess fibro-epithelial and bone tissue which forms the tuberosity to facilitate the construction and placing of a denture.

maxillary-mandibular planes angle (MxMnPA) The cephalometric angle measured between the maxillary plane and the mandibular plane. Normal is 27 degrees plus or minus 4.

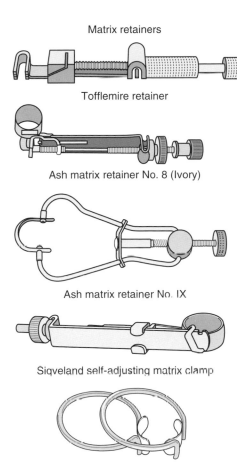

Matrix retainers

Tofflemire retainer

Ash matrix retainer No. 8 (Ivory)

Ash matrix retainer No. IX

Siqveland self-adjusting matrix clamp

Ring retainer

maxillectomy Surgical resection of part (partial) or all (total) of the maxilla.

maxillofacial Relating to the face and maxilla.

maximum intercuspal contacts Tooth contacts in the maximum intercuspal position.

maximum intercuspation The complete intercuspation of opposing teeth independently of the position of the condyles.

maximum permitted dose Upper limit of a radiation dose received by a person during a specified period. Ionizing radiation may cause somatic or genetic injury to individuals either by a concentrated high dose or by accumulated small doses over a period of time.

McKesson prop *See* mouth prop.

McSpadden compactor *See* compactor.

MDD Medical Devices Directive.

mean A minimal average. The sum of all observations divided by the number of observations.

measles Infectious virus disease characterized by fever and a rash, which usually appears after 4 days. Koplik's spots (q.v.) may be seen in the mouth in the early stages. Incubation period 10–14 days. Complications include lung and ear troubles.

measure Size or quantity of something found by measuring.

meatus A canal or orifice. *External auditory m.* The outside passage into the middle ear, passing through the temporal bone.

mechanical amalgamator Equipment, generally electrically powered, that vibrates amalgam alloy and mercury together for a controlled time to form amalgam. Other materials, such as cements and composite fillings, can also be mixed by this method.

mechanical stimulus Any substance, such as wax, that is chewed in order to stimulate a flow of saliva.

Meckel's ganglion *See* ganglion, sphenopalatine.

medial Relating to the middle.

median 1. In the midline of the body. 2. Near the midline of the dental arch. *M. palatine cyst.* Developmental cyst arising in the median fissure of the palate. *M. plane. See* mid-sagittal plane. *M. rhomboid glossitis. See* glossitis.

medicament Any healing drug or medicine.

medicated Impregnated with a medicinal substance.

medium 1. A middle quality or degree of intensiveness. 2. Any substance by which something is transmitted. 3. An environment. *Separating m.* Substance used to coat surfaces to facilitate their clean separation.

medulla The inner cancellous bony layer, also called the *marrow.*

meiosis Cell division during maturation of the cells in which each daughter cell nucleus retains half of the chromosomes of the parent cell.

melaena Black tarry faeces resulting from haemorrhage in the alimentary tract.

melanin Dark-brown to black pigment contained in the epithelial cells of the skin, hair and retina.

melanoma Pigmented mole that has become malignant.

Melkersson–Rosenthal syndrome Soft diffuse swelling of the lower lip, often erythematous, associated with facial paralysis and fissured tongue (*see* orofacial granulomatosis).

membrane Thin layer of tissue acting as a lining or covering or connecting two structures. *Basement m.* Non-cellular, thin transparent layer situated below the epithelium of mucous membranes and secreting glands. *Cell m.* Thin delicate structure enclosing a cell. It regulates the passage of substances into and out of the cell from the surrounding environment. *Mucous m.* Membrane covered by epithelium, lining the oral cavity and all tubular organs. *Periodontal m. See* periodontal ligament. *Synovial m.* Connective tissue membrane lining a synovial joint and producing the synovial fluid lubricant.

membranous Relating to a membrane.

meniscectomy Surgical removal of an intra-articular disc, e.g. from the temporomandibular joint.

meniscus 1. Crescent-shaped film seen on the surface of a liquid column and occurring because of the influence of capillarity. 2. Fibrocartilaginous, crescent-shaped structure that cushions the articulation of two bones.

mental 1. Relating to the mind. 2. Relating to the chin. *M. foramen.* Foramen in the body of the mandible through which passes the mental branch of the inferior dental nerve.

menton 1. *Soft tissue*—lowest point of the soft tissue of the chin. 2. *Hard tissue*—lowest point of the bony outline of the chin.

mepivacaine (Scandonest®) An amide local anaesthetic that is used in dental anaesthesia. It is provided as a 2% solution with 1:100,000 epinephrine (adrenaline) as the vasoconstrictor or as a 3% plain solution.

mercaptan Basic ingredient of polysulphide impression materials.

mercury (quicksilver) Liquid, heavy, silvery white metal that is purified by distillation for dental use. It is mixed with amalgam alloy to form amalgam. It is poisonous and emits toxic vapour if left in a warm room. It should not be handled. Any waste amalgam should be stored in sealed jars containing water or a commercially available disposal jar and kept in a cool place.

mercury poisoning *Acute m.p.* Symptoms are vomiting and abdominal pain followed by ulceration of the stomach wall and colon, with kidney inflammation. *Chronic m.p.* Characterized by oral manifestations such as a metallic taste, increased salivation, gingivitis and ulceration showing greyish-blue lines at the gingival margins, painful tongue and loosening of the teeth. May also be accompanied by degeneration of the peripheral nerves and the central nervous system.

mesenchymal Relating to mesenchyme.

mesenchyme Embryonic connective tissue capable of developing into many kinds of connective tissue including bone and cartilage as well as blood and lymphatic tissue.

mesial Towards the midline. Refers to the surfaces of the teeth in the dental arch that face towards the midline. *M. drift.* Gradual movement of all teeth mesially, which occurs naturally with age. Also the movement of a tooth or teeth distal to the socket of an extracted tooth which may drift mesially in the absence of a bridge or orthodontic space maintainer. *M. surface.* In anatomy, any surface of an organ situated towards the midline (or the mid-sagittal line).

mesiodens Supernumerary tooth usually malformed and lying in the midline of the anterior maxilla between the central incisors.

meso- Prefix denoting middle or intermediate.

mesoderm Middle germ layer of an embryo, between the ectoderm and the endoderm. From it are derived the bones, cartilages, muscles, fibrous connective tissue, cardiovascular and lymphatic systems, dermis, gonads, kidneys, spleen, upper genital and urinary tracts, the cortex of the suprarenal gland and all the connective tissue elements of all organs and tissues.

metal Any element with the following properties: ductility, fusibility, hardness, lustre, malleability and being a good conductor of heat and electricity. *Base m.* A metal whose constituent elements are neither precious (q.v.) nor noble (q.v.). *M. ceramic restoration.* A restoration having a metal substructure onto which a ceramic veneer is fused (*see* crown, porcelain bonded; V.M.K.®). *Noble m.* A metal that cannot be readily dissolved by acid, nor oxidized by heat alone. *Non-precious m. See* base m. *Precious m.* A metal containing primarily gold, silver and elements of the platinum group. *See also* alloy, m. base, semi-precious m., casting alloy.

metastasis Transfer of a malignant cell from one part of the body to another through the blood vessels or lymph channels to form a secondary lesion.

metastatic Relating to metastasis.

meter 1. Apparatus or instrument for measuring a physical quantity by direct reading. 2. Suffix used in the formation of names of automatic measuring instruments, e.g. thermometer, barometer. 3. *See also* metre.

methohexitone sodium White powder (to be mixed with sterile water) presented in a rubber-capped bottle. Used as an intravenous anaesthetic agent either alone for a short operation, in advance of an inhalation anaesthetic (such as a mixture of oxygen and nitrous oxide) or intermittently in small incremental doses.

methylmethacrylate Monomer from which polymethylmethacrylate (PMMA) (q.v.) is produced. *See* monomer.

$$CH_2 = C - C - O - CH_3$$
$$| \quad ||$$
$$CH_3 \, O$$

metre (m) SI unit of length equal to 100 centimetres or 1000 millimetres. It is equivalent to about 39.4 inches. It is defined as 'the length of the path travelled by light in vacuum during time interval 1/299792458 of a second'.

metronidazole (Flagyl®) An antibiotic active against anaerobic bacteria used in the treatment of spreading odontogenic infections, acute ulcerative gingivitis and pericoronitis in conjunction with local hygiene measures. It is administered orally, intravenously or as a gel (Elyzol®) that is placed in periodontal pockets.

miconazole An antifungal drug used to treat oral fungal infections. Trade name is Daktarin®.

micro- Prefix meaning small.

micro-abrasion *See* acid–pumice micro-abrasion.

microbiological examination Taking and investigation of microbiological specimens, e.g. sampling a root canal using sterile paper points.

microbiology The scientific study of micro-organisms.

microbrush Swedish brush, like a small bottle brush, used to remove plaque from the interproximal areas of the teeth.

microcracks *See* crazing.

microcrystalline wax Synthetic wax that resembles natural wax in its physical characteristics and is used in the production of modelling waxes. Obtained by the fractional distillation of crude oil.

microdontia Condition in which the teeth are abnormally small, especially the maxillary lateral incisors and the third permanent molars.

microglossia Condition in which the tongue is abnormally small.

micrognathia Underdevelopment of the mandible and/or the maxilla.

microleakage Passage of liquids, micro-organisms and ions between a restoration and the walls of its cavity preparation.

micromotor Miniature electric motor to which a handpiece is fitted.

micron (μ) One-thousandth of a millimetre.

micro-organism Organism too small to be seen with the naked eye, e.g. bacteria, viruses and protozoa. *Commensal m.-o.* Micro-organism that lives in the body without normally causing disease. *Pathogenic m.-o.* Micro-organism that may cause disease.

microscope Optical instrument used to magnify small objects. *Binocular m.* Microscope with two eyepieces thus enabling objects to be seen in perspective. *Electron m.* Microscope in which a beam of electrons replaces the beam of light of a simple microscope, enabling magnification up to 500 000 times to be achieved. *Vernier (micrometer) m.* Microscope mounted on a movable slide and used to measure accurately the dimension of small objects.

microscopic So small that it can only be seen through a microscope.

microstomia Condition in which the mouth is unusually small.

MICRR Multiple idiopathic cervical root resorption.

midazolam (Hypnovel®) A benzodiazepine drug that is used in dentistry as an intravenous sedative agent. It is supplied in vials of 10 mg in either 2 ml or 5 ml of solution.

middle-third fracture *See* fracture.

mid-sagittal (median) plane Imaginary plane passing through the midline of the body dividing it into left and right halves.

migraine Severe periodical headache often preceded by an aura. May be accompanied by nausea and vomiting.

migration 1. Abnormal movement or drifting of teeth due to the inflammatory process of periodontitis (q.v.). 2. Movement of leucocytes through blood vessel walls. 3. Normal physiological drift of a tooth.

Mikulicz's disease Disease of the major salivary glands characterized by a hyperplasia of the lymph nodes within the gland.

milk teeth Deprecated lay term for the primary or deciduous dentition (q.v.).

milled bar Metal bar that has been milled or ground to have flat sides which serve as a means of retention for a prosthesis. Prevents rotation of the prosthesis about the bar.

milli- Prefix meaning one-thousandth part.

milli-ampere (mA) One-thousandth of an ampere. In radiography, the unit of current measurement passing from the cathode to the anode, and determining the quantity of radiation emitted by the tube.

milligram (mg) One-thousandth of a gram.

millilitre (ml) One-thousandth of a litre.

MIMS Monthly Index of Medical Specialties. A monthly publication containing the drugs that are currently available for prescription in the United Kingdom.

mineral trioxide aggregate (MTA) Material based on building cement increasingly being used in surgical and non-surgical endodontics, especially in the treatment of open apices and repair of perforations.

mineralization The addition of mineral matter to the body tissues.

miniature handpiece Handpiece with a small head and chuck allowing easy access into a small mouth.

minimal carious lesion Early lesion into dentine, comprising a dark-stained central pit with dark dentinal caries shining through translucent enamel with decalcification of the enamel lined walls of the pit. Usually treated using a preventive resin restoration (PRR). *See* PRR.

minimum The lowest possible amount or limit.

minor connector *See* connector.

miscible Able to be mixed so as to form a homogeneous substance.

Misuse of Drugs Act Act of Parliament aimed at checking the unlawful use of drugs that are liable to induce dependency or cause harm if not used properly and as advised. These drugs are known as 'controlled drugs' and include the following: cocaine, diamorphine (heroin), dipipanone (Diconal®), hydrocodone, hydromorphone, methadone (Physeptone®), morphine, opium, oxycodone, pethidine and phenazocine (Narphen®).

Mitchell's trimmer Multi-purpose hand instrument with spoon-shaped end and an angled pointed blade, triangular in section.

mite Extremely small animal. *Acarus m.* Mite that causes skin diseases such as scabies.

mitosis Division of cells into two identical daughter cells, each with the same number and type of chromosomes as the parent cell.

mitral valve Heart valve situated between the left atrium and the left ventricle to ensure the one-way flow of blood.

mixed dentition Dentition consisting of primary and permanent teeth during the period when the primary teeth are being shed.

mixed parotid tumour Slow-growing adenoma of the parotid gland. A benign growth of epithelial origin which may become malignant. Treatment is by excision.

mixed saliva *See* whole saliva.

mixing pad Pad of treated paper sheets on which powders, liquids or pastes may be mixed.

mixing slab Rectangular slab, usually of glass or glazed pottery, on which dental materials are mixed. One surface may be ground. When cooled, the thickness of the slab retains its cool condition, allowing for a slower mixing and setting time.

mixing time That part of the working time (q.v.) required to complete a satisfactory mix of the components of a material. The manufacturer's instructions for the mixing time of their products should be followed carefully.

mobile unit (or cart) Assembly of instruments that can be moved.

mobility 1. Capable of movement or free flow. 2. In dentistry, the looseness of a tooth. A numerical periodontal index of mobility may be charted according to the degree of mobility of each tooth.

mobility test Diagnostic test to determine the degree of mobility of one tooth in relation to its supporting structures.

model A replica A three-dimensional shape representing a likeness of an existing object. In dentistry, a cast, i.e. a positive and accurate reproduction of the dentition and adjacent structures. *M. base former.* Flexible mould used to form an acceptable base shape for plaster of Paris models, especially orthodontic models. *M. cement.* Deprecated term for sticky wax (q.v.).

modelling wax (pink wax) *See* wax.

modifier An agent that alters or changes a material without transforming it.

modiolus Point distal to the corner of the mouth where several facial muscles converge and which stabilize the cheeks and lips.

molar Posterior grinding tooth. There are eight primary molars, two in each quadrant, and 12 permanent molars, three in each quadrant. The upper molars normally have three roots and the lower molars have two roots. The permanent most posterior molars tend to have fused roots. They have broad multicuspal occlusal surfaces.

molariform Having a molar shape.

mole Lay term for a pigmented blemish of the skin.

molecular Relating to molecules.

molecule Smallest mass of substance able to keep its independent existence and characteristic properties.

molten metal sterilizer *See* sterilizer.

mongolism An archaic term for Down syndrome (q.v.).

moniliasis *See* candidiasis and thrush.

monitoring 1. Constant observation. 2. In radiology, the use of measuring instruments to determine whether a place or a person's radiation exposure is within permissible limits.

monitoring badge Device containing a film that determines whether a person is receiving an excessive exposure to ionizing radiation. The badge should be worn between the neck and the groin whenever exposure to X-rays is likely and should be assessed at regular intervals.

mono- Prefix meaning single or one.

monoamine An amine containing only one amino group.

monoamine oxidase inhibitors (MAOI) A group of antidepressant drugs which may dangerously enhance the effects of other drugs (e.g. anaesthetics, barbiturates, tranquillizers, opioids and alcohol), leading to a drop in blood pressure, coma and sometimes death. Patients who are taking any of these anti-depressants are advised to avoid eating cheese, Marmite®, Bovril®, broad beans, yoghourt and other foodstuffs which may cause severe symptoms. Coffee also may cause hyperexcitability in such cases.

monobloc *See* appliance, Andresen a.

monocyte Large white blood cell with clear cytoplasm and a single large nucleus. Monocytes are capable of phagocytosis and constitute about 5% of all leucocytes. Of equal size or larger than granular leucocytes.

monocytic Relating to monocytes.

monomer 1. Simple molecule of low molecular weight that can be bound to a similar molecule to form a polymer. 2. In dentistry, it refers to methyl methacrylate, a clear liquid with a characteristic smell which can be mixed with polymer powder to make a dough which polymerizes, hardens or cures, to form acrylic. Used in the construction of dental prostheses and appliances.

monosaccharide A simple sugar that is the end-result of digestion of carbohydrates such as starches and disaccharides, e.g. glucose, fructose.

Monson's curve *See* curve of Monson.

Moon's probe Blunt, flat-handled probe used to explore sinuses.

Moon's teeth *See* tooth.

Moore's mandrel Split stud mandrel (q.v.) with latch-type end to its shank for contra-angled handpieces or smooth-end shank for straight handpieces. Used with discs and wheels.

morbilli *See* measles.

morphology The study of the shape or form of objects.

mortar Glass receptacle with ground glass internal surface used with glass pestle to mix substances, by hand.

mosquito artery forceps *See* forceps.

motile Capable of spontaneous movement.

motivation In dentistry, inciting a person to wish to achieve and maintain a good standard of dentistry and oral hygiene.

motor nerve *See* efferent nerves.

motor neurone Efferent neurone consisting of nerve cells, dendrites and axons (nerve fibres), that controls the contraction and relaxation of muscles.

mottling Surface marking of teeth caused by fluorosis (q.v.) or by drugs such as tetracycline.

mould 1. To shape. 2. Hollow shape in which materials are cast or set. 3. General

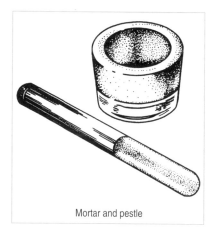

Mortar and pestle

term describing the growth of fungi. *M. chart.* An illustration of tooth moulds available from a particular artificial tooth manufacturer. *M. guide.* A mounted selection of artificial teeth available from a particular manufacturer.

mounting 1. Attaching a plaster cast to an articulator. 2. Placing radiographs in a display card. *M. rings/plates.* Metal or plastic devices used to attach casts to an articulator (q.v.). *See also* split cast m.

mouth gag Two-handled instrument used to prise and hold the mouth open during an anaesthetic. It has a ratchet device to maintain the opening. The two blades are set at right angles so that they may be applied between the teeth and/or edentulous ridges. Mostly used while a mouth prop is being changed from one side to the other. Examples: Mason, Ferguson, Doyen and Ackland.

mouth guard Flexible sports appliance worn during contact sports to protect the teeth from trauma.

mouth mirror Reflecting surface designed for intra-oral use and enabling the dental surgeon to see areas indirectly and to direct light into dark areas. Also used to hold the cheek and tongue away from the operating area. The mirror head unscrews from the handle. They are numbered according to size and are of three types: those reflecting from their front surfaces, those reflecting from their back surface and magnifying mirrors.

mouth prop Prop used during an anaesthetic to maintain the mouth in an open position. *Hewitt's metal props* and *McKesson rubber props* are in sets of three on a chain. The *Lane centre prop* is spring loaded and hinged so that its connecting bar may be swung from one side to the other without being removed from the mouth.

mouthwash Medicated solution for cleansing the mouth.

MRI (magnetic resonance imaging) An imaging modality based on the alignment and spin of hydrogen ions in a strong magnetic field and their movement following applied radiofrequency wave pulses.

mucin Major constituent of mucus, found in saliva and made up of many proteins, acting as a lubricant during swallowing. The daily output varies from person to person and from time to time. It tends to make the saliva 'ropey'.

mucobuccal fold The area of flexure of the mucous membrane between the maxilla or the mandible and the cheek.

mucocoele (mucus retention cyst) Collection of mucus within the tissue arising from a salivary gland. May be due to blockage of a salivary duct.

mucodisplacement impression See impression.

mucogingival Relating to gingival and alveolar mucosa. *M. complex (dentogingival complex)*. Generic term for anything that entails both gingivae and alveolar mucosa. Includes the oral epithelium, the gingival crest and sulcus, the junctional epithelium, the complex network of collagen fibres including the periodontal ligament, the alveolar bone and the attached gingivae. *M. junction*. Irregular line indicating the meeting of the alveolar mucosa and the attached gingiva. *M. surgery*. Surgery conducted on the gingivae to improve or modify defects in shape, position or amount.

mucoperiosteal flap See full-thickness flap.

mucoperiosteum Periosteum with an overlying, firmly attached mucosal layer. Seen in the hard palate and gingiva.

mucopolysaccharidosis I See Hurler's syndrome.

mucosa Layer of epithelium covering or lining the oral cavity. Often termed the *oral mucosa*.

mucosal Relating to mucous membrane.

mucosal grafting vestibuloplasty (archaic) Surgical deepening of the gingival sulcus by introducing a free mucous membrane graft.

mucostatic impression See impression.

multi- Prefix meaning many.

multicellular An organism characteristically consisting of many cells.

multilocular Having many compartments as found in a multilocular cyst.

mumps (parotitis) Virus infection of one or both parotid salivary glands occurring mostly in children. Accompanied by painful swellings, it may cause inflammation of the sex glands in males and result in sterility.

murmur Cardiac sounds produced by the turbulence due to pathologically damaged valves.

muscle Tissue, composed of minute fibres, that contracts or shortens when stimulated by a nerve impulse. *M. attachments*. Deprecated term for abnormal fraenum (q.v.). *M. reposition*. Surgical procedure to move a muscle attachment into a more acceptable functional position.

muscle trimming See border moulding.

muscles of mastication Muscles concerned with mastication are: masseter, temporalis, lateral pterygoid and medial pterygoid, all innervated by the mandibular branch of the trigeminal nerve. Other muscles of mastication are: the buccinator muscle, the tongue, the anterior belly of the digastric muscle, the mylohyoid muscle and the orbicularis oris.

muscular tissue Tissue composed of cells that can contract. There are three types. *Cardiac m.t.* Striped heart muscle. *Involuntary m.t.* Plain or unstriped, not controlled by will but responding to the autonomic nervous system. *Voluntary* or *striped m.t.* Can be controlled at will and effect movement. Found attached to bones and includes the muscles of mastication, the tongue and the facial muscles.

mutans streptococci A collective term used to describe a group of bacteria with characteristics similar to *Streptococcus mutans*. It comprises two human species, *S. mutans* and *S. sobrinus*, and a variety of animal species including *S. rattus, S. downei, S. cricetus, S. ferus* and *S. macacae. m.s.* is also referred to as the *Streptococcus mutans* group.

mutually protected occlusion *See* occlusion.

myalgia Muscular pain.

mycosis Disease caused by a fungus, e.g. ringworm.

mylohyoid muscle Thin sheet of muscle running the whole length of the mylohyoid ridge on the lingual surface of the body of the mandible. The two mylohyoid muscles from each side of the mandible join to form the floor of the anterior part of the mouth. Supplied by the mylohyoid branch of the inferior alveolar nerve.

mylohyoid ridge Bony ridge running along the internal surface of the body of the mandible providing attachment for the mylohyoid muscle. The ridge separates two hollows: the upper and more anterior depression against which the sublingual salivary gland lies, and the lower and more posterior depression that accommodates the submandibular salivary gland. When the alveolar bone becomes absorbed following extractions, the ridge becomes more superficial and is often a source of pain from the pressure of complete dentures.

mylohyoid ridge reduction Surgical removal of the mylohyoid ridge that may be affecting the comfortable fitting of a complete denture.

myocarditis Inflammation of the muscular walls of the heart and may be acute or chronic.

myofunctional appliance An orthodontic appliance, can be removable or fixed, that attempts to influence the growth of the maxilla and mandible in order to correct a malocclusion. *See* appliance.

myoma Benign growth of muscle tissue.

myositis Inflammation of a voluntary muscle.

myx- (myxo-) Prefix denoting mucus.

myxoedema Hypothyroidism caused by underactivity of the thyroid gland resulting in diminished activity of cells throughout the body. Severe form results in dry skin, brittle hair, swollen face and puffy eyelids, dull expression and general muscular weakness.

myxoma Benign soft tissue growth of fibrous tissue

N

naevus (nevus) A birthmark—a developmental, clearly defined pigmented lesion of the skin or oral mucosa.

nanotechnology Technology at the atomic or molecular scale. Nanotechnological advances in dentistry have exploited the atomic or molecular properties of materials and led to the development of newer materials with better properties.

narco- Prefix denoting stupor or narcosis.

narcotic Drug that induces a state of almost trance-like natural sleep—one of the controlled drugs, for example morphine derivatives, heroin, pethidine. Not used in normal dental procedures.

nares External orifices of the nose; the nostrils.

naropharynx Area where the nasal cavity runs backwards to join the pharynx. Shut off by the soft palate during deglutition.

Naropin® *See* ropivacaine.

nasal Relating to the nose. *N. cavity.* Air passage bounded by the orbit above, the hard palate below, the inner walls of the maxillary sinuses and divided by the nasal septum. *N. concha.* Any of the three thin, scroll-like turbinate bones that form the sides of the nasal cavities.

nasion Both a hard and soft tissue anatomical landmark. *Bony n.* Most anterior point of the frontonasal suture as seen on a lateral skull radiograph. *Soft tissue n.* Deepest point of concavity between the nose and forehead in the midline. *See* Appendix 10.

naso- Prefix denoting nose.

nasolabial cyst Developmental cyst arising in the soft tissues beneath the nasolabial fold.

nasopalatine Relating to the nose and palate. *N. cyst* (incisive canal cyst). Developmental cyst arising from the nasopalatine duct epithelium. *N. canal.* Canal leading from the nasopalatine or incisive foramen. The nasopalatine afferent nerve from the mucosa and gingivae of the anterior part of the hard palate runs through the incisive foramen and the canal, later to join the maxillary branch of the trigeminal nerve.

nasopharyngeal intubation Technique of passing a flexible tube into the nasopharynx through the nose.

nasotracheal Pertaining to the technique of passing an anaesthetic tube through the nose and trachea.

natal teeth *See* tooth.

natural dentition *See* dentition.

nausea Feeling sick and having the inclination to vomit.

near parallelism Feature of inlay and crown preparations in which the opposing surfaces or walls are only very slightly tapered (i.e. very nearly parallel to each other), thus allowing the insertion of the restoration and also providing maximum retention.

nebulizer A device that converts a liquid into a fine stream. A nebulizer may be used to deliver drugs such as salbutamol (q.v.) in the emergency treatment of asthma.

neck 1. That part of the body between the head and the trunk. 2. Any constricted portion of an organ or structure. 3. That part of the tooth where the crown joins the root. 4. The thinner area below the condylar process of the ramus of the mandible.

neck strap (cervical strap) Form of orthodontic headgear designed to fit around the neck only.

necro- Prefix denoting dissolution or death.

necrosed Refers to tissue that is dead and has no blood supply.

necrosis Death of a group of cells within a circumscribed area.

necrotic Relating to necrosis.

necrotizing ulcerative periodontitis *See* periodontitis.

needle Sharp device for suturing or puncturing. *Injection n.* Hollow needle of various gauges and lengths, used for injection purposes. Most medical syringes have push-on Luer fittings (q.v.) while dental needles have threaded hubs. *Suture n.* Steel needle, either triangular or round in cross-section, used for the insertion of sutures. May have an eye for the suture material or be eyeless, when the material is fixed into the hollow end.

needle holder Hinged metal instrument with scissor handles, ratchets and serrated blades to grip suture needles without allowing any rotation.

needle point tracing Arrow point tracing produced extra-orally. *See* tracing.

neo- Prefix meaning new.

neohesperidine DC Intense sweetener, approx. 1500-1800 times sweeter than sucrose. *See* sweetener.

neomycin Wide-spectrum antibiotic.

neonatal Referring to the newborn, generally applied to the first month of life. *N. line.* Line seen under the microscope as an exaggerated incremental line in the enamel and dentine of the primary teeth and the first permanent molar. It is a sign of metabolic upset at or about the time of birth. *N. teeth. See* tooth.

neoplasia New growth or tumour. Abnormal mass of tissue growing at an unusual rate in which all growth is progressive and uncontrolled. May be benign or malignant and slow or fast growing. Treatment consists of radiotherapy, chemotherapy or excision.

neoplasm Abnormal swelling or tumour of the tissue. Classified according to the tissue from which it arises or by its behaviour.

neoplastic Relating to a neoplasm.

nephritis Inflammation of the kidney.

nerve Microscopic, cord-like structure of nerve fibres that convey impulses between the central nervous system (CNS) and some other body organ, tissue or system. Depending upon their action nerves are known as sensory (afferent), motor (efferent) or mixed. *Sensory nerves* bring information from the various nerve endings to the brain and spinal cord. *Motor nerves* transmit impulses from the brain and spinal cord to the body and its muscles. *Mixed nerves* are composed of both motor and spinal sensory nerves. They transmit impulses in both directions at the same time. These types of nerves are known as the *peripheral nervous system* as distinguished from the *central nervous system*, which consists of the brain and spinal cord. Twelve pairs of cranial nerves arise directly from the base of the brain. The spinal nerves arise directly from the spinal cord. *Anterior superior dental n.* Afferent nerve from the upper central and lateral incisor and canine teeth, passing upwards to join the maxillary division of the trigeminal nerve in the infra-orbital canal. *Greater palatine n.* Nerve descending through the greater palatine foramen, running forwards in a groove in the palate to the mucous membrane of the palate. Gives rise to the lesser palatine nerve which passes through the lesser palatine foramen to supply the soft palate and its mucous membrane. *Long buccal n.* Afferent nerve running from the mucosa and outer alveolar plate, in the region of the molar and sometimes premolar teeth, obliquely across the anterior border of the ramus of the mandible between the mucous membrane and the buccinator muscle. It ascends between the two heads of the pterygoid muscle to join the mandibular nerve. *Mandibular n.* One of the three divisions of the *fifth cranial* or *trigeminal nerve*. Nerve fibres run from the skin of the lower lip and chin and the mucous membrane of the lower lip and gingivae to the mental foramen through which, as the mental nerve, it passes to join the main branch. The incisive nerve from the lower incisor teeth runs back through the body of the mandible to emerge at the mandibular foramen. It then runs deep to the ramus in front of the condyle to a foramen at the base of the skull through which it passes to the brain. The mandibular division is joined by the long buccal sensory nerve and the lingual nerve. Efferent fibres from the brain branch off the mandibular nerve to the muscles of mastication and the salivary glands. *Maxillary n.* Division of the trigeminal nerve. Afferent fibres from the eyelids, nose and upper lip pass through the infra-orbital canal of the maxilla via the infra-orbital foramen. Here they are joined by afferent nerve fibres from the anterior, middle and posterior superior dental nerves from all of the upper teeth. The greater palatine and nasopalatine afferent nerves from the soft palate join the maxillary nerve via the sphenopalatine ganglion as it leaves the infra-orbital canal. *Mental n.* Afferent nerve arising from the skin of the lower lip and chin, and mucous membrane and gingivae between the second premolar tooth and the midline of the dental arch. It passes through the mental foramen as the incisal nerve to join the mandibular nerve. *Middle superior dental n.* Afferent nerve from the first and second upper premolars and part of the first permanent upper molar. It runs upwards to the infra-orbital canal, to join the maxillary division of the trigeminal nerve. *Nasopalatine n.* Afferent nerve arising from the mucous membrane of the anterior part of the hard palate and gingivae of the adjacent teeth. It ascends through the anterior palatine foramen running back to join the sphenopalatine ganglion and through this to the maxillary division of the trigeminal nerve. *N. block. See* analgesia, block. *N. cell. See* neurone. *Posterior superior dental n.* Afferent nerve running from the palatal and distobuccal roots of the first molar and all roots of the second and third molars passing backwards through the posterior aspect of the maxilla to join the maxillary division of the trigeminal nerve. *Trigeminal n.* Fifth and largest of the 12 cranial nerves. It divides into three main branches or divisions; the OPHTHALMIC, the MAXILLARY, which receives nerve impulses from all of the upper teeth, and the MANDIBULAR BRANCH, which receives nerve impulses from all of the lower teeth and anterior two-thirds of the tongue, also sending efferent impulses to the salivary glands and the muscles of mastication. *Vasoconstrictor n.* Efferent nerve that causes blood vessels to constrict. *Vasodilator n.* Efferent nerve that causes blood vessels to dilate. *Vasomotor n.* Efferent nerve that can cause dilatation or constriction of blood vessels.

nerve block *See* analgesia.

nerve cell *See* neurone.

nerve fibre *See* axon.

nerve trunk Cord-like arrangement of nerve fibres from which many branches take origin.

nervous 1. Excitable, agitated. 2. Relating to nerves. *N. tissue. See* tissue. *See also* parasympathetic n. system and sympathetic n. system.

network Structure composed of interconnected filaments. Also called a *reticulum*.

neur- (neuro-) Prefix denoting nerves or nervous system.

neural Relating to nerves or a nerve.

neuralgia Severe pain arising from an afferent nerve pathway. *Trigeminal n. (tic douloureux).* Condition of unknown origin giving rise to severe facial pain along the distribution of the fifth cranial (trigeminal) nerve.

neuralgic Relating to neuralgia.

neurapraxia Traumatic injury to a nerve resulting in a temporary loss of sensation or paralysis.

neurectomy Excision of a nerve.

neurilemmoma (schwannoma) Tumour arising from connective tissue covering the sheath of a nerve.

neuritic Relating to neuritis.

neuritis Inflammation of a nerve.

neurofibrils Delicate fibres running through the cytoplasm of nerve cells and extending into the axons and dendrites.

neurofibroma Tumour of peripheral nerves arising from connective tissue elements.

neurone A complete nerve cell—the basic functional unit of the nervous system. Contains the nucleus, surrounding cytoplasm, the dendrites (q.v.) and the axons (q.v.).

neutral Neither acid nor alkaline. *N. zone.* Area within the mouth in which the opposing forces of the cheeks, lips and tongue are said to be in equilibrium.

neutrophil A phagocytic polymorphonuclear leucocyte.

nevi Plural of nevus.

nevus *See* naevus.

niacin Nicotinic acid. Water-soluble vitamin found in meat, bread, flour, vegetables, fruit and milk. Lack of niacin in the diet leads to a deficiency disease called pellagra.

nickel-titanium Synonym NiTi. Highly flexible alloy of nickel and titanium with shape memory and resistance to cyclic fatigue fracture. Applications include flexible orthodontic archwires and endodontic instruments.

nigrities *See* tongue, black hairy.

nitrogen Colourless, tasteless, odourless gas that forms about four-fifths of the atmospheric air.

nitrous oxide Inhalation anaesthetic agent in the form of a gas that is rapidly absorbed into the bloodstream. Supplied in light blue cylinder and used in combination with oxygen. Smaller bottles are sized A–E, the larger ones F–H. Size D = 900 litres, size F = 1360 litres and size G = 3400 litres.

node Small mass of tissue in the form of a swelling.

nodule Small elevated area of the skin.

noma *See* cancrum oris.

non-accidental injury (NAI) Injury resulting from child (or elderly person) physical abuse. Physical abuse is one of four forms of abuse generally recognized in vulnerable groups. The other three are emotional abuse, sexual abuse and neglect.

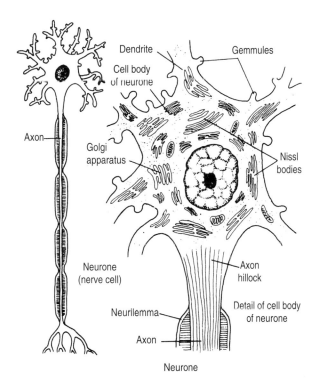

Axon

Dendrite

Cell body of neurone

Gemmules

Golgi apparatus

Nissl bodies

Neurone (nerve cell)

Axon hillock

Neurilemma

Axon

Detail of cell body of neurone

Neurone

non-anatomic teeth *See* tooth, non-anatomic, cuspless.

non-gamma 2 amalgam alloy *See* alloy, high copper amalgam.

non-nucleated Without a nucleus.

non-screen film Direct action film in which the emulsion is more sensitive to radiation than to light.

non-union Complication of bone fractures in which the bone fails to heal.

non-vital pulp therapy Strictly, any endodontic treatment that leads to successful retention of a tooth with a non-vital pulp. Generally restricted to the treatment of primary teeth with non-vital pulps in which disease is managed by chemical agents rather than shaping, cleaning and filling of the pulp space.

non-working side contacts (balancing contacts) Contacts between the mandibular and maxillary teeth or of the denture bases on the non-working side, or posteriorly in a protrusive position.

norm A fixed standard.

normal saline *See* saline.

normal solution *See* isotonic.

normality Condition of being normal.

normo- Prefix denoting normality.

notation System of signs, notes, figures and symbols that convey information in abbreviated form to others who understand them. In dentistry, a charting system using a dental formula and recognized abbreviations, signs and symbols. *See* Appendix 3.

NP New patient.

NSAID Non-steroid anti-inflammatory drug.

nuclear Relating to a nucleus.

nucleated Possessing a nucleus.

nuclei Plural of nucleus.

nucleus 1. The central part around which others gather. 2. Controlling part of a cell. A densely packed rounded structure embedded in cytoplasm. It contains large quantities of DNA (q.v.) thought to be the control centre of the cell and its reproduction.

NUG Necrotizing ulcerative gingivitis. *See* gingivitis.

Nurofen® *See* ibuprofen.

nursing bottle caries *See* rampant caries and early childhood caries.

nutrient Nourishing food.

nutrition Process by which food is broken down and assimilated into the body to provide it with nourishment for growth, metabolism and repair.

NYD Not yet diagnosed.

Nystan® *See* nystatin.

nystatin (Nystan®**)** An antifungal agent used to treat oral fungal infections.

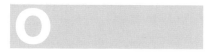

object-to-film distance (OFD) Distance from the object being radiographed to the film.

oblique Inclined, slanting. *O. lateral projection.* Extra-oral radiographic projection that demonstrates the mandibular and maxillary teeth with minimal superimposition of the contralateral side. *O. line.* Thickened line where the horizontal body of the mandible and the alveolar process merge into the ascending ramus. *O. occlusal projection.* Occlusal radiographic projection in which the central ray is directed obliquely to the teeth. *O. ridge.* Ridge of enamel, joining the antero-internal or mesiolingual cusp on the occlusal surfaces of all upper molar teeth to the posterobuccal cusp.

obliteration Complete removal.

obtund To dull or blunt pain or touch sensations.

obtundent Pain-relieving agent, e.g. oil of cloves.

obturate To obliterate or close an opening. In endodontics: to fill a root canal.

obturator Device for closing any abnormal opening or cleft such as a cleft palate or a fistula between the oral and nasal cavity.

occipital bone Unpaired bone of the skull situated at the posterior aspect of the cranium. Bounded by the parietal and the temporal bones. At the base of the skull, the large foramen magnum conveys the spinal cord to the brain.

occipito- Prefix referring to the occiput (q.v.).

occipitofrontal Relating to the occipital and frontal bones. *O. projection.* Radiographic technique for demonstrating the skull and jaws in the coronal plane.

occipitomental projection (standard) Radiographic technique for demonstrating the facial bones and the maxillary sinuses. The orbitomeatal line is tilted at 45° to the plane of the film and the central ray is projected through the occipital bone perpendicular to the film.

occiput Back of the skull or the head.

occlude To close or shut, as when the occlusal surfaces of the mandibular teeth are closed on the maxillary teeth.

occluded gas Gas dissolved in molten metal and which, when released on cooling and solidification of the metal, causes porosity.

occluding surfaces Those surfaces of the natural or artificial teeth that make contact with those of the opposing jaw.

occlusal Refers to the surfaces of teeth or their replacements that make contact with those of the opposing jaw. *O. adjustment*, *correction* or *equilibration*. Adjustment, usually by grinding, that is made to improve occlusal contact. *O. analysis*. Study made of the occlusal contacts of opposing teeth. *O. clearance*. *See* interocclusal clearance. *O. face height*. *See* o. vertical dimension. *O. film*. Radiographic film, 57 × 76 mm in size, that can be used intra- or extra-orally, preferably in a cassette with intensifying screens. It is wrapped similarly to an intra-oral film and may also be placed along the occlusal plane to give a view, taken from below, of the mandible. *O. indicator wax*. Wax used to register the occlusal relationship between mandibular and maxillary teeth. *O. overlay appliance*. Appliance having a component covering the occlusal or incisal surfaces of the teeth or both. *O. path*. Path of movement of one occluding surface, relative to another. *O. plane (plane of occlusion)*. Imaginary line touching the incisal surfaces of the upper incisors and the tips of the cusps of the posterior teeth. 'Plane' is a misnomer as the 'line' is usually curved. *O. plane guide*. Device used to determine the occlusal plane during denture construction. *O. prematurity*. A contact between opposing teeth occurring before the planned intercuspation. *O. radiograph* or *projection*. Radiograph

obtained by placing the film along the occlusal plane. *O. registration*. Recording of jaw relationships, usually by means of heat-softened wax occlusal rims attached to temporary or permanent denture bases. *O. rehabilitation*. Modification of the occlusal relationships by grinding the crowns of teeth and fitting inlays, crowns and bridges. The aim is to improve the functional harmony of the dentition and the associated musculature. *O. reshaping*. *See* selective grinding. *O. rest*. Rest, usually of metal, that is placed on the occlusal surfaces of certain teeth to maintain the occlusal level of a prosthesis. *O. rim*. Occluding surface formed of a mouldable material such as wax, which is attached to a temporary or permanent denture base. Intended to record jaw relationships and indicate tooth positions. Previously called a *bite block* or *bite rim*. *O. splint*. *See* o. overlay appliance. *O. surfaces*. Those surfaces of molars which, in normal occlusion, meet the corresponding surfaces of the opposing teeth. *O. table*. Total amount of surface provided for occlusion by natural or artificial teeth. *O. trauma*. Trauma to the teeth or their supporting structures caused by the opposing teeth. *O. vertical dimension*. Any vertical dimension when the teeth or occlusal rims are in contact. The Willis gauge (q.v.) may be used to record this measurement but is subject to inaccuracies as it has to be placed on soft tissues.

occlusally approaching clasp Clasp originating on the occlusal side of the survey line.

occlusion 1. Process of closing or being closed. 2. Any contact between teeth of opposing arches and usually referring to their occlusal surfaces. 3. Static relationship between maxillary and mandibular teeth during maximal intercuspation. *Balanced o.* A state in which the teeth of complete dentures, or the natural teeth, meet overall without any one tooth causing interference with the occlusion or balance of the prosthesis or dentition. *b.* Simultaneous contact of the occluding surfaces of the teeth on both sides of the mouth in various positions of closure. *Centric o. (intercuspal o.).* Position of centric jaw relationship in which there is maximum intercuspation of the teeth. *Eccentric o.* Any lateral, protrusive or retrusive occlusion other than centric. *Edge-to-edge o.* Occlusion in which the anterior teeth of the jaws meet along their incisal edge when the teeth are in centric occlusion. *Ideal o.* Occlusion in which every tooth, with the exception of the lower central incisor and the upper third molar, occludes with two teeth in the opposing arch and is based on the shape of the unworn teeth. *Mutually protected o.* An occlusal arrangement in which the posterior teeth prevent excessive contact of the anterior teeth in maximum intercuspation (q.v.) and the anterior teeth disengage the posterior teeth in all mandibular movements. *Normal o.* Occlusion that satisfies the requirements of function and aesthetics but in which there may be minor irregularities of individual teeth. Present when the upper and lower teeth are well aligned and the cusps of the posterior teeth slot in between the opposing lower teeth. The upper and lower incisors just touch each other with a minimum of overlap, on closure. *O. rim. See* occlusal rim. *O. wear.* Loss of tooth substance on opposing occlusal surfaces as a result of abrasion (q.v.) or attrition (q.v.). *Traumatic o.* Any occlusion of the teeth that is injurious to the oral or related structures, teeth or periodontium.

oculomotor Refers to those muscles that control eye movement. *O. nerve.* Third cranial nerve that controls the movement of the oculomotor muscles.

odds ratio Measure of how likely it is that a disease, condition or effect will occur, for example in a test group receiving an intervention or particular treatment compared with a control group. An odds ratio of 1 means that an intervention has had no effect. An odds ratio of more (less) than 1 means that the effect of the intervention or treatment is greater (less) than the control group

odontalgia Toothache.

odontoblast Specialized cell lying on the periphery of the dental pulp and which is primarily responsible for dentine formation.

odontoblast process Protoplasmic process of the odontoblast present in the dentinal tubules and responsible for the formation of dentine.

odontoclast Cell believed to be involved with the process of root resorption.

odontogenic Relating to the origin and development of the teeth. *O. keratocyst.* Developmental cyst arising from odontogenic epithelium.

odontogeny Origin and formative development of the teeth.

odontome Abnormal mass of calcified dental tissue, e.g. neoplasms and malformation arising from dental tissues, such as adamantinoma.

odontoplasty A procedure to reshape the contour of the crown or root (or both) of a tooth or the anatomy of the fissure of a tooth in order to provide a contour that allows improved plaque control and oral hygiene. The term may also be used when modifying sharp edges on teeth which may cause soft tissue and tongue lesions.

oedema Effusion of excess fluid into the soft tissue spaces thus causing a swelling. May be due to obstruction of a vein, certain heart diseases, inflammation and allergic reactions.

oesophagus Tube of about 25 cm in length that passes behind the trachea, heart and lungs and conveys food and drink from the pharynx to the stomach.

OFD *See* object-to-film distance.

OHI Oral hygiene index. *See* index.

oil Liquid not miscible in water and generally combustible. Oils are classified as animal or vegetable, volatile and mineral. *O. of cloves* or *clove o.* An oil consisting of 85–90% eugenol distilled from cloves. It is obtundent, antiseptic and deodorant. *O. of eucalyptus.* Oil from the Australian gum or eucalyptus tree.

olfactory Relating to the sense of smell.

olfactory nerve The first cranial nerve concerned with the sense of smell.

oligodontia Developmental absence of 6 or more teeth. *See* hypodontia.

-ology Suffix meaning the study of, e.g. bacteriology.

-oma Suffix denoting tumour, e.g. carcinoma.

oncology The study of tumours.

onlay (overlay) Metal, ceramic or composite restorations designed to cover the occlusal and/or incisal surfaces of teeth. *O. graft. See* graft.

opacifier Substance used to reduce the translucency or transparency of a material and make it more opaque. Metal oxides are used to opacify dental porcelains.

opacity State of being opaque. The opposite of transparency. *Dental o.* Tooth surface defect due to increased sub-surface porosity of enamel or dentine.

opalescent Having a milky appearance like an opal.

opaque Not allowing the passage of light.

open bite (open occlusal relationship, apertognathia) Failure of some opposing teeth to occlude when other teeth are in maximum intercuspation. May be due to a congenital, developmental or acquired deformity; to dislocation of the temporomandibular articulation; to fracture and/or malunion of a fracture.

operative dentistry Branch of dentistry defined as 'that branch of dentistry which relates to diagnosis, prognosis or treatment of teeth with vital or non-vital pulps; to the maintenance or restoration of the functional and physiological integrity of the teeth as this applies to the adjacent hard and soft tissue structure of the oral cavity'. (Definition taken from *Glossary of Operative Dentistry Terms*, 1st Edition, issued by the Academy of Operative Dentistry.)

operculectomy Surgical removal of an operculum.

operculum 1. Any structure resembling a lid or cover. 2. Hood or flap of gingival tissue overlying the crown of a partially erupted tooth.

OPG® (Orthopantomograph) The registered trade mark of Siemens Co. The abbreviation has become accepted usage for a panoramic radiograph. *See also* panoramic tomography.

ophthalmic Relating to the eye.

opiate Sedative preparation containing opium or one of its derivatives.

opioid Means opiate-like and refers to drugs that have the pharmacological properties of opiates.

opportunistic pathogen A micro-organism which is normally harmless but which may cause disease under certain conditions or if it gains access to sites in the body usually denied, e.g. *Staphylococcus epidermidis* which normally resides on the skin may cause infective endocarditis if it gains access to the bloodstream.

opsonic Relating to opsonin.

opsonin Antibody that causes bacteria to become vulnerable to phagocytosis (q.v.).

optic Relating to vision.

optic nerve The second cranial nerve, concerned with sight.

optimum The most favourable.

or- (oro-) Prefix meaning of the mouth.

oral Relating to the mouth. *O. flora.* Micro-organisms normally residing in the mouth. *O. fluid. See* whole saliva. *O. hygiene index (OHI). See* index. *O. hygiene.* Maintenance of oral cleanliness by removing bacterial plaque with brushes, dental floss and other special instruments. *O. mucosa.* Layer of epithelium and subjacent connective tissue lining the oral cavity. *O. rehabilitation.* Restoration of the form and function of the masticatory arrangements to as nearly normal as possible. *O. screen.* Myofunctional appliance used to exert pressure in the upper labial segment by displacing the lips from their resting position. *O. seal.* Seal of the oral cavity effected by the soft tissues without any conscious effort. May be at the anterior end (ANTERIOR SEAL) or the posterior end (POSTERIOR SEAL) or both. *See also* seal. *O. stereognosis.* Ability to recognize the shape of an object placed in the mouth purely by intra-oral tactile information. *O. surgery.* That part of dental surgery which includes the diagnosis and surgical treatment of the diseases, injuries and defects of the jaws and associated structures.

Oraqix® A topical anaesthetic for use in periodontal pockets. It is a 5% mixture of lidocaine and prilocaine. It is used to reduce the discomfort of periodontal scaling.

orbicular Circular or rounded.

orbicularis oris Muscle of facial expression that encircles the mouth and joins with the buccinator muscle. It is the sphincter muscle of the mouth.

orbit The eye socket. Formed by the frontal, ethmoid, lacrimal, maxillary, sphenoid and zygomatic bones.

orbital Relating to the orbit. *O. blow-out fracture.* Fracture of the orbital floor, possibly with the displacement of orbital tissue into the maxillary sinus.

orbitale Lowest point on the infra-orbital region. *See* Frankfort plane and Appendix 10.

orbito-meatal line Imaginary line between the external auditory meatus and the outer canthus of the eye.

organ A part of the body designed to perform a particular function or functions.

organic 1. Pertaining to the organs and their structure. 2. In chemistry, relating to compounds of carbon. 3. Arising from an animal or vegetable organism. 4. Opposite of synthetic, e.g. organic chemicals.

organic matrix 1. Organized structure such as the intercellular substance of a tissue which constitutes the basic background of a tissue. 2. *See* enamel matrix.

organism An organized body showing the characteristics of life.

ORIF Open reduction internal fixation. *See* fixation.

orifice An opening or entrance. *O. enlarger (O opener)*. Endodontic instrument used to enlarge the openings of root canals to improve access.

origin The starting point; the source. In anatomy, a more fixed end or attachment of a muscle as distinct from its insertion.

oro-antral fistula Abnormal epithelialized connection between the oral cavity and the maxillary sinus.

orofacial granulomatosis (OFG) A chronic granulomatous inflammatory condition of the lips and oral mucosa which may be of hypersensitivity origin. *See* Melkersson–Rosenthal syndrome.

ortho- Prefix meaning straight or normal.

orthodontic Refers to the correction of irregularities in teeth. *O. appliance. See* appliance. *O. band*. Retaining device for fixed orthodontic appliances. Made of stainless steel strip, adapted to fit individual teeth. *O. band tape*. Stainless steel or precious metal tape, obtainable in various sizes and grades, used in the construction of fixed orthodontic appliances. *O. elastic band*. Rubber or latex elastic band used to apply forces to the teeth through appliances attached to the teeth. *O. face-bow*. That part of an extra-oral traction appliance placed between the headgear or cervical strap and the intra-oral orthodontic appliance. *O. ligature*. Soft stainless steel wire used to connect the arch or bow of a fixed orthodontic appliance to brackets either fixed onto bands or cemented to the teeth. *O. scissors. See* scissors, crown. *O. screw*. Device with a screw thread which is inserted into an orthodontic appliance. When turned it may bring together or separate portions of the appliance. *O. tape. See* o. band tape. *O. welder*. Specialized electric spot welder used with orthodontic materials. *O. wire*. Corrosion-resistant wire used in the construction of orthodontic appliances. May be round, square or oval in cross-section, usually constructed from stainless steel or a nickel-titanium alloy.

orthodontics That branch of dental science concerned with the study of the growth, development and infinite variations of the face, jaws and teeth, including dentofacial abnormalities and their corrective treatment.

orthodontic separator A wire, spring or rubber band used to separate teeth prior to orthodontic band placement.

orthodontic therapist Member of the dental team who is able to undertake orthodontic procedures under the prescription of a dentist or orthodontist.

ortho-ethoxybenzoic acid cement *See* EBA cement.

orthognathic Pertaining to the malposition of the bones of the jaw. *O. surgery*. Surgical correction of craniofacial disharmonies by repositioning either segments of the mandible or maxilla or the entire jaws, in order to achieve a more acceptable function.

orthograde root filling Root filling normally carried out in a root canal through the coronal access cavity. *See also* retrograde (root-end) filling.

orthopaedics Branch of surgery dealing with deformities of the skeletal system. The correction of deformities of children and the treatment of diseases of muscles, bones, joints and traumatic injuries.

orthopantomograph (OPG®) *See* panoramic tomography.

orthophosphoric acid *See* phosphoric acid.

Orthodontic appliances

Removable

Functional (Twin block)

Fixed

osmosis Passage of liquids or fluids through a semi-permeable membrane.

osmotic Relating to osmosis.

osseo-integration is defined as the direct bone-to-implant fixture interface which will provide a foundation to support a prosthesis.

osseous Bony.

ossicle A small bone.

ossification Formation of bone or a bony substance. The conversion of a tissue into a bony tissue.

ostectomy Division of a bone at two lines and removal of the intervening segment.

osteitis Inflammation of the bone.

osteo- Prefix meaning bone.

osteo-arthritis Chronic inflammation of the joints of the elderly, especially males.

osteoblast Bone-forming cell.

osteoblastoma Benign vascular giant cell tumour producing osteoid tissue and immature bone.

osteoclast Bone-destroying cell with a large multi-nucleus.

osteocyte Osteoblast cell embedded within the bone matrix.

osteo-ectomy (archaic) Removal of some of the supporting alveolar bone from around the root of a tooth in order to correct an imperfect bone contour around the root.

osteogenesis Bone formation which may take place within a membrane, e.g. the skull bones. *O. imperfecta.* Bone disease, usually present at birth, characterized by extreme fragility and porosity of the bones with an increased risk of fracture.

osteology The study of bone and bones.

osteoma Benign tumour of bone.

osteomalacia Generalized condition in which bone softening occurs due to lack of vitamin D, giving rise to poor calcification.

osteomyelitis Osteitis affecting bone and its marrow, resulting in its destruction.

osteopath Person who practises bone manipulation and treats bone conditions. Often not medically qualified.

osteopetrosis (Albers–Schönberg disease) Hereditary progressive bone disease in which there is continuous formation of bone without concurrent normal resorption of bone, resulting in a diffuse sclerosis. Also known as *marble bone disease.*

osteoplasty (archaic) Surgical reshaping of the alveolar process to achieve as closely as possible the ideal architectural design of a healthy periodontium.

osteoporosis Hereditary condition in which the deficient formation of bone gives rise to brittle bones. Radiographically the appearance of such bone is less dense than normal bone.

osteoradionecrosis Necrosis of bone, following radiation therapy, due to a reduction in blood supply and infection.

osteosynthesis *See* fixation, internal skeletal.

osteotome Bone-splitting instrument with a sharp, shaped blade. Used with a mallet to cleave bone or split teeth.

osteotomy Sectioning of a bone without appreciable loss of substance. *Maxillary* or *mandibular o.* The surgical exposure and fracturing of the maxilla or of the mandible at a predetermined plane in order to correct its position or its form.

otalgia Pain in the ear caused by a dental stimulus. Earache.

OTC Over the counter, i.e. medicaments available for purchase which do not require a prescription.

outline (outline form, cavo-surface margin or line angle) Boundary of a restoration or preparation at its junction with the tooth surface.

outpatient Person who receives treatment on a single occasion or at a series of attendances but is not admitted to a bed in a hospital ward.

OVD Occlusal vertical dimension.

overbite Overlap of the upper incisors over the lower incisors in the vertical plane.

overclosure Reduced distance between the upper and lower teeth or occlusal rims.

over-denture *See* denture.

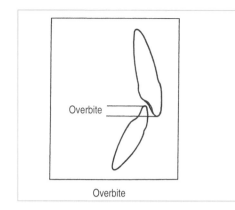

Overbite

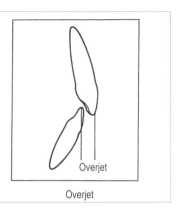

Overjet

over-eruption Vertical migration of a tooth beyond its proper position in normal dental arches. Generally caused by absence of an opposing occlusal force because of the loss of a contacting tooth from the opposite arch. *See also* intrusion.

overgrowth Overall increase in the size of a tissue by an increase in either the size of its cells or in their number.

overhang Excess restorative material projecting beyond the preparation or cavity margin thus causing a shoulder beneath which plaque may accumulate or food may lodge.

overjet (horizontal overlap) The projection, in a horizontal plane, of teeth, usually the incisors, in one arch beyond the teeth of the opposing arch.

overlapping 1. Imbricated, like tiles on a roof. 2. In radiography, a distortion of a radiological tooth image in which the structures of one tooth are superimposed on those of another.

overlay *See* onlay.

oxidation Combination of a substance with oxygen.

oxidized cellulose Prepared, haemostatic cellulose used to pack a tooth socket in the event of severe or persistent haemorrhage, e.g. Surgicel®.

oximeter An instrument for determining, photoelectrically, the oxygen content of blood.

Oxycel® *See* oxidized cellulose.

oxygen Colourless, odourless gas constituting one-fifth of the earth's atmosphere. Stored under pressure in various sized cylinders painted black with white tops.

oxyhaemoglobin Oxygenated haemoglobin as found in arterial blood.

oxyphosphate cement *See* zinc phosphate cement.

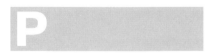

P

pacemaker Battery-driven electrical device that controls or paces the contraction of heart muscle by pulsed electrical stimulation, regulating the heart rhythm. Such regulation may be upset by the use of high-frequency or ultrasonic equipment on a patient fitted with a pacemaker.

pachy- Prefix denoting thickening or thickened.

pachyglossia Abnormal thickness of the tongue.

pack 1. To fill or press into a cavity. 2. Dressing inserted into a wound to reduce or arrest haemorrhage. *Periodontal p.* Dressing designed to protect a wound created by periodontal surgery, to encourage healing. *Pressure p.* Sterile folded gauze pressed into a wound to arrest haemorrhage. *See also* cyst pack; throat pack.

packing 1. Filling a plaster mould in a metal flask with a plastic material which is then processed to make a prosthesis.

paed- (paedo-) Prefix denoting child.

paediatrics Branch of medicine dealing with children's diseases.

paedodontics, paediatric dentistry or children's dentistry Branch of dental science concerned with the oral health of children.

Paget's disease Chronic disease of bones occurring in the elderly and affecting the skull and facial bones, which become enlarged and their structure becomes disorganized.

pain Unpleasant sensation caused by injury or disease, ranging from mild discomfort to excruciating agony. *Referred p.* Pain arising from a particular organ yet felt in an adjacent area.

paint In pharmacology, a liquid preparation that is applied to the skin or mucous membranes, and contains antiseptic, analgesic or other drugs.

palatal Pertaining to the palate or palatine bone. *P. arch.* In orthodontics, a heavy-gauge wire between bands on posterior teeth and used to reinforce orthodontic anchorage. *P. bar.* A major connector of a maxillary partial denture that crosses the palate and unites the bilateral parts of the prosthesis. *P. retractor. See* finger spring. *P. spring. See* finger spring. *P. surface.* That surface of all upper teeth which faces the tongue.

palate Roof of the mouth, separating the mouth from the nasal cavity and consisting of the hard and soft palate at its posterior border. *Cleft p. See* cleft. *Hard p.* Formed by the processes of the maxillae and palatine bones, fused in the midline during development, and covered by mucous membrane, the mucosa being exceptionally tough and having rugae on its external surface. *Soft p.* Movable fold of mucous membrane that tapers towards the back of the mouth to form the uvula (q.v.).

palatine Relating to the palate. *P. bone.* One of a pair of L-shaped bones that contribute to the hard palate, the nasal cavity and the orbit.

palato- Prefix denoting palate.

palatoplasty Surgical correction of a palatal defect such as a cleft palate.

pali- (palin-) Prefix denoting recurrence or repetition.

palladium Rare metal in the platinum group which is white, ductile and malleable. Its chief dental use is as a constituent of casting gold alloys.

palliative Medicine or treatment that alleviates but does not cure disease.

pallor Paleness; lack of skin colour due to reduced blood flow or lack of skin pigments.

palpable Able to be felt by touch.

palpate To feel. A swelling or fracture may be palpated as an aid to diagnosis.

palpation Part of the diagnostic procedure entailing the examination of a part of the body by careful feeling with the hands and fingertips.

palpitation Awareness of an abnormally rapid or irregular heart beat.

palsy Archaic word for paralysis, inability to move, lack of muscle function. *Bell's p.* Unilateral paralysis of the facial muscles supplied by the seventh cranial nerve (facial). Condition of unknown origin and sudden onset. The patient is unable to whistle and tends to dribble. Recovery is often spontaneous.

pan- (panto-) Prefix denoting all or generalized.

panacea Medicine or treatment said to be a cure for all diseases and conditions.

pancreas Gland lying behind the stomach. It secretes (1) enzymes and digestive juices that enter the small intestine to mix with the partially digested food from the stomach and (2) the hormone insulin (q.v.).

pancreatic juice Digestive enzymes produced by the pancreas and ducted into the duodenum.

pandemic Widespread epidemic disease.

panoramic Complete view. *P. film.* In radiography, a type of extra-oral radiographic film used to provide a radiograph of the dental structures. *P. radiography.* A radiographic technique where the X-ray source is placed inside the mouth in order to obtain a radiographic image of the mandibular and/or the maxillary dental arches. *P. (rotational) tomography.* A technique of obtaining a radiograph which incorporates an image of the mandibular and maxillary dental arches. It is obtained by moving the X-ray source simultaneously and in the opposite direction to the film whilst the patient remains stationary. A panoramic radiograph is sometimes referred to as an 'orthopantomograph' (OPG®) or a 'panorex', after the trade name of the machine used to obtain the radiograph.

pantogram A pantographic tracing (q.v.).

pantograph Complex of tracing devices attached to the mandible and the maxilla in order to obtain a record of mandibular movements in three planes.

pantographic tracing A three-dimensional graphic record of mandibular movements as registered by the styli on the recording tables of a pantograph (q.v.).

paper points Absorbent, tapered cones of paper for drying root canals in endodontic treatment.

papilla Small elevation of tissue. *Gingival p.* That part of the gingiva which occupies the interproximal space.

papillary Relating to a papilla. *P. hyperplasia of the palate.* Chronic inflammatory hyperplasia of the palate seen as closely grouped papillary projections. *P. bleeding index (PBI). See* index.

papillectomy Surgical removal of an interdental papilla.

papilloma Benign neoplasm or local overgrowth of the skin, e.g. a wart.

papillomatosis *See* papillary hyperplasia of the palate.

Papillon–Lefèvre syndrome Syndrome characterized by alveolar bone destruction in both the primary and the permanent dentitions, by inflammatory gingival enlargement and by deep pocket formation and various skin lesions.

papular Relating to a papule.

papule Raised spot or pimple forming part of a skin rash.

PAR Peer assessment review. An orthodontic index for measuring the occlusion before and after treatment in order to ascertain the improvement resulting from treatment.

para- Prefix meaning beside, beyond, against or near.

paracetamol Analgesic tablet used as an alternative to aspirin for patients who are sensitive to aspirin or who suffer from gastric ulceration. Normal dosage is one or two 0.5 mg tablets taken 4-hourly as necessary.

paradental cyst Deprecated term for lateral periodontal cyst (q.v.).

paradontal Sited near or close to a tooth.

paraesthesia Abnormal sensation of numbness, tingling or burning. Sometimes described as a 'pins and needles' sensation.

paraffin wax *See* wax.

parafunctional A movement that is distorted or beyond normal function, e.g. bruxism (q.v.) or jaw clenching.

parallax Apparent alteration in the relative positions of two objects when viewed from different positions. The technique is used in radiography to assess the buccolingual relationship of roots and unerupted teeth.

paralleling technique Periapical radiographic technique in which a film holder is used to align the film parallel to the long axis of the tooth and also to allow the central ray to pass perpendicular to the plane of the film. *See* Appendix 10.

parallelometer Instrument designed to ensure that preparation surfaces or prosthetic structures are parallel to one another.

paralysis Loss of sensation and power of movement of any part of the body. *P. agitans. See* Parkinson's disease.

paralytic Person afflicted with paralysis.

paranasal sinus Air-filled space, lined with mucous membrane, within some bones of the skull.

paraplegia Paralysis of the lower limbs and trunk. All parts below the point of lesion in the spinal cord are affected. May have a sudden onset because of injury to the spinal cord or develop slowly as a result of disease.

paraplegic Relating to paraplegia.

parasite An organism which gains benefit by living in or on a second organism which is harmed in the process.

parasympathetic nervous system Part of the autonomic nervous system (q.v.) that controls the life sustaining organs of the body under normal conditions.

parathyroid Gland located beside the thyroid gland. *See* gland.

parenteral Descriptive of drug administration other than by the digestive tract, e.g. subcutaneous or intravenous injections.

paresis Weakness or incomplete paralysis.

parietal bone One of the two quadrilateral bones forming the sides and roof of the skull.

Parkinson's disease (paralysis agitans) Disease due to a brain lesion and causing a tremor of limbs and a shuffling gait. The muscles of the face and body become rigid.

paronychia A whitlow; an inflammation and swelling in the tissues around a finger or toenail.

parotid gland *See* gland.

parotitis *See* sialoadenitis.

paroxysm A sudden spasm or seizure.

partial anodontia Deprecated term for hypodontia (q.v.) or oligodontia.

partial denture Denture provided for a dental arch in which one or more teeth remain. *See also* denture.

partial thickness flap Surgical flap consisting of epithelium and connective tissue but not the periosteum, which is left undisturbed on the bone.

partial veneer crown *See* crown.

passive Not active. In orthodontics or prosthetics, refers to a spring or clasp which exerts no tension. *P. eruption*. Apical migration of the gingiva thus increasing the clinical crown without there being an active eruption of the tooth.

paste In pharmacy, a semi-solid preparation that is applied externally.

patch test A skin test to detect sensitivity to drugs or other substances to which a person may be allergic and to certain infections.

patent Open, exposed or unobstructed.

path- (patho-) Prefix denoting disease.

path of insertion (path of placement) Direction followed by a prosthesis on insertion. The path is from the first contact of a removable prosthesis with the supporting tissues until it is completely seated.

path of insertion and withdrawal Path along which a prefabricated restoration (e.g. crown) may be inserted into, and withdrawn from, a preparation.

pathogen Micro-organism causing disease. There are four main types: bacteria, viruses, fungi and protozoa.

pathogenesis The mechanism of disease development.

pathogenic Harmful. Causing disease. Describes disease-carrying micro-organisms that harm humans, e.g. pathogenic bacteria.

pathological Caused by disease.

pathological fracture Fracture of a bone weakened by disease. May occur in the mandible as the result of an enlarged cyst.

pathology The study of disease.

-pathy Suffix denoting disease.

patient Historically, a person who suffers patiently; in dentistry, a person who suffers from dental disease and requests treatment.

patrix The male portion of a precision attachment that interlocks with the matrix.

pattern A form, generally in wax, that is made to be invested and so produce a mould for the 'lost wax' casting technique (q.v.).

PBI Papillary bleeding index. *See* index.

PCR Plaque control record.

PDI Periodontal bleeding index. *See* index.

pearl *See* enamel, pearl.

pedicle Stem structure that remains attached to the parent body. *P. graft* or *flap. See* graft.

peduncle Connecting stem-like structure.

pedunculated Having a stalk or pedicle.

peer A person of equal rank, ability, experience and qualifications. *P. review*. A retrospective examination, by one or more persons of equal rank, of another person's work or publications.

peg lateral *See* tooth, conical.

pellet Small pill or granule, e.g. cotton wool p.; gold foil p.

pellicle 1. Thin layer of membrane, skin or any other substance. 2. In dentistry, a thin film or membrane of salivary proteins deposited on teeth shortly after cleaning, and which cannot be completely removed by tooth-brushing. It contains no organisms at this stage and covers most of the crown of the tooth. When it has been invaded by micro-organisms it is then called plaque (q.v.).

pemphigus Generic term for any of a number of skin diseases marked by successive outbreaks of bullae (q.v.).

Penbritin® *See* ampicillin.

penetration Piercing deeply to make a hole.

-penia Suffix denoting lack or deficiency.

penicillin Antibiotic produced by certain moulds (*Penicillium*) cultured on media and also produced synthetically. Discovered by Fleming in 1929 and developed by Florey and Chain in 1941. Administered by injection (intramuscularly or intravenously), orally (in liquid or tablet form) or topically (in pastes and ointments). Certain people present allergic reactions to it which may be mild or serious, e.g. anaphylactic shock, which can be fatal.

penumbra Partial or imperfect shadow about an image of an object. In radiography, it is influenced by the size of the focal spot (q.v.) and may be modified by alteration in the focus-to-subject and object-to-film distance.

pepsin Enzyme found in gastric juices. It partially digests proteins in an acid solution.

per- Prefix meaning throughout or through.

per-alveolar wiring (archaic) Method of immobilizing a fractured maxilla by the use of stainless steel wire which traverses the alveolar process. The projecting ends are then passed over a splint and tightened. The technique is useful in the treatment of fractured edentulous jaws.

percolation Deprecated term for micro-leakage (q.v.).

percussion Method of diagnosis by tapping a tooth, teeth or an implant to elicit the degree of sensitivity of supporting tissues (periodontal or bone) or any change from normal in the sound produced.

percutaneous Having the ability to pass through unbroken skin.

perforation Hole in an object. In endodontics, procedural error in which a hole is created in a tooth or root during root canal treatment. *Lateral p.* Puncture hole created in the side of a root. *Furcal p.* Hole created in the floor of a pulp chamber. *Strip p.* Long, narrow hole created in the wall of a root by over-enlargement of the root canal.

peri- Prefix meaning around.

periapical Refers to the area around the apex of a tooth. *P. abscess. See* abscess, periapical. *P. curettage. See* apical curettage. *P. projection.* In dental radiography, intra-oral technique for demonstrating the anatomy of the tooth and the adjacent supporting bone. *P. radiograph. See* p. projection.

pericarditis Inflammation of the pericardium.

pericardium Smooth membranous sac enveloping the heart.

perichondrium Fibrous membrane covering cartilage, except at joint ends, and consisting of an outer layer of dense connective tissue and an inner layer responsible for new cartilage formation.

pericision Sectioning of fibres of the periodontal ligament as an adjunct to the orthodontic movement of teeth.

pericoronitis Acute inflammation of the soft tissue surrounding the crown of a partially erupted tooth.

peri-implantitis Inflammatory reactions with loss of supporting bone in the tissues surrounding a functioning implant.

perikymata Grooves on the surface of enamel running at right angles to the long axis of the tooth where the enamel striae of Retzius reach the surface.

perimolysis A pattern of tooth surface loss in which the occlusal cusps of posterior teeth are particularly affected.

PerioChip® *See* controlled delivery device.

periodontal 1. Relating to the supporting structures of a tooth. 2. Pertaining to the periodontium. *P. curette. See* periodontal instruments. *P. cyst.* Cyst of inflammatory origin around the root (usually the root apex) of a pulpless tooth.

periodontal disease Inflammatory disease of the supporting tissues of the teeth. One of the most common diseases of modern civilization. In advanced cases, the patient complains of mobile teeth, teeth drifting apart, spontaneous gingival bleeding, recurrent abscess formation, difficulty in eating due to pain and mobility of teeth, sensitive teeth when being cleaned and halitosis. *P.d. index. See* index.

periodontal dressing (or pack) Dressing designed to protect a wound following periodontal operations and to promote healing.

periodontal fibres *See* Sharpey's fibres.

periodontal flap operation Lifting of a gingival flap to gain access for thorough instrumentation of the root surfaces to remove tooth deposits and infected cementum from the tooth surface.

periodontal hoe *See* periodontal instruments.

periodontal index *See* index, periodontal.

periodontal instruments Instruments used to remove plaque, calculus, debris and stains from teeth, and in the treatment of periodontal disease. *Electrosurgery unit.* Diathermy apparatus using high-frequency electric currents. May be BIPOLAR, when the current passes between the tips of two electrodes, or UNIPOLAR, when the patient holds one electrode and the current passes from another electrode to the gingivae. *Gingivectomy knife.* Knife designed for gingivectomy procedures, e.g. Blake's, Fish, Fox. BLAKE'S UNIVERSAL G.K. Hand instrument with thin handle ending in a screw device to hold the tip portion of a scalpel blade at an angle to the handle. A small hexagonal spanner or key operates the screw when changing the blades. The projecting, non-cutting part of the blade is snapped off by pliers. Used in sets of four to cover all angles of approach to the gingivae. FISH G.K. Single-ended hand instrument with a fixed, double-edged sharp blade set at an angle to the handle. *Jacquette hand scaler.* Sickle-shaped end with sharp edges on both sides of its cutting blade. Usually in sets of three and used to remove calculus from a tooth surface. *Periodontal curette.* Universal or area specific. Hand instruments with hollow ground blade like a spoon-shaped excavator. Used to plane root surfaces. *Periodontal file.* An instrument with multiple, straight cutting edges used either for crushing calculus (to make removal with other instruments easier) or for removing overburnished calculus. *Periodontal hoe.* Hand

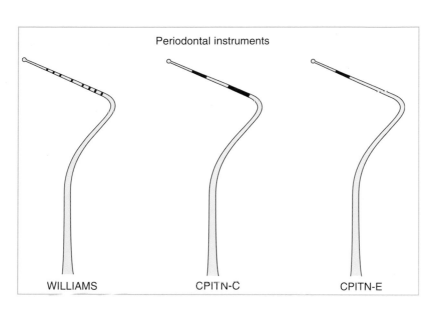

Periodontal instruments

WILLIAMS   CPITN-C   CPITN-E

instrument with small blade at right angles to the shank; usually in sets of four. Used with a pulling motion. *Periodontal probe.* Blunt-ended graduated probe used to measure the depth of a periodontal pocket. *Pocket marking forceps.* Left and right forceps with pin on one blade to perforate the side of a pocket and thus mark its depth. *Pocket measuring probe. See* periodontal probe. *Push, watchspring, Guy's* or *Cushing scaler. See* scaler. *Ultrasonic scaler. See* ultrasonic.

periodontal ligament Connective fibrocellular tissue that attaches the cementum of a tooth root to the alveolus. Contains blood vessels, nerves and fibres that support the tooth in its socket, so allowing slight mobility. The main groups of bundles of collagen fibres forming the ligament are the oblique, apical, cervical, transseptal, inter-radicular and circular. Chronic periodontitis causes destruction of the ligament, loss of bone and hence increased mobility of the tooth. Previously known as the *periodontal membrane.*

periodontal membrane *See* periodontal ligament.

periodontal pack *See* periodontal dressing.

periodontal pocket Pathological deepening of the gingival crevice.

periodontal space Radiolucent zone seen on a radiograph between the cementum and the alveolar bone.

periodontal–endodontic procedures Treatment involving both the periodontal and pulpal tissue, necessary because of a combined lesion.

periodontics Branch of dental science concerned with the study and treatment of diseases and conditions of tissues surrounding and supporting the teeth and gingivae.

periodontitis Inflammation of the periodontal ligament and supporting teeth tissues with ensuing loss of bone and the periodontal ligament. Caused by bacteria. It is the main cause of loss of teeth in adults. *Aggressive p.* (juvenile periodontitis, early-onset periodontitis). A relatively uncommon disease having an onset, classically, around adolescence. May be localized, usually affecting incisors and molars, or more generalized. Progression of the disease is usually rapid. *Necrotizing ulcerative p.* Possible sequela of longstanding NUG but with involvement and necrosis of the alveolar bone as well as the overlying gingiva. Has been associated with specific micro-organisms such as *Porphyromonas gingivalis* and *Prevotella intermedius* and systemic medical conditions such as HIV infection. *Prepubertal p.* A form of periodontitis which affects the primary dentition and is often associated with syndromes such as Papillon–Lefèvre or leucocyte deficiency syndrome.

periodontium Those tissues that invest and support the teeth: alveolar bone, periodontal ligament, gingivae and cementum.

periodontology The study of the healthy and diseased periodontium.

periodontosis Deprecated term for aggressive periodontitis.

Periostat® A subantimicrobial dose of doxycycline that may be given as an adjunct to root surface instrumentation in the treatment of periodontitis. Appears to exert its effect by inhibiting collagenase enzymes that are in part responsible for the destruction of the periodontal tissues.

periosteal Pertaining to or composed of periosteum. *P. elevator.* Hand instrument, usually double ended, used to separate the periosteum from the underlying bone.

periosteum Tough fibrous membrane covering the surface of bone, and forming a strong union with tendon and ligaments. It supplies blood vessels and nerves to the bone and aids its growth.

peripheral 1. Relating to the periphery. 2. The furthermost edge from the centre of an object. *P. nervectomy.* Accidental or surgical cutting of the terminal distribution of a nerve trunk. *P. nervous system. See* nerve. *P. seal.* Deprecated term for *border seal. See* seal.

periphery Boundary of a surface or area.

peristalsis Rhythmic muscular contractions that propel foodstuffs and waste products along the intestines of the alimentary tract.

permanent (secondary) dentition The 32 teeth present in an adult mouth and consisting of four incisors, two canines, four premolars and six molars in each jaw.

permeability Degree to which a fluid can pass through a wall or membrane from one structure to another.

permeable Not impassable. Allowing the passage of fluids, etc.

permeate To penetrate or pass through and spread into every part.

pernicious Indicating a fatal issue. Destructive or injurious. *P. anaemia (Addison's anaemia).* So called because it was inevitably fatal before the introduction of vitamin B12 treatment.

peroral Administered through the mouth.

pertussis Whooping cough.

Peru balsam *See* balsam.

pestle Glass rod with ground surface used in a mortar to provide a homogeneous mixture of solids.

petechiae Skin rash of small purplish haemorrhagic spots.

petit mal *See* epilepsy.

Peutz–Jegher's syndrome (hereditary intestinal polyposis) Rare

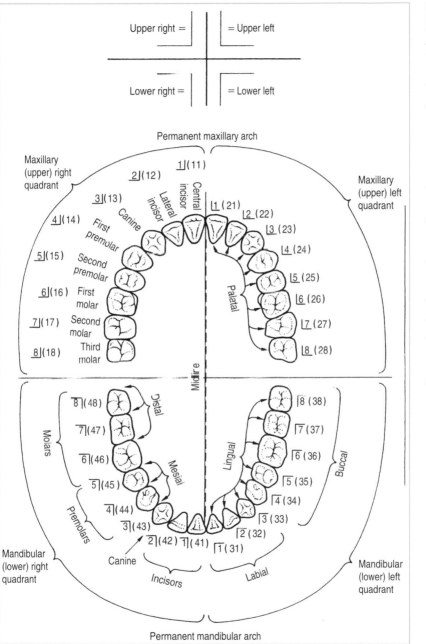

Upper right = | = Upper left

Lower right = | = Lower left

Permanent maxillary arch

Maxillary (upper) right quadrant

Maxillary (upper) left quadrant

1|(11)
2|(12)
3|(13)   Central incisor
4|(14)   Lateral incisor
          Canine
          First premolar
5|(15)   Second premolar
6|(16)   First molar
7|(17)   Second molar
8|(18)   Third molar

|1 (21)
|2 (22)
|3 (23)
|4 (24)
|5 (25)
|6 (26)
|7 (27)
|8 (28)

Palatal

Midline

Molars

8|(48)   Distal
7|(47)
6|(46)
5|(45)   Mesial
4|(44)
3|(43)
2|(42) 1|(41) |1 (31)

Premolars

Canine

Incisors

|8 (38)
|7 (37)
|6 (36)
|5 (35)
|4 (34)
|3 (33)
|2 (32)

Lingual

Buccal

Labial

Mandibular (lower) right quadrant

Mandibular (lower) left quadrant

Permanent mandibular arch

183

inherited disease characterized by melanin pigmentation of the face, oral mucosa, hands and feet and by intestinal polyps seen at operation. Frequent episodes of abdominal pain and marked borborygmi (q.v.) may also occur.

PFM Porcelain fused to metal.

pH Measure of the hydrogen ion concentration and so of the relative acidity or alkalinity of a fluid. Expressed numerically from 1 to 14; 7 is neutral, below 7 is acid and above 7 is alkaline. Enamel destruction takes place at 5.5 and below although enamel treated with fluoride is not destroyed until 5.2.

phag- (phago-) Prefix denoting eating or phagocyte.

-phagia Suffix denoting eating.

phagocyte Any cell that ingests microorganisms, other cells or foreign bodies.

phagocytosis Process whereby white blood cells such as polymorphonuclear leucocytes and the larger lymphocytes such as monocytes and eosinophils ingest foreign matter such as infective dead bacteria and cells, etc., into their cytoplasm. These white cells are found in great numbers in inflammatory exudate. *See also* macrophage.

phantom head A manikin or simulator. Model of the head on which either artificial or extracted teeth are set up in order allow students or clinicians to experience dental operative procedures.

pharmaco- Prefix denoting drugs.

pharmacology Branch of medical science concerned with the action, properties and characteristics of drugs.

pharmacopoeia Authoritative publication on drugs and their use.

pharyngeal Relating to the pharynx.

pharyngitis Inflammation of the pharynx. Commonly known as a *sore throat*.

pharynx That part of the back of the mouth that is lined with mucous membrane, leads to the oesophagus and communicates with the nasal cavity, larynx and ears through the Eustachian tubes. Consists of the nasopharynx, oropharynx and laryngopharynx.

Phenergan® *See* promethazine hydrochloride.

phenol (carbolic acid) Derived from coal tar and formerly used as an antiseptic and disinfectant.

phenytoin sodium Drug with anticonvulsant properties used in cases of epilepsy, e.g. Epanutin®. Long-term use leads to gingival hyperplasia.

phial (vial) Small glass container for storing medicines or poisons.

phleb- (phlebo-) Prefix denoting vein or veins.

phlegm Lay term for sputum (q.v.).

phobia Pathological, intense fear of a particular event, place or thing. Any abnormal fear or aversion.

phoenix abscess *See* abscess.

phonation Flow of air passing through the vocal cords and which produces sound, later modified into speech as it passes through the air passages.

phonetic Relating to speech sounds.

phosphate-bonded investment material High temperature investment material. Silica, magnesium oxide and ammonium phosphate react on mixing with water to form magnesium ammonium phosphate.

phosphorescence Luminescence persisting after a period of irradiation.

phosphoric acid 1. Main constituent of the liquid component of many dental cements. 2. *See* Acid etchant.

phot- (photo-) Prefix denoting light.

photon Quantum of electromagnetic energy.

physi- (physio-) Prefix denoting normality or nature (as opposed to a pathological state).

physiological Relating to physiology. Normal as opposed to pathological.

physiology The study of normal bodily functions.

physiotherapy Treatment by natural forces such as heat, light, electricity and massage.

PI Plaque index. *See* index.

pickling Process in which a hot metal is placed in acid to remove surface oxides and other impurities. *See* acid bath.

PID (position indicating device) *See* beam guiding instrument.

Pierre Robin syndrome Congenital disease characterized by mandibular underdevelopment and backward displacement of the tongue so that swallowing and breathing may be obstructed.

piezograph Form moulded by the cheeks, lips and tongue in edentulous areas of the mouth during the construction of dentures.

pigment Colouring. *See also* fluorescent agent.

pigmentation Colouring produced in the body by the deposition of pigment.

pilocarpine Drug used to increase sweating and salivary secretion and as eyedrops to reduce intra-ocular pressure.

pin 1. Pin-shaped projection from the fitting surface of a cast restoration to increase retention. It fits into a tapered or cylindrical pinhole in the tooth substance which is part of the preparation. 2. Metal pin or wire that is cemented into a prepared pit in the dentine of a tooth preparation or threaded and then screwed into position in the pinhole, or held in place by friction grip. Used to retain a restoration that is placed over a pin or pins while in its plastic state. 3. Long slender metal rod used to immobilize bone fragments in fracture cases. *Incisal guide p. See* guide pin. *Self-threading p.* A threaded pin screwed into a prepared hole in dentine to enhance retention. *P. fixation. See* fixation. *P. teeth. See* tooth.

pin ledge restoration Cast-metal restoration covering the lingual surface of an incisor or canine and retained by pins slotting into small ledges cut in the tooth preparation.

pink spot Term used to describe the pink-hued area on a crown of a tooth that is undergoing internal resorption. The pink hue is due to the hyperplastic vascular tissue visible through the resorbed enamel and dentine.

pink wax Obsolescent term for modelling wax. *See* wax.

pinlay Cast-metal inlay or onlay that has additional retention by virtue of a pin or pins on its fitting surface.

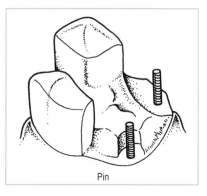

Pin

pit 1. In anatomy, a hollow or depression in an organ. 2. In dentistry, a small depression in the enamel of a tooth.

pit and fissure sealant Material, usually resin, which may or may not contain fillers and colouring matter, used to seal the developmental pits and fissures in enamel surfaces as a preservative measure.

pituitary Relating to the pituitary gland.

pituitary gland *See* gland.

PJC (porcelain jacket crown) *See* crown.

placebo (Latin—I will please) Medicine of no curative value given to placate a patient or as an inactive agent in a controlled clinical trial.

plane 1. A level or flat surface defined by 3 points. 2. An imaginary line dividing the body into flat sections in one direction. *Bite p. See* bite. *P. of cut. See* focal plane. *P. of occlusion. See* occlusal plane. *Sagittal p.* A plane that bilaterally bisects a symmetric body. *See also* Frankfort p.

planes of reference Planes that locate landmarks from which anatomical and cephalometric measurements can be made.

planing *See* root planing. In dentistry, the instrumentation of root surfaces to remove subgingival tooth deposits and necrotic cementum.

plaque In dentistry, a specific but highly variable and tenacious film composed of 70% micro-organisms and 30% matrix. Clinically it occurs supragingivally and subgingivally and may also be found on other solid surfaces such as restorations and oral appliances. The causal factor of dental caries and periodontal disease when in combination with other factors over a period of time. *P. control.*

The removal of plaque by brushing and the use of floss, silk, tape, interdental brushes and other instruments to maintain oral hygiene and cleanliness. *P. index. See* index, plaque, and index, plaque score.

-plasia Suffix denoting development or formation.

plasma Clear, straw-coloured liquid making up 55% of the blood and in which red and white cells and platelets are suspended. Can clot blood by producing fibrin which enmeshes the blood cells. Contains plasma proteins, inorganic salts, gases, nutrients, waste matter from the body, enzymes and hormones.

plaster knife Hand-held knife, usually with a wooden handle, used to trim plaster of Paris models.

plaster of Paris Calcium sulphate hemihydrate ($CaSO_4\frac{1}{2}H_2O$) powder which when mixed with the correct proportion of water sets to a hard white solid. Used extensively in the dental laboratory for moulds and models and occasionally as an impression material (q.v.). *P. of P. headcap.* Headband of gauze and plaster of Paris into which various attachments can be incorporated. Used to immobilize maxillary fractures. Use now largely superseded.

plastic 1. Capable of being shaped or moulded, e.g. mixed amalgam prior to setting. 2. Common term for methyl methacrylate (acrylic).

plastic point Tapered plastic pin of various sizes, sometimes used in conjunction with wax patterns for crown and inlay work. The pin burns out during the casting process.

plastic surgery Branch of surgery dealing with the reconstruction and/or replacement of deformed or damaged parts of the body.

plasticizer Substance added to plastic materials to increase their softness and flexibility.

-plasty Suffix denoting plastic surgery.

plate *Bone p.* Perforated plates usually made out of titanium which are secured across the fracture line of a bone with screws in order to achieve fixation. *Mini b.p.* Small plates of varying thicknesses (usually ≤ 2 mm) and lengths usually used to fixate maxillofacial fractures. *Compression b.p.* Perforated metal plate designed to exert a compressing force at the site of a fracture. *Buccal p.* Term used to describe the buccal cortex of alveolar bone.

platelet (thrombocyte) The smallest blood cell. Platelets are disc-shaped with a fragile membrane and tend to stick to damaged or rough surfaces. They are concerned with the coagulation of a blood clot. Normally 250 000 per cm^3 of blood.

platinum Naturally occurring greyish white precious metal that does not tarnish in air. Used in combination with gold as an alloy for casting purposes and as platinum foil matrix in the construction of porcelain crowns. *P. foil.* See foil. *P. matrix.* Matrix of a platinum foil that is burnished onto a crown preparation model. Wet porcelain powder is then applied to it and baked in a furnace to form a porcelain crown or inlay.

pledget Small quantity of cotton wool, gauze or sponge compressed into a ball.

-plegia Suffix denoting paralysis.

pleura Membrane lining the thorax and investing the lungs.

pleural cavity Cavity between inner pleura attached to the lung and outer pleura attached to the thorax wall.

plexiform Resembling a plexus.

plexus A network. Usually refers to veins and nerves.

pliers Two-handled instrument designed to grip, bend, hold or cut wires and metal strips. *Adams' p.* Pliers with solid tapered beaks that form a four-sided pyramid when closed. Used to adjust removable orthodontic appliances and to bend and form modified arrowhead (Adams') clasps. *Light wire-bending p.* Pliers with short beaks, one conical and one pyramidal. Used for bending small wires and springs. *Arrowhead clasp forming p.* Used to form arrowhead wire clasps of orthodontic appliances. *Band contouring p.* Used for contouring and adapting bands. There are several patterns, e.g. Adams'. *Band removing p.* Used to remove orthodontic bands from teeth. The longer beak is placed on the occlusal surface of the tooth and the shorter one levers off the band by its cervical edge. *Band splitting p.* Pliers used to remove orthodontic bands by cutting them. *Bird beak p.* Similar to the light wire-bending p. but with shorter beaks. *Bracket removing p.* Similar to band removing p. Used to remove orthodontic brackets bonded to teeth. *Howe's p.* Pliers with slender flat beaks terminating in a comma shape with serrated surfaces and meeting only at the tips. Used for tying and bending orthodontic ligature wires. *Ligature and pin cutting p.* Used for cutting orthodontic ligatures and arch-retaining pins. *Ligature locking p.* Used in edgewise orthodontic technique to tighten a ligature when opened. *Martthew's p.* Wire-bending pliers with one conical beak closing into a hollow-ground beak. *Nance loop closing p.* Used to form parallel-sided wire loops. They have flat, thin beaks stepped down in size towards their tips. *Snipe nosed p.* Pliers with square-nosed flat beaks used for wire bending. *Spring-forming p.* Orthodontic wire-bending pliers with one conical and one pyramidal beak. *Triple beak p.* Pliers with a single beak opposing two beaks, used to place bends in orthodontic wire. *Tweed arch bending p.* Pliers with flattened blades that are parallel when gripping orthodontic wire. Used for square and rectangular wires. Another pattern forms loops or curves in such wires. *Universal p. See* Adams' p. *Weingart p.* Similar to Howe's p. but with curved offset beaks.

plug A mass that closes an opening.

plugger 1. Hand instrument, usually double ended, with a round- or oval-shaped end, either serrated or plain. Used to plug and condense amalgam into a cavity preparation. 2. Single-ended hand instrument used to plug and condense gutta percha in a root canal.

plumbago *See* graphite.

Plummer–Vinson syndrome (or anaemia) Syndrome associated with an iron deficiency anaemia and characterized by cracks and fissures in the corner of the mouth, a smooth, red, painful tongue with papillary atrophy and dysphagia.

plunger cusp A cusp that forces food interproximally between teeth in the opposing arch.

PMA (index) Papillary, marginal and attached gingiva index. *See* index.

PMMA *See* polymethylmethacrylate.

pneum- (pneumo-) Prefix denoting the lungs, respiration or the presence of air or gas.

pneumonia Inflammation of the lung.

pneumothorax Presence of air or gas in the pleural cavity.

-pnoea Suffix denoting breathing.

PNS *See* posterior nasal spine.

pocket *See* periodontal pocket. *P. marking forceps. See* periodontal instruments. *P. measuring probe. See* periodontal probe.

pogonion Orthodontic cephalometric landmark defined as the most prominent bony point of the chin. *Soft tissue p.* Most anterior point on the soft tissue outline of the chin when a patient is viewed in profile. *See* Appendix 10.

point A small area, a sharp end. *Contact p.* Deprecated term for contact area (q.v.). *P. 'A'. See* subspinale. *P. angle.* Point on a tooth where three surfaces meet. *P. 'B'. See* pogonion.

poison Any substance which, when applied externally to the body or taken internally, causes injury to any part of or the whole body.

poliomyelitis Acute viral disease sometimes involving the central nervous system with accompanying paralysis. May be controlled by vaccines.

polished surface Any surface of a denture, usually polished, that is in contact with the lips, cheeks and tongue, but excluding the occlusal surfaces. The greater the polish, the less the tendency for foreign bodies to stick to the surface.

polishing Production of a smooth glossy surface. *P. paste.* Used for cleaning and polishing surfaces of teeth and restorations. A blend of fine abrasive particles containing bonding agents, flavouring and colouring matter. The term *prophylactic paste* is not recommended. *P. strip. See* abrasive strip.

pollen Airborne product of flowers that is capable of sensitizing some people to allergic reactions. *P. count.* Published index of the amount of pollen in the air.

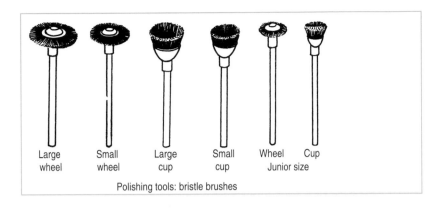

| Large wheel | Small wheel | Large cup | Small cup | Wheel Junior size | Cup |

Polishing tools: bristle brushes

poly- Prefix denoting many or much.

polyacrylic acid A polyacid formed by the polymerization of acrylic acid. In a 40% aqueous solution it is used as the liquid phase of glass ionomer and zinc polycarboxylate cements.

polyantibiotic creams or pastes Cream or paste containing more than one antibiotic and used in septic root canals during endodontic treatment.

polycarbonate A thermoplastic material derived from carbonic acid. Used to produce crown forms by injection moulding.

polycarboxylate cement *See* zinc polycarboxylate (q.v.).

polychromatic Multicoloured.

polydactylism Congenital abnormality in which more than 10 fingers and toes are present.

polydimethylsiloxane Silicone used in the manufacture of silicone impression material (q.v.).

polyether impression material *See* impression material.

polymer 1. Chemical substance made up of very large molecules and consisting essentially of recurring structural units. 2. In dentistry, powder ingredient of acrylic resin.

polymerization 1. The forming of a compound of high molecular weight by joining together similar molecules of low molecular weight. 2. Curing of a mixture of polymer powder and monomer liquid to form an acrylic resin.

polymethylmethacrylate (PMMA) Acrylic powder formed by the polymerization of methylmethacrylate and used in the manufacture of acrylic resin teeth and denture bases.

polymorphonuclear leucocyte *See* white blood cell.

polyneuritis Inflammation of many nerves at the same time.

polyol Polyhydric alcohol. Many polyols have a sweet taste and low fermentability by oral micro-organisms. They are often included in sugar-free foods, confectionery and medicines as a bulk sweetener.

polyp (polypus) Tumour arising from any mucous membrane. *Pedunculated p.* Polyp attached to the mucosa by a slender pedicle. *Sessile p.* Polyp with a broad base.

polysaccharide Carbohydrate yielding 10 or more monosaccharides on being hydrolysed. They do not taste sweet or dissolve in water, e.g. starch.

polysulphide impression material *See* impression material.

polytetrafluoroethylene *See* Teflon®.

polyvinylchloride Vinyl polymer historically used for maxillofacial prostheses.

PoM Prescription-only medicines. Drugs available only on medical and dental prescription.

pontic That part of a bridge which replaces the crowns of missing teeth. The suspended portion consists of one or more units made of metal, porcelain, composite or acrylic resin or a combination of metal with one of these.

porcelain In dentistry, a ceramic material made of kaolin, feldspar, silica and various pigments. Used to restore the form and function of a natural tooth and to make inlays, crowns, bridge pontics and teeth for dentures. May be high, medium, or low fusing according to the temperatures at which it is fired in an electrically heated furnace. *Aluminous p.* Contains a significant amount of alumina to provide increased strength. *Core p.* Contains a large proportion of alumina to provide extra strength and opacity to the core of the construction on which the covering porcelain is baked. *Dentine p.* Translucent pigmented porcelain used to form the body of a porcelain crown and provide the overall shape and colour. *Enamel p.* Porcelain powder applied to the outer surface of a porcelain crown during the baking process to provide translucency and pigmentation, as in natural teeth. *Glazing p.* Clear, low-fusing porcelain used to produce a thin glossy surface on a ceramic restoration. *P. bonded crown. See* crown. *P. jacket crown (PJC). See* crown.

Stain p. Low-fusing porcelain containing various metallic oxides, which is fired on to porcelain work to produce individual characteristics of colour and surface markings. *Vacuum-fired p.* Range of ceramic materials of various types fired in a furnace under vacuum conditions in order to minimize air bubbles and produce a stronger end-product.

porcelain teeth Artificial teeth made of porcelain, the anterior teeth being secured to the denture base by pins. Now largely superseded by acrylic teeth.

porion An orthodontic landmark defined as the most superior point of the bony external auditory meatus. *See also* Frankfort plane. (*See* Appendix 10.)

porosity Condition of a material such as metal, porcelain or plastic having minute holes or voids on the surface or in its substance.

porous 1. Having many pores. 2. Able to be permeated by fluids or air.

position indicating device (PID) *See* beam guiding instrument.

post 1. Prefix meaning following, behind or after. 2. In dentistry, a tapered or cylindrical rod that is cemented into a root canal as a retention for a core or post crown. *P. crown. See* crown. *P. dam. See* seal, posterior palatal.

post and core Integral retention portion of a post crown having a post to fit the root canal and a core shaped as a crown preparation.

post mortem Strictly, after death but loosely applied to the examination of a cadaver by a pathologist.

posterior Located at the back, behind or to the rear. *P. bite block.* Platform of acrylic polymer attached to a baseplate and placed over the occlusal surface of posterior teeth. *P. bite plane. See* p. bite

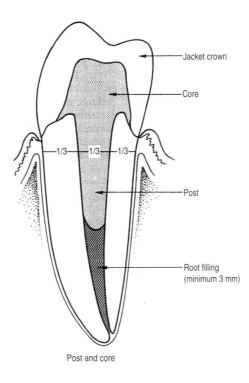

Post and core

block. *P. capping. See* p. bite block. *P. nasal spine (PNS).* Tip of the posterior spine of the palatine bone. *P. oral seal. See* seal. *P. palatal seal. See* seal. *P. superior dental nerve. See* nerve. *P. teeth.* Premolar and molar teeth.

postero-anterior projection In radiography, a technique for demonstrating the skull in a coronal plane by directing the X-ray beam from the posterior aspect of the patient towards the anterior. *See* Appendix 10.

postoperative Following a surgical operation.

postprandial After a meal.

potash alum *See* potassium aluminium sulphate.

potassium aluminium sulphate (alum, potash alum, aluminium potassium bis sulphate) Chemical used in an aqueous solution to accelerate the setting reaction of gypsum products.

potassium bifluoride Deprecated term for potassium hydrogen fluoride (q.v.).

potassium fluoride Chemical constituent of fluxes used in soldering.

potassium hydrogen fluoride (potassium hydrogendifluoride) Substance used in the manufacture of silver solder fluxes.

potassium sodium tartrate *See* sodium potassium tartrate.

potassium sulphate Chemical used to accelerate the setting time and reduce the setting expansion of gypsum plasters and investments.

potential Existing but not yet active.

potential difference The difference in electrical pressure (voltage) between two points in an electrical circuit. If there is no difference then no current runs between these points.

potentiation Effect of one drug on the action of another such that their combined action, when administered together, is greater than the sum of their effects when given separately.

pour resin *See* pourable denture base resin.

pour-type resin *See* pourable denture base resin.

pourable denture base resin (pour, pourable or pour-type resin) Specially formulated denture base material that flows and fills a mould under gravity.

pourable resin *See* pourable denture base resin.

power (statistical power) Measure of the strength of a study to be able to, for example, reliably detect a true difference rather than a difference due to chance.

power-operated syringe Syringe activated by a mechanism or by gas pressure.

ppm Parts per million.

practice The utilization of one's acquired knowledge in a particular profession, trade or art. *P. administration* or *management.* The establishment, organization and operation of the business aspects of a dental practice. *Private p.* A practice in which the dentist is independent of any outside policy or financial control.

prandial Relating to a meal.

pre- Prefix denoting before or preceding.

pre-adjusted appliance *See* appliance.

pre-amalgamated amalgam alloy Alloy containing a mixture of high copper amalgam, to which spherical silver copper particles and conventional lathe cut amalgam alloy are added.

precancerous Tending to become malignant.

precision attachment Interlocking mechanical device, one part of which is fixed to an abutment either intra- or extracoronally, while the other is integrated into a bridge or a denture in order to provide retention and/or support to the appliance.

preclinical 1. Occurring before the onset of a disease and before clinical symptoms can be detected. 2. Period in training of medical and dental students before they have contact with patients.

precursor That which precedes another; a forerunner. In medicine, an advance sign or symptom that warns of further complications.

predentine Dentine that has not yet calcified and is found on the actively forming dentine surface between the calcified dentine and the odontoblast cells.

predisposing To influence in advance. *P. factors.* Factors that increase the development of a disorder or disease.

prefabricated attachment Commercially manufactured precision attachment.

preformed band *See* band.

preformed metal crown (PFMC) *See* crown.

pregnancy epulis Pyogenic granuloma that may occur during pregnancy.

pregnancy gingivitis *See* gingivitis.

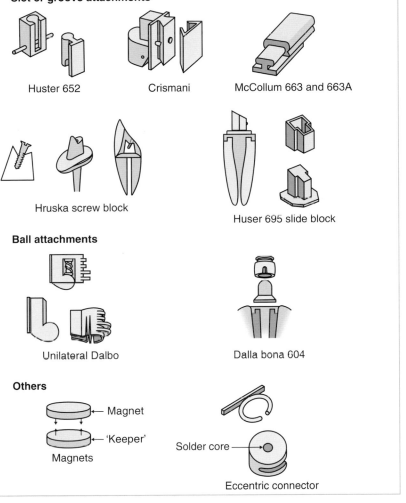

Precursor
Slot or groove attachments

Huster 652   Crismani   McCollum 663 and 663A

Hruska screw block

Huser 695 slide block

Ball attachments

Unilateral Dalbo   Dalla bona 604

Others

Magnet

'Keeper'   Solder core

Magnets

Eccentric connector

pregnancy hazards If dental treatment is essential during pregnancy it should be carried out during the middle trimester and especially not in the 3rd month. The patient should not be placed horizontally in the chair, radiographs should be avoided unless essential. Patients should avoid contact with German measles and must not be exposed to halothane vapour. Tetracycline should not be prescribed. Intravenous and inhalational sedation are best avoided in early pregnancy.

pregnancy tumour Deprecated term for pregnancy epulis (q.v.).

prehension Power of grasping or seizing.

premalignancy Any developmental or acquired change in a tissue that is capable of becoming malignant.

premature Happening before the usual or proper time.

premature contact (initial contact) *See* contact, premature.

premaxilla That part of the maxilla in which the incisor teeth develop and erupt. Considered as part of the maxilla in humans but a separate bone in other mammals.

premaxillary Situated anteriorly to the maxilla.

premedication The administration of a sedative drug prior to treatment to allay apprehension and thus facilitate subsequent management of the patient.

premolar One of eight permanent teeth which succeed the primary molars, two in each quadrant and lying immediately distal to the canine. They have two cusps and are used for grinding food. In over 70% of cases the upper first premolar has two roots placed buccopalatally, the bifurcation of the roots occurring anywhere between the neck and the apex. The roots are usually of similar size, flattened mesiodistally. There may be three roots, the buccal one being bifurcated. The other premolars normally have one root. There are no premolars in the primary dentition.

preoperative Before operation. Generally refers to the treatment, such as sedation, given before the administration of a general anaesthetic and a surgical operation.

preparation 1. The process of making ready. 2. In dentistry, *cavity or tooth preparation* is the removal of carious and weakened tissue from a tooth and the shaping of sound tissue to accept and retain a temporary or permanent restoration. 3. A medicament.

prescription Written directive concerning the composition, quantity and method of administration of drugs, signed by a qualified person.

prevalence The proportion of a population that has a condition or disease at a point in time.

preventive dentistry Community- or patient-based measures taken to prevent the incidence of dental decay or caries. Includes fissure sealing, fluoride therapy, oral hygiene instruction, dietary analysis and advice and regular review. Collectively these measures are known as 'The Pillars of Prevention'.

preventive resin restoration (PRR) Restoration used to restore minimal carious lesions, usually less than 2 mm in depth using a bonded filled composite resin to replace enamel/dentine plus fissure sealant to obturate the remaining vulnerable fissure system on the tooth surface.

prilocaine hydrochloride Citanest®. An agent less toxic than lignocaine or procaine used in local anaesthetic solutions. Marketed as Citanest in a 3% solution with 0.03 IU/ml felypressin as a vasoconstrictor or as a 4% plain solution.

primary 1. The earliest in time or order. 2. Principal. 3. In radiography, the radiation emanating directly from the focal spot. *P. cell.* Initial body cell formed after conception which multiplies and develops to become specialized cells forming tissues and organs. *P. closure.* Immediate closing of a wound or incision by suturing, etc. *P. dentine.* Dentine present when the tooth is fully formed. *P. dentition. See* below. *P. impression. See* impression, primary. *P. lesion. See* lesion.

P. occlusal trauma. Injury caused to a tooth or teeth, with normal periodontal support, due to adverse occlusal forces.

primary dentition Dentition which starts to erupt about the age of 6 months and is complete at about 2½ years, after which it is gradually replaced by the permanent dentition. When complete it consists of 20 teeth, which start to calcify before birth: one central and one lateral incisor, one canine and two molars in each quadrant. Primary teeth are usually whiter and softer, and have a relatively thin enamel covering with proportionally much larger pulp chambers than their permanent replacements. The crowns are more bulbous and the cusps are generally well worn before the teeth are shed. They are smaller than their successors except for the molars which are larger than the premolars replacing them. The first upper and lower primary molars are unlike any other teeth, each having a very bulbous crown and four cusps. The upper molar has three widely splayed roots while the lower has two widely divergent roots.

primary herpetic gingivostomatitis Common cause of severe oral ulceration in children, caused by the herpes simplex type 1 virus. *See* herpes.

primate spacing Diastema (q.v.) present in some deciduous dentition between the mandibular canine and first molar and the maxillary lateral incisor and canine.

primer Changes the nature of the tooth surface prior to bonding.

primordial cyst *See* odontogenic keratocyst.

principal fibre *See* fibre.

prism Solid geometrical shape with similar equal and parallel ends.

p.r.n. Abbreviation of Latin phrase 'pro re nata', as the occasion arises, or repeat when necessary. Used in prescription writing.

pro- Prefix denoting before or a precursor to.

probability (p) value Shows whether a particular result in a research study or trial was due to a true difference or the result of chance. A value of <0.05 for p is statistically significant.

probe (explorer) Sharp-pointed hand instrument used to explore teeth and restoration surfaces in order to detect caries, overhanging edges and other defects. May be single or double ended. *Periodontal p. See* periodontal instruments.

procaine An ester local anaesthetic no longer available in dental local anaesthetic cartridges. It has been replaced by amide agents such as lidocaine in dental local anaesthetic formulations.

process 1. Prominence or outgrowth of any part. 2. Very fine microscopic extension of a cell. 3. Procedure whereby a denture base resin is polymerized (or cured) in a mould.

proclination Sloping of anterior teeth in a labial direction.

prodromal Denoting those signs and symptoms heralding the onset of an illness, e.g. headache, fever, malaise, vertigo.

productive Inflammatory state of a lesion leading to formation of new tissue.

profile Side view, especially of the face.

prognathism Protrusion of the lower jaw beyond the normal distance from the cranial base.

prognosis Forecast of the course and duration of a disease or results of a treatment.

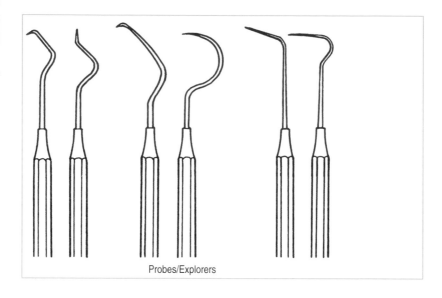

Probes/Explorers

prokaryote An organism lacking an internal membrane, structurally discrete nucleus and other subcellular compartments, e.g. bacteria.

prolapse Downward displacement of an organ or tissue from its normal site. *P. of antral mucosa.* Protrusion of the antral mucosa through an oroantral fistula into the oral cavity.

proliferate To grow by the multiplication of similar cells.

proliferation Growth of a tissue by multiplication of its similar cells.

promethazine hydrochloride (Phenergan®) Sedative antihistamine which acts for up to 12 hours. Of value in nasal allergy, urticaria and rashes associated with drug allergies. Widely used as an anti-emetic and useful for patients with an overactive vomiting reflex.

promoter *See* accelerator.

prone Lying face downwards.

prop Instrument used, generally during an anaesthetic, to maintain the mouth in an open position. Often in sets of three (of different sizes) joined together by a safety chain, e.g. Hewitt or McKesson.

prophylactic 1. Pertaining to the prevention of disease. 2. Agent that prevents the development of a disease or condition. *P. odontotomy.* Elimination of pits and fissures in tooth enamel to prevent caries. *P. paste.* Deprecated term for polishing paste (q.v.). *P. treatment. See* treatment.

prophylaxis 1. The art or technique of preventing disease. 2. In dentistry, the use of measures to prevent the onset of diseases of the teeth and soft tissues. Sometimes loosely used to describe the scaling, cleaning and polishing of teeth. *P. cup. See* rubber cup.

propofol (Diprivan®) An intravenous anaesthetic agent that is also used as an intravenous sedative in dentistry. Infusion can be controlled by the operator, patient or by feedback from the target organ.

proprietary drug In pharmacology, the trade name of a drug, generally followed by the symbol®.

proprioreceptor Sensory end-organ that provides information about the movement and position of the body. Found chiefly in the muscles, tendons, joints and ears.

prostaglandins One of a group of hormone-like substances found in a wide variety of body tissues and fluids.

prosthesis Artificial restoration of a part of the body that is congenitally missing, has been destroyed accidentally or removed surgically. *Cosmetic p.* Appliance designed to improve a person's appearance. *Dental p.* Fixed or removable appliance to replace one or more missing teeth. *Maxillofacial p.* Designed to restore the contour of the face and/or jaw following injury or surgery.

prosthetic surgery Surgical procedures designed to facilitate the manufacture of dentures and to improve the long-term prognosis of denture wearing.

prosthetics Branch of surgical science dealing with the replacement of an absent part of the body. *Dental p.* Branch of dental science dealing with the artificial replacement of one or more natural teeth or associated structures by a denture or bridge.

prosthion Most anterior point of the alveolar crest in the premaxilla and usually situated between the central incisors.

prosthodontics (prosthetic dentistry) Branch of dental science concerned with removable dental prosthetics. This definition is applicable to the UK only. In other countries prosthodontics may refer to both removable and fixed appliances (i.e. bridge work).

prosthodontist (dental prosthetist) Dental surgeon engaged in the practice of prosthodontics.

protective barrier In radiography, a barrier, e.g. lead or lead glass, placed between the operator and the focal spot to reduce the absorption of radiation to permissible levels.

protein Complex compound of amino acids and source of the body's nitrogen requirements. Obtained from meat, poultry, fish, eggs, cheese, milk, peas, beans and whole cereal. Proteins usually contain carbon, hydrogen, oxygen, potassium, nitrogen and sulphur. They are essential to the structure and function of the body.

proto- Prefix denoting first, primitive or precursor.

protocol A plan for a scientific investigation or treatment.

protoplasm A semifluid, jelly-like, transparent, granular substance within a cell membrane surrounding its nucleus.

protozoa Single celled eukaryotic organisms showing some of the characteristics of animals. Traditionally classified as a subkingdom of the Animal Kingdom, more recently protozoa have been grouped with some algae in the Kingdom Protista. Some protozoa can cause disease in humans, e.g. *Giardia, Cryptosporidium* and some amoebae.

protrusion 1. Thrusting forward movement of the mandible. 2. Malposition of the teeth of one jaw relative to the other jaw.

protrusive interocclusal record Interocclusal record made with the mandible in a protruded position by means of thin wax films or registration pastes.

protrusive record Record of the protruded relationship of the mandible relative to the maxilla.

provisional restoration Generic term for a temporary restoration, either intra- or extracoronal, designed to provide stabilization of a tooth prior to the next stage of treatment, e.g. temporary crown or temporary filling.

proximal The deprecated term for approximal (q.v.). *P. cavity. See also* approximal cavity. *P. surface. See* approximal surface.

PRR Preventive resin restoration. Technique used to restore a minimal carious lesion, using a combination of filled composite resin and fissure sealant.

pruritus Itching caused by a local irritation.

pseud- (pseudo-) Prefix denoting false or of superficial resemblance. *P. pocket.* Deprecated term for periodontal pocket (q.v.).

psychic stimulus Any stimulus, other than the presence of food in the mouth, that results in salivation.

psychologist Person who studies normal and abnormal mental processes, development and behaviour.

psychosomatic Referring to the inter-relationship of the body and the mind. *P. illness.* Illness with bodily symptoms of emotional or mental origin.

pterygoid Wing shaped.

pterygoid muscle One of two muscles on each side of the face. The *lateral pterygoid* is short and cone shaped with two heads attached to the sphenoid bone, running backwards as it diminishes in size, to be attached to the anterior aspect of the condyle of the mandible, the capsule of the temporomandibular joint and its disc. It assists in opening the jaw, protruding it and pulling it towards the opposite side. The *medial pterygoid* is square shaped and thick, attached to the internal aspect of the ramus of the mandible, low down between the angle of the mandible and the mandibular foramen. Its other end has two heads, the largest being attached to the sphenoid bone and the smaller one to the posterior surface of the maxilla. Its action is to close the jaw, protrude it and pull the mandible to the opposite side. The pterygoid muscles are supplied by the mandibular branch of the trigeminal nerve and the external carotid artery.

pterygo-maxillare (PTM) Lowest point of the outline of the pterygo-maxillary fissure.

PTFE Polytetrafluoroethylene. *See* Teflon®.

PTM *See* pterygo-maxillare.

ptosis Drooping or prolapsed eyelid.

ptyal- (ptyalo-) Prefix denoting saliva.

ptyalin Deprecated term for amylase (q.v.).

ptyalism Condition in which there is an excess of saliva in the mouth, due to excessive secretion or inability to swallow.

pulmo- (pulmono-) Prefix denoting the lungs.

pulmonary Pertaining to, or affecting the lungs. *P. artery.* Artery that carries deoxygenated blood from the right ventricle of the heart to the lungs. *P. collapse.* Collapse of part or all of the lung due to an obstruction of the airway. *P. embolism.* Embolus detached from a blood vessel may be circulated in the bloodstream provided the vessels through which it passes are increasing in size. When the vessels decrease in size it may become impacted. A large embolus may cause death immediately or within hours. *P. vein.* Large vein conducting oxygenated blood from the lung to the left auricle or atrium.

pulp 1. Soft mass of tissue. 2. In dentistry, soft tissue lying within the dentine of a tooth and containing fibres, cells and structures such as blood vessels, sensory nerves and lymphatics. These vessels pass through the apical foramen of the tooth or through accessory canals. *Indirect p. capping.* Technique of pulp capping when the pulp is not overtly exposed. *P. abscess. See* abscess. *P. canal.* Canal running within the dentine of a tooth from the coronal portion of the tooth to the apex. *P. cap* Wound dressing placed on the dentine floor of a deep cavity (*indirect pulp cap*) or in direct contact with pulp tissue (*direct pulp cap*) with the intention of preserving pulp vitality and promoting defensive tertiary dentine deposition. Examples include calcium hydroxide cement and MTA. *P. capping.* Application over an exposed vital pulp of one or more layers of protective and/or therapeutic material, e.g. calcium hydroxide, which promotes the production of reparative dentine. *P. cavity.* Cavity within the dentine of the tooth that contains the dental pulp. *P. chamber.* Cavity within the crown of a tooth that contains the dental pulp. *P. cornu* (or *horn*). Horn-shaped extension of the pulp cavity extending in towards the cusp or the incisal margins. *P. extirpation.* Complete removal of the contents of the pulp chamber and root canal. *P. horn. See* p. cornu. *P. mummification.* Application of a medicament to the pulp remnants to render them inert and preserve them in an aseptic state. *P. stone (denticle).* Calcified area within the substance of the dental pulp. *P. surface.* That surface of the tooth cavity which overlies the pulp. *P. sensitivity test.* Diagnostic aid involving the application of an electrical, thermal or mechanical stimulus to the crown of a tooth in order to indicate the excitability of the pulp. The test is not necessarily indicative of the vitality of the pulp. *Vital p.* Pulp in which the blood supply is intact. Vitality is elicited by stimulation of the nerve endings within the pulp which are present if the blood supply is intact.

pulpal Relating to the pulp.

pulpectomy *See* pulp extirpation.

pulpitis Inflammation of the dental pulp. *Reversible p.* Clinical diagnosis of pulp inflammation which may resolve if causative factors are eliminated. *Irreversible p.* Clinical diagnosis of pulp inflammation which is unlikely to resolve if causative factors are eliminated.

pulpotomy Removal of the coronal part of a vital pulp in order to preserve the underlying radicular portion. *Partial (superficial) p.* Removal of the coronal 2-3 mm of infected pulp tissue after pulp exposure. *Coronal p.* Removal of all pulp tissue from the coronal pulp chamber.

pulsate To beat rhythmically as does the heart.

pulse Wave of increased pressure throughout the arterial blood system caused by contraction of the left ventricle of the heart. Can be felt in any superficial artery, e.g. radial artery in the wrist.

pumice Abrasive used in polishing dentures and consisting of various silicates obtained from lava.

punch *See* rubber dam punch.

puncture 1. To pierce with a pointed object. 2. The hole produced by puncturing.

purpura Disease or condition characterized by a skin rash resulting from bleeding into the skin from small blood vessels.

pus Thick, yellow semi-liquid substance resulting from an inflammatory reaction and consisting of blood and tissue fluid, dead and living bacteria, white blood cells and dead tissue cells. *Staphylococcus aureus* or *pyogenes* is the main pus-forming micro-organism. Pus appears in a cavity in which there has been tissue destruction.

push scaler *See* scaler.

pustular Relating to a pustule or pustules.

pustule Small infected vesicle containing pus.

putrefaction Rotting or decomposition of tissues accompanied by a foul odour.

py- (pyo-) Prefix denoting pus.

pyaemia Blood poisoning in which there is a general secondary infection forming multiple abscesses in several locations.

pyogenic Any organism or other agent that produces pus.

pyorrhoea Former and often lay term for gingivitis or chronic periodontitis (q.v.).

pyramidal fracture *See* Le Fort classification.

pyretic Relating to a fever.

pyrexia *See* fever.

pyro- Prefix denoting heat.

pyrogen Substance that produces a fever.

pyrogenic Relating to that which produces a fever.

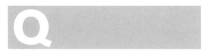

q.d., q.d.s. or q.i.d Abbreviation of Latin phrase 'quater in die', i.e. 4 times a day. Used in prescription writing.

quadrangular Having four angles.

quadrant A fourth part. In dentistry, one half of each dental arch, the dividing line being the midpoint of the arch. There are thus four quadrants—the upper left and right and the lower left and right.

quadrate Square shaped, having four equal sides and four right angles.

quadri- Prefix meaning four.

quadricusped Having four cusps.

quality (of ionizing radiation) In radiography, the relative energy assessment based on penetrating power.

quality factor Factor measured in terms of linear energy transfer to express the biological effectiveness of different types of radiation. Used in the calculation of dose equivalents.

quantum Unit of energy associated with electromagnetic radiation.

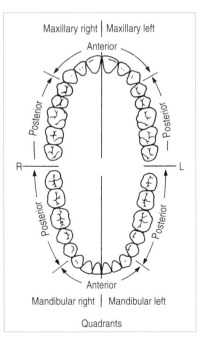

Quadrants

quarantine Period of isolation imposed on a person who might spread a contagious disease.

quartz Crystalline substance occurring naturally as silica. Used in investment materials as a refractory material, in some composite filling materials and in some light sources.

quenching Sudden cooling of a hot metal in a cool liquid in order to temper it.

quicklime *See* lime.

quicksilver Rarely used name for mercury (q.v.).

quiescent Relates to a disease that is in an undetectable or inactive period.

Quincke's oedema *See* angioneurotic oedema.

quinsy (peritonsillar abscess) Acute inflammation of the tonsils and surrounding tissues causing dysphagia, swelling of the soft palate, pain in the throat and pyrexia.

R

RA Relative analgesia. *See* analgesia.

racemose Resembling a bunch of grapes on the vine.

rad (radiation absorbed dose) Obsolescent unit for measuring the amount of energy absorbed from a radioactive source. The preferred SI unit is the gray (q.v.) (1 rad=0.01 gray).

radial Associated with the radius. *R. pulse.* Pulse of the radial artery at the wrist felt by the fingertips.

radiation Emanation of energy from a source. The most usual form is that of photons in the form of radio waves, X-rays or gamma rays. Radiation causes damage to living tissues. *Absorbed dose of r.* Amount of radiation absorbed by the tissues (SI unit of measure is the gray). *R. burn.* Severe skin damage caused by exposure to ionizing radiation, either of high dosage for a short period or of small dosage over an extended period of time. *R. caries. See* caries, radiation. *R. hazard.* Ionizing radiation in high doses can cause damage to the body tissues (somatic damage). Exposure (of lesser doses), especially to the sex glands, can cause changes in the hereditary characteristics contained in the genes (genetic damage). Protective measures include staying out of the surgery during radiography, and the patient wearing a rubber- or plastic-covered lead apron during exposure to X-rays. *R. injury.* Injury due to ionizing radiation which may be SOMATIC, affecting the body tissues in the form of burns, loss of digits, nausea and vomiting, or GENETIC, affecting the offspring of parents whose reproductive cells have been exposed to lower doses. *R. necrosis.* Tissue death caused by radiation. *R. sickness. See* r. injury. *R. therapy.* Early treatment of malignant growths and some skin diseases by radium, X-rays and radio active isotopes.

radical Relating to treatment that cures by completely removing the cause.

radicular Relating to the root or roots of a tooth. *R. cyst. See* cyst. *R. fracture.* Fracture of the root or roots of a tooth.

radio- Prefix denoting radiation or radio-active substance.

radio-active Having the power of radioactivity.

radiograph Roentgenogram, roentgenograph. Processed film showing an image of an object that has been exposed to X-rays. *See also* cephalometric r.

radiographer Person trained to expose patients to localized radiation in order to produce a radiograph for diagnostic purposes.

radiographic Relating to radiography. *R. baseline* or *reference plane*. In skull radiography, the orbitomeatal line. In intra-oral radiography, the occlusal plane of the jaw being radiographed.

radiography Method of making photographic records of various parts of the body by the use of X-rays.

radiologist Medically or dentally qualified person who specializes in the interpretation of radiographs.

radiology Science of the diagnosis and treatment of diseases by the use of X-rays and radiographs. *Diagnostic radiology* includes the study of radiographic films and a visual examination of body structures on a fluorescent screen, or the demonstration of certain body systems by the introduction of radio-opaque chemicals prior to radiological investigations.

radiolucent Permitting partial passage of X-rays. On a radiograph radiolucent areas appear darker than radio-opaque areas.

radio-opaque Resisting the passage of X-rays, e.g. a metal tooth restoration which appears lighter than its surroundings in a dental radiograph. *R. denture base material*. Denture base material to which has been added a radio-opaque substance in order to facilitate the location of the appliance if swallowed, inhaled or implanted in tissues.

radiotherapy *See* radiation therapy.

radium Radio-active element used in the treatment of malignant growths and some rodent ulcers.

rami Plural of ramus.

ramification A branching out; a subdivision of a main structure.

ramify To branch in all directions.

ramus That part of the mandible which is at an angle to its body and carries the coronoid process and the condyle (part of the temporomandibular joint). The masseter muscle is attached to its outer surface.

ranula Retention cyst, usually under the tongue, occurring when a sublingual salivary gland duct or mucous gland is blocked.

raphe Line, crease or ridge in a tissue or organ.

rarefaction Thinning of bone tissue that is sufficient to cause a decreased density of bone to X-rays and is thus recorded as a darker area on the radiographic film.

rash Inflammatory skin lesion commonly associated with infectious diseases, developing at some stage of the disease.

rasp *See* bone file.

RCP Retruded cuspal position.

reabsorb To absorb again, to resorb.

reabsorption Process of absorbing again.

reaction 1. Response to a stimulus. 2. Interaction of substances resulting in a chemical change.

reamer *See* root canal reamer.

reattachment Re-establishment of attachment of the periodontal tissue to the tooth root on which viable periodontal tissue has been retained following surgery or trauma.

rebase Removal and replacement of the denture base without changing the occlusal relationship.

recall system The organization of a method of recalling patients for a periodic dental examination.

receptor Minute organ at the extremities of sensory nerves. Capable of detecting various stimuli such as pressure, touch, taste and temperature changes.

recession In dentistry, the migration of the gingival margin in an apical direction so exposing the root surface of a tooth.

recipe A statement of ingredients. The heading of a prescription by the symbol R meaning 'take'.

reciprocating handpiece *See* handpiece.

record 1. A list of facts or findings relative to a specific condition and recorded in a permanent way. 2. The registration of jaw relations. *Functional r.* A record of the lateral and protrusive movements of the mandible on the occluding surface of the maxillary occlusal rim or other recording surface. *Terminal hinge position r.* A record of the relationship of the mandible relative to the maxilla at the retruded mandibular position.

recrudescence Recurrence of symptoms following an improvement which may have lasted several months; a relapse.

recurrent Occurring again after a period of time.

red blood cell *See* erythrocyte.

reduction Replacement of displaced fractured bone fragments into their correct position, generally just prior to fixation by pins, splints or wiring.

reference plane *See* radiographic baseline.

referred pain Manifestation of pain at a given site when the cause is situated elsewhere. Not an unusual occurrence with the branches of the fifth cranial nerve.

refined carbohydrate Sugar and white flour product on which the lactobacillus acts to form lactic acid. Found in biscuits, cakes, sweets, jams and cereals with sugar.

reflex Involuntary reaction produced automatically and immediately in response to a stimulus, e.g. the knee jerk, blinking, retching.

refractory 1. Not readily responding to treatment. 2. Substance resistant to heat. 3. Mineral suitable for lining furnaces and investing materials for casting moulds.

regeneration The repair or renewal of pathologically lost tissue. In dentistry, regeneration techniques are used for the augmentation of alveolar ridges and in guided tissue regeneration (q.v.).

regional analgesia *See* analgesia.

registration Act of registering, making an entry or record. *See also* occlusal registration.

registration paste Dental material used to physically record the occlusion of a dentate mouth, partially dentate mouth, or alternatively the occlusal surfaces of registration blocks. Usually the material will be applied in a plastic form and will set to a rigid or semi-rigid state.

regression Returning, following a remission to a former condition.

regressive Relating to regression. Subsiding.

regurgitation The backward flow of partially digested foods from the stomach via the oesophagus to the mouth.

rehabilitation Restoration to normal form and function. *Occlusal r.* Restoration of the functional integrity of the dental arches by the use of directly placed composite restorations or laboratory constructed onlays, inlays, crowns, bridges and partial dentures.

reimplantation *See* replantation (preferred term).

reinfection Further infection by the same causative organism.

reinforced zinc oxide-eugenol cement Zinc oxide-eugenol cement (q.v.) that has been reinforced by the addition of a polymeric and/or an inorganic filler in the powder, e.g. EBA cement, or by the addition of a solution of a polymer in the eugenol liquid.

relapse To drift back into a former state of ill health. In orthodontics, to return towards the original state of malocclusion following correction.

relative analgesia *See* analgesia.

relaxant Drug or other agent that brings about muscle relaxation or relieves tension.

reliability Measure of a study's or experiment's reproducibility, i.e. its ability to produce the same result if repeated. It is a reflection of how well a study has been designed.

relief 1. Lessening of pain or distress. 2. Reduction of pressure on a specific area below a denture base. *R. area.* Area defined on a plaster model to relieve pressure on underlying tissue. Tin foil is swaged onto this area, and is removed from the processed denture before finishing, to provide a space between the mucosa and a denture. *R. chamber.* Recessed area on the fitting surface of a denture obtained by the use of a tin foil spacer.

reline To add a material to the existing base of a denture in order to improve its fit.

remineralization Restoration of mineral salts to a tissue, e.g. calcium salts to enamel or bone.

remission Temporary relief from an illness, either spontaneously or as a result of treatment.

remittent Increasing and decreasing at periodical intervals.

removable appliance Orthodontic appliance that can be removed from the mouth by the patient.

renal Pertaining to the kidneys.

Rendu–Osler–Weber disease *See* hereditary haemorrhagic telangiectasia.

reni- (reno-) Prefix denoting kidney.

repair 1. Natural process to restore normal tissue function, e.g. healing of fractures, diseased and necrosed tissues. 2. In prosthetics, a prosthesis that has been repaired.

reparative dentine Similar to secondary dentine (q.v.) but laid down more rapidly over a period of time as a repair tissue.

replaced flap Flap of tissue that has been replaced in the preoperative position.

replantation Replacement of a tooth in its socket following deliberate or traumatic avulsion.

replication A repetition or copy.

report A written description of the examination, clinical findings and proposed treatment.

reproducibility *See* reliability

resect To remove part of a tissue or organ.

resection Excision of an organ or other tissue or structure.

residual cyst *See* cyst.

residual ridge Bone and covering tissue that remain after the extraction of teeth.

resin 1. Substance that is secreted naturally by certain plants and insects, e.g. rosin, or produced synthetically. 2. Uncompounded polymeric material used in the manufacture of plastics. *Acrylic r.* General term for the resinous material of the various esters of acrylic acid. Its chief use is in the manufacture of dentures and synthetic resin teeth. *Autopolymerizing r.* A resin whose polymerization is initiated by a chemical activator and without the application of heat. The preferred term is *cold curing acrylic r. Composite r.* Hard, durable, strong filled resin used for tooth-coloured restorations. The filler may consist of finely powdered glass or quartz crystals. *Epoxy r.* A synthetic resin characterized by the reactive epoxy or ethyloxyline groups. It is resistant to moderate heat and chemicals and is used as an adhesive and in the manufacture of dies. *R. bonding (Bonding r.).* Unfilled resin used to assist the adhesion of restorative materials to tooth structure. *See* adhesive. *R. cement.* Any of a group of filling or cementing materials that may be filled or unfilled and marketed in single-, dual- or multi-component systems.

resin modified glass ionomer cement *See* glass ionomer cement.

resistance form Design feature of a tooth preparation that imparts strength to a restoration and the tooth when under load.

resolution Process of returning to normal following an inflammatory reaction.

resolve To return to normal following an inflammatory reaction.

resorb To take up or absorb again, to undergo resorption.

resorption Removal of tissue by pathological or by normal physiological

processes. In dentistry, the removal of the calcified parts of teeth and jaws. *Alveolar r.* The reduction in size of the residual ridges of the mandible and maxillae following the extraction of teeth.

respiration Gaseous interchange between the tissue cells in the lungs (alveoli) and the atmosphere. The act of breathing by which oxygen is absorbed and carbon dioxide exhaled to produce energy. *Artificial r.* Respiration which is maintained by artificial means, e.g. mouth-to-mouth resuscitation.

respirator 1. Apparatus connected to a patient to ventilate the lungs. 2. Protective screen fitted over the mouth and nose.

respiratory Relating to respiration.

respiratory arrest Cessation of respiratory function. Follows respiratory failure and may be the result of lack of oxygen or paralysis of the respiratory muscles. Air or oxygen-rich air must be administered immediately after removal of any obstruction of the airway.

respiratory centre Area of the brain that controls the acts of inspiration and expiration to ensure regular breathing.

respiratory system Body system by which air passes into and out of the lungs, allows the blood to absorb oxygen and eliminates carbon dioxide and water.

respiratory tract Route by which air containing oxygen enters the lungs and leaves containing carbon dioxide. Consists of the nose and nasal cavity, the mouth, larynx and trachea leading to the bronchi of the lungs. Secondary functions of the respiratory tract are the production of speech in the larynx and the sense of smell.

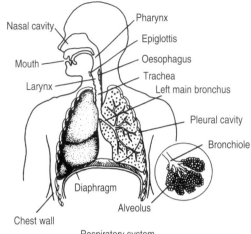

Nasal cavity
Mouth
Larynx
Pharynx
Epiglottis
Oesophagus
Trachea
Left main bronchus
Pleural cavity
Bronchiole
Diaphragm
Alveolus
Chest wall

Respiratory system

response Reaction to a stimulus.

rest 1. Natural state of relaxation. 2. Component of a partial prosthesis resting on the occlusal, lingual, cingulum or incisal surface of a tooth to resist a vertical load. *R. face height. See* r. vertical dimension. *R. jaw relation.* Relationship of the mandible to the maxilla when the former is in the rest position. *R. position of the mandible.* Natural position assumed by the mandible when the mandibular musculature is in a relaxed state and the patient is in an upright position. *R. seat.* That part of the tooth that has been prepared to receive a rest. *R. vertical dimension.* Vertical dimension (q.v.) when the mandible is in the rest position.

resting flow Salivary flow that occurs normally in the absence of exogenous stimulation.

restoration End-result of dental procedures carried out to restore the form, function and appearance of teeth.

restorative dentistry General term for dental care provided to establish a stable and healthy functional dentition. Covers conservative, periodontal, prosthetic, orthodontic, endodontic and surgical procedures.

restorative material Material used to restore the form and function of a tooth.

Resusci bag® Folding bag with face-piece used in continuation of mouth-to-mouth resuscitation at the rate of 15–20 times per minute. *See also* Ambu bag®.

resuscitation 1. Bringing back to life of a person who is apparently dead, collapsed or shocked. 2. Restoration of normal breathing and pulse. *Cardiopulmonary r.* The restoration of cardiac output and pulmonary ventilation following cardiorespiratory arrest.

resuscitator Apparatus used to force air and/or oxygen-enriched air into the lungs.

retained teeth Primary teeth that are retained beyond their normal time of exfoliation.

retainer 1. In prosthetics, an attachment such as a clasp which retains a partial denture against dislodging forces. 2. In orthodontics, a passive removable appliance or device cemented to teeth which maintains their position following active orthodontic treatment. *Bonded r.* In orthodontics, use of a wire or other structure bonded directly to teeth in order to retain their position following orthodontic tooth movement. *Essix r.* A clear, thin vacuum-formed retainer used in orthodontics. Can also be used to correct mild malocclusions. *Hawley r.* An orthodontic removeable appliance used to retain the tooth position achieved following orthodontic treatment. The design is a labial bow with Adams' clasps for retention. 3. Restoration cemented to an abutment tooth and serving as the retention for a bridge. *Matrix band r.* See matrix band.

retarder Substance that slows down a chemical reaction such as the setting of plaster of Paris or alginate impression materials.

retching Involuntary spasmodic but ineffectual attempt to vomit. May be caused by stimulation of the soft palate or the posterior third of the tongue.

retention 1. In prosthetics, the resistance of a prosthesis to dislodgement along the natural path of displacement (usually vertical). *Direct r.* Retention obtained for a partial denture by the use of clasps or attachments to resist its dislodgement. *Indirect r.* Retention obtained by extending a partial denture base to provide a class II lever. 2. In orthodontics, the use of a removable or fixed retainer. An alternative term for fixation (q.v.). *Acid etch r.* Retention for certain filling materials provided by etching or roughening the enamel surface of a tooth by the use of dilute acids. *R. form.* Any design feature of a tooth preparation that prevents displacement

of a restoration. *R. mucocoele.* Pathological collection of mucus within the soft tissues and arising from a salivary gland. May be due to extravasation from a gland or a duct or to retention within a duct. *See also* index, retention.

retentive arm Flexible component of a prosthesis that engages in an undercut of a tooth to provide retention. *See* clasp.

reticular Relating to a lace-like substance. Net-like.

reticulocyte Earliest stage in the growth of a blood cell in circulating blood. One per cent of all red blood cells are reticulocytes.

reticulo-endothelial system System of protection against infection, destruction of red blood cells too old to function properly, and the storage of fat substances. Unlike other endothelial cells the cells of the system are phagocytic and found in great numbers in the lymph glands, liver, spleen and bone marrow. Its vessels consist of a network of reticular fibres enmeshing cells. The cells ingest micro-organisms, dust particles and antigenic substances so that they can stimulate lymphocytes to produce immunity responses. Alternatively called the *macrophage system.*

reticulum A network.

retinol Vitamin A, concerned with vision in dim light and bone formation. Occurs in most green plants, especially carrots.

retract To draw back.

retraction Drawing back or shortening of tissue. In orthodontics, the moving back of one or more teeth into a better position by the use of an appliance. *R. cord.* Thin friable cord impregnated with a vasoconstrictor and placed in the gingival crevice to facilitate accurate impression taking of inlay and crown preparations.

retractor 1. Instrument used to hold the cheeks, tongue or soft tissues away from the site of operation in order to improve vision and access and to protect them during surgical procedures, e.g. cheek retractor, tongue retractor, flap retractor, tissue retractor, lip retractor. 2. *R. spring*. In orthodontics, a spring used to move teeth distally. *See also* finger spring.

retro- Prefix meaning backwards or behind.

retroclination Leaning backwards. In dentistry, lingual or palatal inclination of anterior teeth.

retrognathia Underdevelopment of the mandible and/or the maxilla.

retrograde Directed backwards. *R. (or reverse) root filling*. Filling inserted into the apical end of a root during root-end surgery. *See also* apicectomy.

retromolar pad Pad of soft connective tissue found distal to the last molar in the lower jaw.

retruded Situated behind or away from. *R. arc of closure*. Arc formed by the movement of any joint on, or attached to, the mandible when the condyles are in their most posterior position. *R. axis*. Hinge axis in the retruded jaw relation. *R. contact position*. Position of the mandible on first tooth contact on the retruded arc of closure. *R. hinge axis. See* r. axis. *R. jaw relation*. The position of the mandible on its retruded arc of closure where the condyles are in the most posterior position.

retrusion 1. Condition of being sited behind the normal position. 2. In dentistry, the most posterior position of the mandible.

reverse bevel *See* bevel.

reverse bevel incision *See* inverse bevel incision.

reverse curve (anti-Monson curve) Imaginary curve of the occlusal surfaces of the posterior teeth that is convex upwards and lies in a coronal plane.

reverse curve of Spee A bend commonly placed into orthodontic archwires to flatten an occlusal plane.

reverse horizontal overlap (reverse overjet) Tooth relationship, in intercuspal occlusion, where the buccal maxillary cusps and/or the incisors are placed lingual to the buccal mandibular cusps and/or incisors.

reverse overjet *See* reverse horizontal overlap.

reversed Towne's projection Modified Towne's projection (q.v.) used to demonstrate the frontal bones. Used in dental radiography to demonstrate the mandibular condyles in a coronal plane.

reversible Able to change in either direction. *R. hydrocolloid impression material. See* impression material.

reversion Returning to a previous position.

revert To return to a former condition or habit.

review General appraisal of past events or of a subject. A reconsideration of facts.

rhesus factor Antigen factor present in the blood cells of about 85% of people, who are said to be *rhesus positive*. The remaining 15% who lack this factor are said to be *rhesus negative*.

rheumatic fever Acute condition exhibiting fever, inflammation and pain in the joints. May also damage the delicate heart lining resulting in endocarditis (q.v.).

rheumatism Generalized term for any condition causing pain and stiffness of muscles and joints and of unknown origin.

rhin- (rhino-) Prefix denoting the nose.

rhinitis Inflammation of the mucous membrane lining of the nasal cavity.

rhinorrhoea Persistent watery mucous discharge from the nose, as in the common cold.

rhizotomy Surgical cutting of a nerve root, generally for the relief of pain such as that caused in a persistent tic douloureux (q.v.).

RI Retention index. *See* index.

riboflavin British Pharmacopoeia name for what was formerly known as vitamin B_2. Yellow crystalline powder concerned with the metabolism of living cells.

ribosome Granular content of a cell containing RNA (q.v.) whose function is to produce proteins.

rickets Deficiency disease caused by lack of vitamin D which gives rise to bone deformities and poor tooth calcification. Treated by adequate doses of vitamin D and ultraviolet or sunlight.

Ricketts appliance *See* appliance.

ridge A projecting structure, a crest. *Alveolar r.* That part of the alveolus and mucosa that remains following the extraction of teeth. *Fibrous r.* Excessive fibrous tissue that has replaced the bone of the crest of the ridge. *Flabby r.* Flabby tissue that has replaced the bone of the ridge crest. *Marginal r.* Ridge forming the outer margins on the occlusal surface of a premolar or molar, or the lingual surface of an anterior tooth.

Oblique r. Ridge running obliquely across the occlusal surface of a maxillary molar.

rigor Severe attack of shivering, usually accompanying acute pyrexia.

rim Outer border or edge of that which is roughly circular. *See also* occlusal rim.

Ringer's solution Physiological isotonic solution containing sodium chloride (common salt), calcium and potassium chloride in sterile water. The principal vehicle for the ingredients of a local anaesthetic solution.

Risdon approach Surgical technique in which the submandibular area is approached through an incision below and behind the angle of the mandible.

risk Probability that an event will occur in the future, or the probability that an individual develops a given disease or experiences a change in health status during a specified interval of time.

risk factor A characteristic, behaviour or exposure with an association to a particular disease.

RNA (ribonucleic acid) Substance present in all living cells and controlling the synthesis of cellular proteins. Similar in composition to DNA (q.v.).

Roach clasp *See* clasp.

Rochette bridge *See* bridge.

rod Slender, straight, round metal bar. *Enamel r.* Near-parallel rod or prism forming tooth enamel.

rodent ulcer *See* basal cell carcinoma.

roentgen Obsolescent unit of radiation exposure now superseded by the kerma (q.v.).

roentgenogram *See* radiograph.

roentgenograph *See* radiograph.

rongeurs (bone-nibbling forceps) *See* forceps.

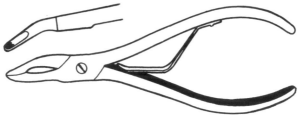

Rongeurs

root 1. In dentistry, that part of the tooth, below the crown, which is normally invested in cementum. 2. In anatomy, the origin of a structure. *Anatomical r.* That part of the tooth covered by, and including, cementum. *Clinical r.* That part of the anatomical root which is attached to the alveolar bone by periodontal ligament. *R. amputation.* Surgical separation and removal of one root from a multirooted tooth while retaining the remaining root or roots. *R. filling.* 1. Filling and sealing of a root canal. 2. Material or combination of materials used to obturate root canals. *R. planing.* Removal of necrotic cementum and planing of root surfaces. *R. resection. See* r. amputation (preferred term). *R. splitting forceps. See* forceps.

root canal Space within a dental root containing pulp which runs from the coronal pulp chamber to the apex of the tooth and is surrounded by dentine. Accessory or lateral canals branch off the main canal to extend to the root surface. *Accessory r. canal.* A branch of the main canal at any point along the root. *R. c. culturing.* (Clinically archaic, largely for research) Method of checking root canals for cultivable micro-organisms by sampling contents. *R. c. dressing.* Temporary filling material placed in a root canal system to eliminate infection, reduce periapical inflammation or induce apexification. Examples include non-setting calcium hydroxide paste, steroid/antibiotic pastes. *R. c. explorer. See* broach. *R. c. file.* Hand-held or engine-driven tool for enlarging root canals in a rasping or planing action. *R. c. filling condenser.* Thin tapered hand instrument with flat end, circular in cross-section, designed to condense materials in root canals. *R. c. filling (McSpadden) compactor.* Rotary instrument which softens root filling materials by frictional heat and condenses them apically into the canal by an Archimedean screw principle. *R. c. filling.* Material employed to fill and seal a prepared root canal. *R. c. preparation.* Shaping and cleaning of a root canal to eliminate micro-organisms and pulp tissue in readiness for filling. *R. c. filling point.* Synonym: *r. c. filling cone.* Tapered cone of material used to fill root canals. 1. *Master r. c. filling point.* Cone of filling material used to seal the apex of the tooth. 2. *Accessory r. c. filling points.* Supplementary cones of material used to fill in canal space around the master r. c. filling point. *R. c. paste carrier (rotary paste filler), lentulo (spiral root canal) filler.* Rotary instrument used to convey fluid materials into a root canal by Archimedean screw action. *R. c. plugger (see* plugger). Tapered instrument with a circular cross-section and flat end for vertical condensation of root filling materials. *R. c. reamer.* Hand-held or engine-driven tool

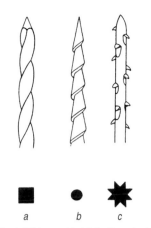

a, 'K'-type file; *b*, 'H'-type or Hedström file; *c*, barbed broach.
Root canal instruments

for enlarging root canals in a rotational motion. *R. c. sealer.* Fluid cement used in root canal fillings. *R. c. spreader.* Tapered instrument with circular cross-section and pointed tip for lateral condensation of root filling materials by a wedge-like action. *R. c. treatment.* Generic term to describe the process of pulpectomy, root canal shaping, cleaning and filling in the preservation of pulpally compromised teeth.

ropivacaine (Naropin®) A long-acting amide local anaesthetic agent.

rosin (colophony) Residue following the distillation of crude turpentine. Used in dentistry as a constituent of certain impression compounds and in varnishes.

rotary instrument Hand- or power-operated instrument that is rotated in order to function, e.g. a bur.

rotary paste filler *See* root canal paste carrier.

rotate To turn around an axis.

rotated oblique lateral projection Modification of the oblique lateral projection (q.v.) in which the position of the mandible is rotated in relation to the cassette. Used to view the incisor, canine and premolar areas.

rotation 1. Force applied to a tooth in order to rotate it about its long axis. 2. Malposition of a tooth due to rotation about its long axis. A qualifying prefix generally indicates the direction of rotation.

rotational tomography Radiographic tomographic technique in which the focal spot and the film move in a circular pattern.

rouge (jeweller's rouge) Finely divided ferric oxide polishing powder used mainly to polish metals.

rouleau Collection of red blood cells piled on each other like coins.

RPD Removable partial denture. *See* denture.

RPP Rapidly progressive periodontitis.

-rrhagia Suffix denoting abnormal or excessive flow or discharge.

211

-rrhoea Suffix denoting discharge or flow from an organ.

rubber base General term for elastic dental impression material.

rubber cup (prophylaxis cup) Flexible rubber cup used in a handpiece with polishing paste to clean and polish teeth and prostheses.

rubber dam Thin sheet of rubber perforated by a punch and clamped over a tooth or teeth to isolate them from the rest of the mouth. A frame keeps the rubber stretched and away from the teeth. It keeps the teeth in question dry and prevents foreign bodies, debris and strong medicaments escaping into the mouth and hence the possibility of inhaling or swallowing them. Also prevents contamination of the field of operation by saliva or micro-organisms. Hypersensitivity reaction to latex has necessitated the development of latex-free alternatives. *R.d. clamp.* Spring clamp applied to grip the cervical area of a tooth to retain rubber dam and in some cases cotton wool rolls. There are different sizes and designs to fit molars, premolars and incisors. *R.d. clamp forceps.* Instrument with self-locking device used to apply and remove rubber dam clamps. *R.d. frame.* Flexible frame used to hold the rubber dam in a taut state, away from the field of operation. *R.d. holder.* Elastic fabric band furnished with clips and placed behind the head in order to hold the rubber dam away from the field of operation. *R.d. ligature.* Length of dental floss tied firmly around the neck of a tooth to retain the rubber dam. *R.d. mask.* Variant of rubber dam consisting of a square of rubber dam attached to a square of tear-resistant paper with two elastic loops that may be hooked around the patient's ears. *R.d. punch.* Instrument used to punch various sized holes in a sheet of rubber dam. *R.d. weight.* Small metal weight clipped to the lower border of the rubber dam to control and stretch it.

rubefacient Agent that causes local reddening of the skin.

rubella *See* German measles.

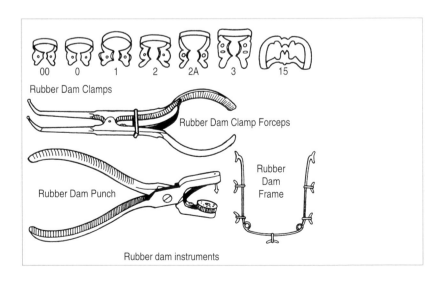

Rubber dam instruments

rudimentary Vestigial. Not completely developed.

ruga Ridge, as of mucous membrane.

rugae Plural of ruga. *R. palatina.* Ridges of mucous membrane found on the surface of the hard palate.

sac A pouch-like cavity.

sacchar- (saccharo-) Prefix denoting sugar.

saccharide One of the carbohydrates which includes the sugars. Divided into mono, di-, trisaccharides, etc.

saccharin Intense sweetener, approx. 500 times sweeter than sucrose. *See* sweetener.

saccular Shaped like a sac.

saddle In dentistry, that portion of a partial denture which rests on the alveolar ridge and carries the teeth. *Bounded s.* A saddle bounded at each end by a natural tooth.

safe-for-teeth Food, drink or confectionery product which does not reduce plaque pH to less than 5.7 and is not dentally erosive.

safe light Light used in a dark-room during the processing of radiographic films in which exposed films may be unwrapped, placed in a film holder and then immersed in developing solution.

sagittal Running anteroposteriorly in the midline. *S. axis. See* axis.

sagittal split osteotomy Surgical technique to correct mandibular prognathism and anterior open bite deformity. The ramus of the mandible is split vertically between two cuts in the cortices, the first through the inner cortex horizontally above the mandibular foramen and the second through the outer cortex at various sites below the mandibular foramen.

salbutamol (Ventolin®) A beta adrenergic agonist drug used to treat asthma. Dentists may need to administer this drug during an asthmatic attack in a patient. It is administered via an inhaler or nebulizer.

saline Relating to or containing salt. *S. solution.* Solution of salt in water. HYPERTONIC S.S. Solution stronger than normal strength HYPOTONIC S.S. Solution weaker than normal strength. NORMAL or ISOTONIC S.S. Physiological 0.9% solution that is isotonic to blood. May be administered intravenously to restore lost blood salts and fluid.

saliva Fluid excreted into the mouth by the salivary glands—parotid, submandibular and sublingual. Assists mastication of food and its digestion by the enzyme amylase. It also plays a part in speech, taste and the natural cleansing of the mouth and oral tissue and has a protective role on the teeth and the gingival and oral mucosa. *S. ejector.* Tube with shaped end or tip through which saliva and other liquids are aspirated from the mouth at low velocity. *See also* whole saliva; artificials Saliva.

salivary Relating to saliva, the glands producing saliva and their ducts. *S. amylase. See* ptyalin. *S. calculus.* Calculus present in the salivary gland or duct. *S. cannula.* Metal or polythene cannula inserted into the duct of the gland to collect saliva. *S. duct.* Duct conveying saliva from a salivary gland to the mouth. Consists of three parts: (*a*) the portion connecting the gland to the striated portion, (*b*) the striated portion that can modify

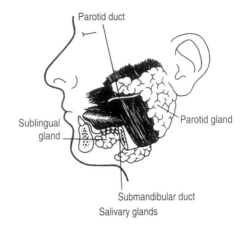

Parotid duct

Sublingual gland

Parotid gland

Submandibular duct

Salivary glands

the composition of saliva, (c) the excretory duct that conveys the modified saliva into the mouth. *S. fistula.* Abnormal passage conducting saliva from a salivary gland or its duct into the mouth or to the skin of the face. *S. gland. See* gland.

salivate To produce a flow of saliva.

salivation The act of producing saliva. The rate of salivation varies during the day; it may be increased by visual stimulation or by certain odours and decreases during sleep.

salmonella Rod-shaped, Gram-negative bacteria belonging to the genus *Salmonella* transmitted through direct or indirect contact with faeces. *S. enteritidis* is a frequent cause of food poisoning via contaminated dairy products and cooked meats. *S. typhi* is the causative organism of typhoid.

salt 1. Compound obtained by the reaction between an acid and a base. 2. Sodium chloride or common salt. *S. sterilizer. See* sterilizer.

sandarac varnish Archaic term. Varnish consisting of a resin dissolved in alcohol and used to provide a thin water-proof film on models and some restorations.

sandwich osteotomy Surgical technique of increasing ridge height by horizontally sectioning the mandible, above the level of the neurovascular bundle, and inserting bone or an allelograph material.

sandwich technique Impression technique in which a light, medium and heavy impression material are used simultaneously to form layers in the set impression.

sanitary pontic Pontic of a bridge designed to be self-cleansing.

sarc- (sarco-) Prefix denoting muscle or fleshy tissue.

sarcoidosis A chronic but benign granulomatous disease of unknown aetiology. Most commonly seen orofacial lesions occur in the salivary glands, particularly the parotid, gingivae, cheeks and floor of the mouth. Also on the skin, eyes, lungs and bones.

sarcoma Malignant tumour arising from connective tissue or its derivatives.

sarcomatous Relating to a sarcoma.

saturated Describes solution to which the addition of any further solute will cause precipitation.

saucer Rounded, hollow depression.

saucerization In surgery, the conversion of a cyst cavity into one with a saucer-like shape.

scab Hard crust of dried blood, serum or pus.

scabies Contagious, irritating skin rash caused by *Acarus scabiei*, a parasitic mite.

scald Burn caused by steam or hot liquid.

scale 1. Flake of dead epidermal cells shed from the skin. 2. In dentistry, to remove deposits of calculus and debris from the teeth.

scaler Instrument for removing calculus and other deposits from the tooth surface. There are five main types. *Curette s.* Hand instrument with a sharp, hollow, ground blade like an excavator used for debridement of periodontal pockets and tooth roots. Usually made in sets of six. *Periodontal hoe s.* Hand instrument with small blade at right angles to the stem. Generally in sets of four and used with a pulling action. *Push, watch spring, Guy's* or *Cushing s.* Hand scaler with thin, chisel-shaped blade, either curved or straight, in line with the handle. Used with a pushing motion. *Trihedral s.* Two main types: sickle and jacquette. Instruments with 2 blades, one either side of the superior surface which ends in a point. Principally used for the removal of supragingival calculus or calculus located just below the gingival margin. *Ultrasonic s.* Scaling instrument whose tip is activated by ultrasonic vibrations and incorporates a water spray. It has several interchangeable tips of different shapes. Theoretically, should not be used on a patient with a pacemaker as it may upset the rhythm of the heart.

scaling Removal of calculus and other deposits from the crown and roots of teeth by means of scalers.

scalpel Originally a sharp cutting blade with flat metal handle in one piece. Now consists of a metal handle with detachable, sterile-packed disposable blades of numbered assorted shapes.

Scandonest® *See* mepivacaine.

scar (cicatrix) Mark left on the skin following the healing of a wound. *S. tissue.* Soft, very vascular connective tissue newly formed during the healing process. It becomes dense fibrous scar tissue with very little blood supply and may contract considerably.

scarlet fever Streptococcal infection causing a scarlet skin rash and possibly serious complications.

scatter Radiation that has been deflected at the surface of, or during its passage through, objects, such as teeth and bone. Care should be taken never to stand in the beam of X-rays and at least 2 metres behind the X-ray source.

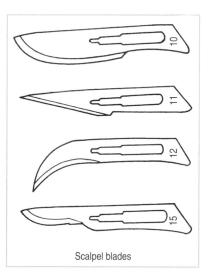

Scalpel blades

Schwann cell Nucleated cell forming the outer aspect of the myelin sheath of nerve fibres. There is one Schwann cell between each node of Ranvier.

schwannoma *See* neurilemmoma.

scissors Cutting instrument with apposed blades and handles on a central fulcrum. *Cross-beak ligature s.* Used in orthodontics for cutting ligature wires, especially against flat or tooth surfaces. *Crown s. (beebee s.).* Scissors with small stout blades, either curved or straight, used to trim copper rings, stainless steel strips or tape and pre-formed metal orthodontic bands. *Gum s. (surgical s.).* Scissors with finer blades that may be curved or straight. *Universal s.* Scissors with straight, broad shearing blades serrated to prevent slip when cutting metals and wires.

scler- (sclero-) Prefix denoting thickening or hardening.

scleroderma A collagen disease of unknown aetiology. Skin and mucous membrane lesions are characterized by progressive hardening and thickening in patches. The periodontal ligament may be affected.

sclerose To harden.

sclerosis Hardening or induration of soft tissue. The term is also applied to bone with an increased calcification.

sclerotic Relating to sclerosis. *S. dentine. See* dentine.

-scope Suffix denoting an instrument used for observation or examination.

scopolamine *See* hyoscine.

screen 1. Partition used for protection. 2. Agent used to intercept injurious agents. *S. film.* Film whose emulsion is more sensitive to light than to radiation. Used in cassettes fitted with intensifying screens. *See also* oral screen.

screw Metal cylindrical object with external or internal spiral thread. *Dentine s.* Screw of various lengths and diameters which is inserted into a matching prepared hole in dentine to provide additional retention for a restoration. *Orthodontic s.* A device used to move one or more teeth as part of a fixed or removable appliance. *Pulpal s.* Tapered screw of various sizes and lengths with a square slotted head. A small finger-held box spanner or cross-sectioned screwdriver is used to insert it into a root-filled pulp canal to provide increased retention for a restoration. *S. post.* Threaded post used in a root-treated tooth to provide retention for a restoration crown or precision attachment.

scurvy Less common vitamin deficiency disease due to a lack of raw fruits and vegetables and hence of vitamin C. Generalized disease affecting connective tissue and bone and causing delayed healing. Seen in the mouth as capillary bleeding from the gingivae accompanied by loose teeth and foetid breath. Treatment is by the administration of vitamin C.

seal Substance used to effect a closure. *Anterior oral s.* Automatic seal of the oral cavity achieved by lip contact or contact with the lower lip and tongue and/or palatal mucosa. *Border s.* Contact of a border of a denture with the soft tissues that prevents the passage of air and thus loss of retention. The term *peripheral seal* is deprecated. *Peripheral s. See* border s. *Posterior oral s.* Seal made by the soft palate and the dorsum of the tongue during speech and swallowing. *Posterior palatal s. (post dam).* Seal at the posterior border of an upper denture.

sealant Substance (usually an unfilled composite resin) used to coat the pits and fissures of a tooth surface to prevent dental caries.

sealer *See* root canal sealer.

seating lug Small component welded to the lingual aspect of an orthodontic band in order to provide a ledge through which pressure may be applied when seating the band onto a tooth.

sebaceous Belonging or relating to sebum. Secreting a greasy, oily or fatty substance. *S. gland. See* gland.

sebum Fatty secretion of sebaceous glands that is protective and water repellent and is usually found in association with hair follicles.

second (s) The SI unit of time and is the duration of 9,192,631,770 periods of the radiation corresponding to the transition between the two hyperfine levels of the ground state of caesium-133 atom.

second impression *See* final impression.

secondary Second in order of time or importance. *S. dentine. See* dentine. *S. dentition. See* permanent dentition. *S. epithelialization vestibuloplasty.* Surgical technique for the deepening of the gingival sulcus when the extended defect is allowed to epithelialize from the adjacent mucosal surfaces. *S. image.* Phenomenon seen in panoramic dental radiography whereby the image of an object on the tube side of the patient is projected onto the opposite side. *S. lesion. See* lesion. *S. occlusal trauma.* Injury to the periodontium caused by physiologically normal occlusal forces on the tooth with a reduced periodontium.

secrete To produce, by secretion, certain chemical substances, such as enzymes, that are useful in further chemical processes.

secretion Action of certain organisms, glands or specialized cells in producing a new substance that passes either into the bloodstream or via ducts to wherever it is required. *Acinar s.* Saliva formed in the acinus that has a similar ionic composition to that of blood plasma and tissue fluid.

secretory Relating to secretion. *S. potential.* Electrical potential change recorded in a salivary gland during stimulation of secretion.

sectional appliance Fixed orthodontic appliance involving a number of teeth in one segment of the jaws.

sectional archwire Archwire fitted to a number of teeth and confined to one section of the dental arch.

sectional denture *See* denture.

sectional impression *See* impression.

sectional root-filling technique Method of sealing the apical portion of a root canal with a portion of core material (e.g. gutta percha) and sealer, leaving the rest of the pulp space unfilled in order to accommodate a post.

sedate 1. Collected, composed, not lively. 2. To administer a sedative to an individual.

sedation Production of a relaxed state. *S. technique.* Method of sedating patients by the use of drugs (e.g. midazolam) to produce a state of depression of the central nervous system without complete loss of consciousness. Verbal contact with the patient is maintained and local analgesics are usually administered to produce analgesia. *Inhalational s.* Sedation delivered via the respiratory system, usually using titrated nitrous oxide and oxygen.

sedative 1. Allaying excitement or irritability. 2. Drug to relieve pain and anxiety, e.g. temazepam, diazepam.

segment A part cut off or separable from others.

segmental surgery Surgical mobilization and repositioning of the alveolar segments of either the maxilla or the mandible together with the teeth in that segment.

selective grinding (spot grinding) Planned adjustment of the occlusal anatomy of teeth by grinding.

self-cleansing area Area of the teeth less liable to accumulate plaque and food debris because of the action of the soft tissues and chewing.

self-curing acrylic *See* resin, autopolymerizing.

self-limiting Relates to a disease that continues for a specific, limited period of time by reason of its own characteristics and not because of external influences.

self-straightening wire Fine stainless steel wire wound onto a labial bow orthodontic appliance as a separate fine-wire bow, to retract incisor teeth.

sella An orthodontic landmark defined as the centre of the sella turcica.

sella turcica Deep depression, said to be in the shape of a Turkish saddle, in the upper surface of the body of the sphenoid.

SEM Scanning electron microscope.

semantic Pertaining to the meaning of words and their changes in meaning.

semi- Prefix denoting half or partly.

semi-adjustable articulator *See* articulator.

semi-lunar valve Half-moon shaped heart valve situated in the ventricular openings to the aorta and the pulmonary artery and which prevents the backflow of blood from the arteries.

semi-permeable Partially permeable. Term generally applied to membranes which, in the process of osmosis, allow the passage of certain molecules but prevent that of others.

semi-precious metal casting alloy Alloy with noble metal content of at least 25% but <75%. Includes low gold content and silver palladium alloys.

sensation Appreciation of an impulse conveyed by an afferent nerve.

sensitive In general, able to feel a sensation; being responsive to or able to transmit a stimulus.

sensitivity Being sensitive to a stimulus.

sensory Relating to sensation.

sensory nerve Afferent nerve conveying sensory impulses from the periphery to the spinal cord and brain.

separating medium Substance used to prevent one surface sticking to another, such as a plaster of Paris cast to the impression material, e.g. soap solution, glycerol, and numerous proprietary preparations.

separating strip *See* abrasive strip.

separating wire Soft brass wire sometimes placed between teeth to separate them prior to the placement of orthodontic bands.

separation In dentistry, the achievement of spacing between teeth in the same dental arch, usually in order to place orthodontic bands.

separator An instrument using a screw force to move teeth apart. Generally, used to obtain a satisfactory contact point in dental restorations.

sepsis Presence in the blood or other tissues of pathogenic micro-organisms or their toxins.

septa Plural of septum.

Septanest® *See* articaine.

septic Relating to sepsis or to a condition caused by sepsis.

septicaemia Presence and multiplication in the blood of micro-organisms and their toxins. Originally called *blood poisoning*. Treatment is by antibiotics.

Septrin® *See* co-trimoxazole.

septum Division or partition, as between the two nasal cavities. *Interdental s.* Bone between the roots of teeth.

sequel Pathological condition resulting from disease.

sequelae Plural of sequel.

sequestration Separation of a part from the whole, e.g. the rejection of necrosed bone by a pathological process.

sequestrectomy Removal of a sequestrum.

sequestrum Piece of bone that has died through loss of blood supply and then separated from the living bone.

serial Series of events, following one another. *S. extractions.* Developed in the 1940s. Planned serial removal of primary and permanent teeth over a period of time to relieve crowding. Is no longer in common practice.

series Events or things of a similar kind, arranged in a regular order.

serous 1. Relating to or resembling serum. 2. Describing saliva which is thin and derived from blood serum. *S. secretion.* Saliva of relatively low viscosity secreted mainly by the parotid gland at a rapid flow rate. It is rich in the enzyme amylase.

serpiginous Possessing a wavy border.

serrated Having a saw-like edge.

serum Clear, thin watery residue of blood from which the blood cells and fibrin have been removed. *S. hepatitis. See* hepatitis.

serumal calculus Deprecated term for subgingival calculus (q.v.).

sessile Having a broadly based attachment as distinct from a peduncle.

setting Hardening, as of plaster of Paris or dental cements. *S. time.* Period of time measured from the start of a mix of a material until it has set. *S. expansion.* The dimensional increase that occurs as various materials harden (or set), e.g. plaster of Paris, dental stone, casting investment.

set-up Deprecated term for trial denture (q.v.) or tooth arrangement.

sevoflurane A volatile liquid anaesthetic that is sometimes used in inhalation sedation.

SFD (source-to-film distance) *See* FFD (focus-to-film distance).

shank 1. Thinner portion of a hand instrument joining the blade to the handle. 2. Non-cutting portion of a bur.

Sharpey's fibres Those portions of the principal fibres of the periodontal ligament that are embedded in root cementum and alveolar bone proper, and which contribute to the anchorage of the tooth.

'sharps' A generic term used to describe the potentially dangerous instruments such as burs, needles, scalpels, endodontic instruments, etc. *S. injury* with an infected instrument puts the recipient at risk of contracting a serious, blood-borne viral infection from infected patients, notably: a 12–20% chance of contracting hepatitis B; a 2% chance of transmission of hepatitis C; and a 0.2% chance of infection from a HIV-infected individual. *S. containers* are receptacles intended to hold the

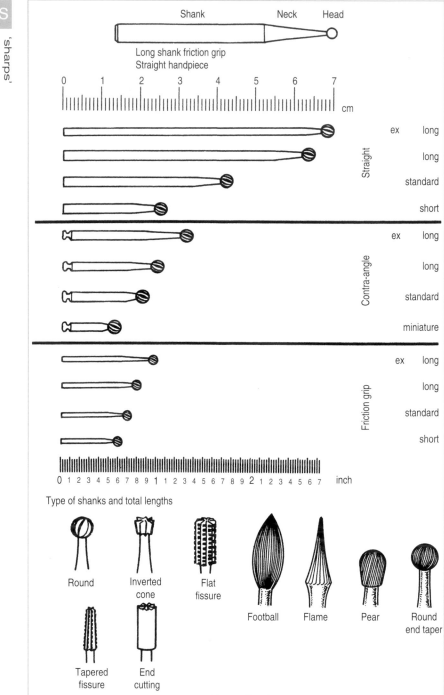

Shank   Neck   Head

Long shank friction grip
Straight handpiece

Straight

ex long
long
standard
short

Contra-angle

ex long
long
standard
miniature

Friction grip

ex long
long
standard
short

Type of shanks and total lengths

Round   Inverted cone   Flat fissure   Football   Flame   Pear   Round end taper

Tapered fissure   End cutting

Types of head

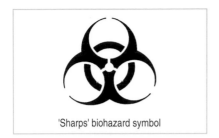

'Sharps' biohazard symbol

potentially infected medical waste. They should be manufactured to B.S. specifications in respect to aperture and closure, resistance to penetration, impact and toppling and should be coloured yellow. They should be marked with the following symbol and marked 'Caution, biological hazard'. Dentists have a legal responsibility to ensure that all waste is disposed of safely.

shears *See* bone, shears.

sheath In anatomy, a layer of connective tissue covering structures such as arteries, muscles and nerves.

shelf life Length of time that a material or drug may be stored without deteriorating and thus remain usable.

shell crown *See* crown.

shellac Natural beetle exudate, occasionally used in the construction of temporary denture bases and impression trays. *See* varnish.

shingles (herpes zoster) Virus infection of the nervous system in which inflammation develops in the sensory ganglion of the cranial nerves or the posterior root ganglions of the spinal nerves. Closely related to the chicken pox virus.

shock Condition in which there is a sudden fall in blood pressure which, if untreated, leads to a lack of oxygen in the tissues and loss of tissue fluid, both

exacerbating the condition. May prove fatal. *Anaphylactic s.* Severe reaction induced by exposure to a substance to which the patient is sensitive. *Delayed s.* Shock which occurs some time after a traumatic experience. *Electric s.* Shock caused by the passage of electric current through the body. *Primary (vasovagal) s.* Occurs instantly from pain, fear or unpleasant sights, as in a faint. The patient should be placed in a prone position, tight clothing loosened and there should be an adequate air supply. *Surgical s.* Shock due to haemorrhage or loss of tissue fluid, as in burns.

short-cone radiography Dental radiographic technique in which the X-ray machine is fitted with a cone that is generally shorter than 20 cm.

shoulder preparation Shelf or shoulder cut around, or partly around, the neck of a tooth to provide a satisfactory thickness of material (e.g. porcelain) for construction of a crown.

shoulder trimmer Hand instrument with a narrow serrated blade used to trim a shoulder preparation and provide a smooth surface.

shrinkage Reduction in volume. *Casting s.* The contraction or volume change that occurs as a molten metal solidifies when cast in a mould.

SI units Système International d'Unitès. Internationally agreed system of units used for scientific purposes. There are seven basic and two supplementary units. All other physical quantities are expressed in derived units consisting of two or more base units.

sial- (sialo-) Prefix denoting saliva or salivary gland.

sialoadenitis Inflammation of the salivary gland. When the parotid gland is involved it is known as *parotitis* (mumps).

221

sialogogue Drug that increases the flow of saliva.

sialogram The technique of producing a sialograph.

sialograph Radiograph of the ducts and acini of the salivary glands following the introduction of radio-opaque material into them. Used to determine whether a gland or duct contains calculus.

sialography Radiographic investigation of the structure and function of salivary glands following the introduction of radio-opaque material into their ducts and acini.

sialolith *See* salivary calculus.

sialorrhoea Profuse salivation, produced reflexly by irritative conditions of the mouth or oesophagus or by certain drugs.

sickle cell anaemia Inherited blood disease in which red blood cells are crescent shaped and unable to transport sufficient oxygen. Prior knowledge of the condition is required if an anaesthetic is to be administered.

sickle scaler *See* scaler.

side shift *See* Bennett movement.

side-effect Effect other than that expected from the normal reaction to a drug.

Sievert (Sv) SI unit of radiation dose when factors of the type of radiation (equivalent dose) and different tissue sensitivity to ionizing radiation (effective dose) are taken into account.

sigmoid notch Notch on the superior border of the ramus of the mandible lying between the condyle and the coronoid process. Also known as the *mandibular notch*.

signs Abnormality recognized by an observer, such as high temperature, sweating or pallor.

Silane Difunctional molecule used to coat filler particles in filled composites, providing link between filler particles and resin matrix.

silica (silicon dioxide) Natural substance found in three forms—quartz, cristobalite and eridymite. *Fused s.* Used widely in dentistry in cements and as a refractory material in investment materials.

silicate cement The first direct tooth coloured filling materials and now rarely, if ever used. Consists of a mixture of fluoride-containing aluminosilicate glass powders, and phosphoric acid causing the cement to set hard. Irritant to pulp, susceptible to erosion and must be kept moist to maintain translucency.

silicon carbide Abrasive powder incorporated in carborundum.

silicon dioxide *See* silica.

silicone Brittle, non-metallic element occurring in amorphous and crystalline forms.

silicone elastomeric impression material *See* impression material.

silicone grease Lubricant containing silicone and used in place of a mineral or vegetable oil.

silico-phosphate cement Silicate cement containing zinc oxide and used for temporary fillings, cementation and die making.

silk ligature Non-absorbable silk thread, used for sutures.

silver Soft white, ductile and malleable metal. *S. casting alloy.* Precious metal casting alloy composed of 95% silver and 5% copper. Used mainly in the construction of cast dental splints in surgical cases. *S. halide.* Metallic salt embedded in a gelatine matrix coating the plastic surface of a radiographic film. *S. nitrate.* Crystalline substance with coagulant, antiseptic and caustic properties. Previously used pure, or in an ammoniacal solution, but seldom used now. When reduced by oil of cloves it produces a black deposit. *S. point.* Thin, conical metal point, mainly composed of silver, used in conjunction with a sealant to obturate the apical foramen at a root canal filling. Made in graded sizes matching reamer and file sizes. Now superseded by gutta percha. *S. solder.* Soldering alloy composed mainly of silver, copper, zinc and tin which melts at a temperature well below that of the metals being soldered.

simple cavity Preparation involving only one surface of the clinical crown of a tooth.

simple (or closed) fracture *See* fracture.

sinus 1. In anatomy, a cavity within a bone or other tissue. 2. Infected tract communication with the skin or with a hollow organ. In dentistry, the formation of a sinus is generally due to the non-vitality and periapical infection of a tooth. *S. balloon.* A rubber or plastic balloon-like device that may be expanded with either a liquid or air and is used to support depressed fractures of the zygoma and/or the maxilla. *Maxillary s. See* maxillary.

sinusitis Acute or chronic inflammation of a sinus caused by bacteria or allergy. Infective material draining from it may lead to inflammation of the bronchi (bronchitis). Sinusitis may cause referred pain from those teeth adjacent to the sinus lining.

sinusoid Resembling a sinus.

Siqveland matrix band holder *See* matrix band.

Sjögren's syndrome Syndrome characterized by the deficient secretion of the lacrimal, salivary and other glands, giving rise to a kerato-conjunctivitis, swelling or atrophy of the salivary glands, a dry mouth and a hoarse voice.

skeletal Pertaining to the skeleton. *S. pattern.* Relationships between the dental bases in the sagittal, vertical and transverse planes. *S. system.* Body system consisting of bones, joints and muscles concerned with movement.

skeleton Bony supporting structure of the body. *S. denture. See* denture.

skia- Prefix denoting shadow.

skin Outer integument or covering of the body, consisting of the epidermis (outer layer) and dermis (thicker, deeper connective tissue layer). *S. dose. See* entrance dose.

skin grafting vestibuloplasty (epithelial or buccal inlay) Surgical deepening of the sulcus followed by grafting a split skin thickness graft to cover the exposed portion of bone.

skin hook Surgical instrument with a fine hook at one end used to grasp tissue during dissecting or suturing.

skull Box-like structure of bone situated on top of the spinal column, containing and protecting the brain, eyes, ears and carrying the upper jaw and attached lower jaw. Consists of two parts—the cranium and the facial part. Its various bones are joined at their edges by bony sutures, which allow for growth. Clothed by two groups of muscles—those of expression and those concerned with mastication. Similar to other bones, the skull stores calcium and produces red blood cells within its bone marrow. *S.-cap.* 1. A type of headgear used as an anchor for the fixation of jaw fractures and also in extra-oral orthodontic therapy. 2. Calvaria (q.v.).

slab *See* mixing slab.

slaking Method of mixing zinc phosphate cement that results in a delayed setting. A small portion of the powder is allowed to remain in the liquid for up to 2 minutes before the main mix takes place.

slide 1. In microscopy, the glass plate on which specimens are mounted for examination. 2. A photographic slide for projection. 3. In gnathology, the short jaw movement that occurs from the moment that the teeth first touch to the time that the jaws come to rest in centric occlusion.

sliding genioplasty Surgical procedure to increase the degree of mental prominence, by detaching the lower border of the mandible and repositioning it more anteriorly.

slit beam radiography Dental radiographic technique in which, by means of slit collimation of an X-ray beam that is aligned perpendicular to the dental arches during radiography, a panoramic view of the jaws is produced.

SLOB Same Lingual:Opposite Buccal rule. *See* parallax.

slough Necrotic tissue separating from living tissue.

small intestine That part of the alimentary canal leading from the stomach to the large intestine. It is responsible for most of the digestion process.

smallpox (variola) A serious contagious disease caused by the variola virus which is sometimes fatal. The disease, characterized by a fever, accompanied by an extensive rash, was declared eradicated in 1980 by the WHO.

smear Substance spread on a glass slide by way of preparation for examination by microscopy. *Cervical s.* A sample of tissue taken from the cervix of the womb. *S.layer.* Thin superficial dentine layer created during cavity preparation consisting of cutting debris and possibly bacteria. May interfere with subsequent adhesive bonding.

smear layer *See* smear.

SN plane A transverse plane through the skull at a level represented by a line drawn on a lateral skull radiograph between the sella and the nasion. *See* Appendix 10.

Snyder's test A test used to predict a patient's susceptibility to caries by determining the concentration of acid-producing bacteria in saliva.

socket Hollow into which another part fits. In dentistry, the cavity in the alveolar bone of either jaw which accommodates the root of a tooth.

sodium chloride (salt) mouthwash Saline mouthwash consisting of one tablespoonful of table salt to one tumbler of warm water.

sodium fluoride paste Paste containing sodium fluoride, kaolin, glycerine and pigments. Applied to sensitive areas on teeth, such as the cervical regions, to reduce sensitivity and harden the enamel.

sodium hypochlorite A colourless, transparent liquid used at a variety of different concentrations (measured as available, or free, chlorine) as a disinfectant and deodorant. In dentistry, used between 1% and 5.25% (free chlorine) to irrigate and disinfect root canals during root canal preparation. Dakin's solution is a dilution (0.5% free chlorine) buffered with boric acid to pH 9.5 and used as an antiseptic to treat infected wounds.

sodium perborate Mouthwash ingredient that releases nascent oxygen, so preventing the growth of anaerobic organisms. Trade name: Bocasan®.

sodium phosphate A chemical used in alginate impression material to delay the reaction between the alginate and calcium sulphate and increase the setting time of the material.

sodium potassium tartrate (potassium sodium tartrate, Rochelle salt) Added to dental plaster to accelerate the setting reaction.

soft liner Soft polymeric material processed onto the fitting surface of a prosthesis to reduce any trauma to the underlying tissues. Usually consists of a synthetic elastomer.

soft palate Movable curtain of tissue extending downwards and backwards into the pharynx from the posterior border of the hard palate. Composed of a fold of mucous membrane whose two layers enclose muscles, glandular structures, blood vessels and nerves. During deglutition it is raised to assist in shutting off the nasal part of the pharynx from the portion below. The uvula (q.v.) hangs from its posterior free border.

soft radiation Less penetrating types of X-rays, beta rays and gamma rays.

sol 1. Colloidal solution in its liquid phase. 2. Abbreviation for a solution.

solder Fusible metal or metallic alloy used to join metal surfaces. When heat is applied to the joint and the solder, which has a lower melting point than the metals to be joined, it melts, runs over the join and hardens on cooling.

soldering Joining of two metal parts by means of solder.

solitary (or unicameral) bone cyst Cyst, within bone, usually without an obvious soft tissue lining.

soluble Capable of being dissolved.

solute Substance dissolved in a solvent to form a solution.

solution Uniform mixture of substances to form a liquid.

solvent Substance with the ability to dissolve another substance, e.g. chloroform and eucalyptus are solvents for gutta percha.

somatic Pertaining to the body as opposed to the mind. *S. effect*. Effect of radiation on the body cells. May be produced by a high dosage of radiation or the cumulative effects of a low dosage over a period of time, e.g. radiation burn (q.v.) and radiation dermatitis.

soporific Drug that induces sleep.

sore 1. Painful. 2. Lay term for any lesion of the skin or mucous membrane. *Canker s.* Aphthae. *Cold s.* Herpes simplex lesions, especially those near the lips. *Denture s.* Ulcer caused by an ill-fitting denture.

sorption Phenomenon of absorption and adsorption or the state in which both phenomena occur at the same time.

source *See* focal spot.

source-to-film distance (SFD) *See* FFD (focus-to-film distance).

space An empty area. *S. loss*. Loss of space in a dental arch when a tooth is lost by extraction or is developmentally absent. *Denture s. See* denture. *Freeway s. See* interocclusal clearance. *Interproximal s. See* interproximal. *Inter-radicular s.* The space between the roots of a multirooted tooth. *Periodontal s.* In radiology, the space seen on a radiograph between the cementum on the tooth root and alveolar bone. *S. maintainer*. Removable or fixed appliance designed to maintain an existing space in a dental arch.

spacer Thin layer of wax or other material interposed between two structures during an impression, in order to allow for a uniform space when it is removed. Used in special trays to allow for a uniform thickness of impression material or over such retention devices as the Dolder bar (q.v.). *S. cone. See* cone.

spasm Sudden involuntary contraction of muscles.

spatula Hand instrument with flat, blunt blade used to mix powders, liquids or pastes on a smooth surface.

spatulate 1. Flat, blunt end. 2. To mix with a spatula.

spatulation Mixing together of various materials with a spatula on a smooth flat surface to form a uniformly consistent mixture.

special tray *See* tray.

specialist One who, after undertaking extensive post-graduate training and then achieving the relevant qualifications, concentrates on a special branch of medicine or dentistry.

specific Particular; clearly distinguished from others. *S. treatment.* A well-established remedy that cures a particular ailment.

speech Sound produced by the passage of air through the vocal cords and modified by the tongue, cheeks, lips and soft palate. Controlled by the speech centre of the brain. *S. therapy.* Treatment by speech therapist for defects and disorders of speech including stammer, brain disorder, cleft palate, severe malocclusion and cases of deafness.

Spencer Wells artery forceps *See* forceps.

sphenoid bone Central, wedge-shaped skull bone situated beneath the brain consisting of a body, greater and lesser wings and processes. It articulates with the temporal, occipital, parietal, frontal, ethmoidal, malar, vomer and palate bones. It forms the posterior wall of each orbit. Through it pass the three nerve trunks from the trigeminal nerve carrying sensations from the face and mouth and supplying the motor nerves of the muscles of mastication and salivary glands. It contains a pair of air sinuses and gives attachment to the internal and external pterygoid and the temporal muscles of mastication.

spherical amalgam alloy *See* alloy.

sphincter Ring of muscle controlling the opening and closing of an orifice.

sphygmomanometer Instrument for measuring arterial blood pressure.

spinal cord Part of the central nervous system running from the base of the brain down through the central canal of the vertebrae.

spine 1. The backbone. 2. In anatomy, a pointed process.

spirillum Bacteria with a rigid helical cell structure. Bacteria belonging to the genus *Spirillum*.

spirochaete Bacteria with a flexible helical structure belonging to the phylum Spirochaetes. Some species are important pathogens, e.g. syphilis (*Treponema pallidum*) and Lyme disease (*Borrelia burgdorferi*). In dentistry *Treponema denticola* is associated with the incidence and severity of periodontal disease.

spittoon Basin attached to a dental unit (q.v.) for mouth rinsing or expectoration.

spleen Ductless organ lying close to the stomach beneath the diaphragm, producing lymphocytes and antibodies. It acts as a reservoir for blood and produces red and white cells in fetal life and white cells in adult life. It destroys spent red blood cells, storing the iron for haemoglobin production. Roughly 11 cm in length and 7 cm in width.

splint 1. Rigid appliance for the fixation of displaced parts. 2. A therapeutic appliance constructed of soft plastic, hard plastic or metal covering the occlusal surfaces of one of the dental arches. *See* occlusal overlay appliance.

splinting 1. Stabilizing one or more loose teeth by splinting them to firm adjacent teeth by means of wires, bands or cast splints made of metal or plastic. 2. Immobilization of fractured bone ends by wiring, pinning or splinting. *See also* fixation. *Flexible s.* Splinting used in avulsion and luxation injuries of teeth. Splint incorporates a flexible wire usually extending to one tooth either side of damaged tooth. *Rigid s.* Used in root fractured teeth where the splint usually extends to two teeth either side of damaged tooth.

split cast mounting In prosthetics, a method of mounting casts on an articulator to facilitate accurate removal and replacement and as a method of checking the accuracy of jaw relations.

split skin graft (Thiersch graft) *See* graft.

sponge gelatin Absorbable gelatin sponge that can be packed sterile into a socket to fill a space or to control haemorrhage.

spoon. Name sometimes given to an excavator (q.v.). *S. denture. See* denture.

spore 1. A form of dormant cell produced by some bacteria under adverse conditions which is very resistant to desiccation, heat, a variety of chemicals and radiation. Also called endospore. Some spore-forming bacteria are important pathogens, e.g. tetanus (*Clostridium tetani*) and anthrax (*Bacillus anthracis*).

2. Small asexual reproductive structures of seedless plants, algae, fungi, and some protozoa.

spot grinding *See* selective grinding.

spot welding Joining of metals at one point by means of pressure and heat generated by the passage of an electric current from a spot welder, without the use of filler metal.

spreader *See* root canal spreader.

spring In dentistry, a bent or coiled metal wire, used to place a force to move teeth or to provide elasticity to a dental appliance. *Auxiliary s. (finger s.).* Small gauge wire attached to arches, bows and removable appliances which applies gentle pressure to one or more teeth. *S. cantilever bridge (s. bridge). See* bridge. *S.-forming pliers. See* pliers.

sprue 1. In dentistry, wire (sometimes hollow), wax or plastic used during the casting process to provide an entrance for molten metal into a mould. It is attached to the wax pattern and the whole invested. When the invested material has set, the sprue is then removed or burnt out during the heating process before casting. 2. Metal that has cooled and become solid in the sprue hole. It has to be cut off from the casting. *S. former.* Conical base into which a casting sprue is fixed prior to investment.

spur Projection, as from a bone. A metal projection from a prosthesis.

sputum Saliva mixed with mucus expelled from the respiratory tract.

squamous Scaly or plate-like.

SSD Source–skin distance.

stability Being stable. Resistance to change. In prosthetics, the resistance of a prosthesis to displacement by functional forces.

stable Not moving, fixed, firmly established, resisting alteration.

Stafne's cavity Developmental invagination in the mandible in which lies the submandibular salivary gland.

stagnation area In dentistry, the opposite of a self-cleansing area (q.v.). Area where debris and plaque accumulate on a tooth and is not easily cleaned either naturally by the tongue or during mastication.

stain Dye or pigment used to provide colour. *Gram's s. See* Gram's staining. *S. porcelain.* Fine pigmented porcelain used to colour a porcelain restoration. *Extrinsic s.* Caused by external agents (e.g. foods or bacteria) which can be removed with cleaning/prophylaxis. *Intrinsic s.* Caused by changes in structure or thickness of dental tissues (e.g. enamel opacities due to increased porosity of enamel), or incorporation of pigments into tooth tissues during or after tooth formation.

stainless steel Alloy steel containing quantities of chromium and other elements. Very resistant to corrosion. Used extensively in orthodontic treatment in the form of wire. *S. s. crown. See* crown, preformed stainless steel.

standard deviation Specific measure of how far from the mean, or average value, a set of results are spread.

standard occipital projection Radiographic technique for demonstrating the maxillary sinus and facial bones.

standard occlusal projection Midline, symmetrical oblique occlusal projection of the mandible or the maxilla.

stannic oxide *See* tin dioxide.

stannous fluoride Form of fluoride used in toothpastes and gels to reduce the incidence of dental caries.

staphylococcal infection Infection with one of several species of *Staphylococcus* bacteria. Staphylococcal infections can affect any part of the body and are characterized by the formation of abscesses.

staphylococci Plural of staphylococcus.

staphylococcus Spherical, Gram-positive bacteria which divide in random planes with incomplete separation of daughter cells to produce clusters of cells similar in appearance to a bunch of grapes (from the Greek *staphyle*). *Staphylococcus aureus* causes a wide range of infections in man and animals and a number of toxin-mediated infections including toxic-shock syndrome and food poisoning. *Staph. epidermidis* is a normal skin commensal but commonly infects prostheses and catheters. Staphylococci are sensitive to many antibiotics, especially penicillin, but many strains have acquired significant resistance. Methicillin-resistant *Staphylococcus aureus* (MRSA) is now common and presents a serious nosocomial infection hazard.

starch Any of the group of polysaccharides that have a large molecule consisting of units of glucose.

stasis Reduction or stoppage in the flow of fluids through vessels.

stat. Give dose immediately.

static At rest, not in motion. *S. mark.* In radiography, an artefact produced by static electricity during film handling. *S. panoramic radiography.* Technique whereby the X-ray source is within the mouth and produces a single radiographic film of the teeth and surrounding structures.

statistical significance Results of a study which for e.g. show a true difference between groups rather than being the result of chance. Results which have a probability value of <0.05 for the statistical test used.

steat- (steato-) Prefix denoting fat.

Steinmann pin (archaic) Stainless steel pin used for fixation in oral surgery.

stellate Star shaped.

steno- Prefix denoting narrow or constricted.

stenosed Narrowed or constricted.

stenosis Permanent narrowing of a hollow structure, as may occur in a blood vessel or salivary gland duct.

Stensen's duct Salivary duct running forwards from the parotid gland to penetrate the buccinator muscle and open into the mouth opposite the upper second permanent molar.

Stephan's curve Curve showing the change of pH of undisturbed plaque with time, originally following a rinse with a glucose solution.

stereograph Instrument to record mandibular movements which allows their reproduction by a series of carved or moulded three-dimensional records.

sterile 1. Infertile, barren. 2. Free of all life forms, especially micro-organisms, and including spores.

sterilization Process of rendering any object sterile. May be achieved by heat (wet or dry), gamma rays or ethylene oxide gas.

sterilize To render free from all life forms, especially micro-organisms.

sterilizer Apparatus for sterilizing objects. *Autoclave s.* Apparatus that sterilizes by heated water vapour under pressure. Downward displacement autoclaves rely on water vapour displacing the air from the container and any packaging whereas prevacuum autoclaves use an initial vacuum to achieve this state which effectively reduces the cycle time of the apparatus. *Chemiclave s.* Similar in operation to an autoclave except for the use of a special solution instead of distilled water. The advantage of this method is that items liable to be damaged by either wet or dry heat can be safely sterilized in this apparatus. *Dry heat s.* Oven-like apparatus used to kill all known bacteria, spores and viruses. Thermostatically controlled and electrically heated. It is only reliable if an uninterrupted timed cycle (160°C for 1 hour) is strictly followed and no instruments are added or removed from the apparatus during the cycle time. Suitable for all metal instruments and those that should be kept dry. Not suitable for plastic and rubber articles and most turbine and mechanical slow handpieces. Cotton wool rolls and paper points may discolor slightly but their absorbency is not greatly reduced. A longer period of time is required for heat to penetrate a metal container. *Ethylene oxide s.* Apparatus in which objects are exposed to ethylene gas for 1 hour at 60°C. Any soft packs treated must not be used for 24 hours in order to allow the poisonous gas to dissipate. *Gamma radiation s.* Apparatus employed industrially to sterilize syringe needles, scalpel blades, suture materials, operating gloves, dressings and disposable syringes, by exposure to gamma-ray radiation for 24 hours. *Glass bead, salt, small steel ball bearings or molten metal s.* Thermostatically controlled, electrically heated small sterilizer containing beads, salt, steel balls or molten metal maintained at 250°C. Small instruments such as those used in endodontic treatment are dipped into it for 10 seconds.

sternum The breast bone. The xiphoid cartilage is its lower extension. The ribs and clavicle articulate on its lateral aspects.

steroid One of a group of chemical substances that includes certain hormones produced in the cortex of the adrenal glands, known as *corticosteroids*, e.g. hydrocortisone and other synthetic drugs, e.g. prednisolone.

steth- (stetho-) Prefix denoting the chest.

Stevens–Johnson syndrome Erythema multiforme (q.v.) characterized by cutaneous lesions of the mouth, pharynx, eyes, nose and genito-urinary orifices.

stick *See* interdental wood point.

sticky wax *See* wax.

stilet *See* stylet.

stimulant Something that produces stimulation.

stimulate To excite into activity.

stimulus Something that rouses an organ or tissue to some special function or activity.

stippled Appearance of healthy gingival tissue whose surface is covered by minute pits. This appearance is often imitated on the buccal aspect of complete dentures.

stippling Producing irregular indentations on a surface.

stitch To pass a needle and suture material through a tissue in order to bring together the wound edges or fix a structure.

stock tray *See* impression tray.

stomach Pear-shaped digestive organ situated in the abdomen and into which food, when swallowed, passes from the oesophagus. The first stages of digestion take place in the stomach where gastric juices containing pepsin and hydrochloric acid are produced, before release at intervals into the duodenum.

stomat- (stomato-) Prefix denoting the mouth or oral cavity.

stomatitis Inflammation of the soft tissues of the mouth. *Aphthous s.* Disease of unknown aetiology characterized by the formation of painful single or multiple mouth ulcers.

stomatology That branch of medicine that studies the function, structure and diseases of the mouth.

stomion Most anterior point of the line of contact of the upper and lower lips in the midline.

-stomy (-ostomy) Suffix denoting opening into an organ or part.

stone 1. Rotary abrasive instrument held in a handpiece, the working end of which incorporates carborundum or similar abrasive mounted on a spindle. 2. A calculus, as found in a salivary duct. 3. The second derivative of gypsum, calcium sulphate hemihydrate $[CaSO_4.H_2O]$ that has been heated to $120\text{-}150°C$ under steam pressure and is used extensively in dentistry to make hard models. Also called Kaffir D. *Pulp s. See* pulp.

strata Plural of stratum.

stratification Arrangement in layers.

stratified Growing or arranged in layers.

stratum Sheet-like arrangement of tissues.

strepto- Prefix meaning twisted.

streptococcal Relating to or caused by a streptococcus.

streptococcal infection Infection in which a streptococcus dominates, e.g. tonsillitis.

streptococci Plural of streptococcus.

streptococcus Spherical, Gram-positive bacteria which divide repeatedly in the same plane with incomplete separation of daughter cells to produce a chain of cells. Various species form an important part of the normal commensal flora of man and animals but some are important pathogens, e.g. *Streptococcus pyogenes* which causes a variety of diseases with a range of severity including tonsillitis, 'strep' sore throat, impetigo and scarlet fever. *S. agalactiae* is an important pathogen of neonates and *S. pneumoniae* causes disease of the middle ear, sinuses, mastoids and lung and is a leading cause of bacterial meningitis.

Streptococcus mutans Bacterium present in plaque and considered to be the prime causative organism of dental caries.

Streptococcus viridans Archaic terminology. Synonymous with 'viridans streptococci', a collective term used to refer to the diverse group of streptococci which normally reside in the mouth. Preferred collective term is 'oral streptococci'.

stress breaker Device intended to relieve an abutment tooth of a load.

stress and tension gauge Gauge used to measure the force exerted by rubber bands and springs.

stria Streak or line; a narrow band.

striated Striped, as of muscle.

striated duct That part of a salivary duct that modifies the salivary composition and is so called because of the striated appearance of its lining cells.

strip Long narrow piece. *Abrasive s. See* abrasive. *Celluloid s.* A clear plastic strip used as a matrix during the placement of tooth coloured restorations in anterior teeth. *Finishing s.* Fine abrasive strip (q.v.) used for smoothing and polishing. *Lightning s. See* separating s. *Polishing s.*

See finishing s. *Separating* (lightning) s. Metal strip carrying coarse abrasives on one side and used to increase the separation between adjacent teeth.

stroke Abrupt cessation of brain function due to a reduction of its blood supply, as in a subarachnoid haemorrhage. Speech disturbances and paralysis (hemiplegia) often follow.

stud attachment Precision attachment having a stud-shaped patrix.

student's alloy Metal mainly consisting of brass (i.e. copper and zinc) and used in teaching casting techniques. Similar in appearance and properties to precious and semi-precious alloy.

study cast (model) *See* cast.

Sturge–Weber syndrome Disease characterized by angiomas (q.v.) of the skin or mucosa and of the jaw and skull bones. There is also vascular abnormality of the meninges with mental retardation and seizures.

stylet 1. Stout wire inserted into the lumen of a catheter or needle to stiffen it during insertion into the body. 2. Fine blunt probe.

stylo- Prefix pertaining to a point.

sub- Prefix denoting under, near or beneath.

subacute Describes a condition that is neither acute nor chronic.

subacute bacterial endocarditis (SBE) *See* bacterial endocarditis.

subcondylar osteotomy Oblique surgical section of the ramus of the mandible below the condyle to reduce mandibular prognathism (q.v.).

subcutaneous Beneath the skin. Underlying the layers of epithelium or epidermis.

S

subgingival Beneath the gingiva. *S. calculus. See* calculus.

subgingival curettage Removal of the junctional epithelium and the epithelial lining of a periodontal pocket, often accompanied by scaling and root planing.

subjective Describing symptoms felt by the patient, such as pain, etc.

sublingual Beneath the tongue.

sublingual bar Major connector of a mandibular partial denture that is placed on the floor of the mouth.

sublining Thin layer of non-irritant cement or vanish placed beneath a cement lining.

subluxation Incomplete dislocation. In dentistry, minor injury to a tooth and periodontal ligament in which the tooth is mobile but not displaced.

submandibular Below the mandible.

submarginal calculus *See* calculus.

submaxillary Below the maxilla.

submental Below the chin.

submento-vertex projection Radiographic projection used to demonstrate the base of the skull and the zygomatic arches. *See* Appendix 10.

submergence (infra-occlusion) Failure of a tooth to maintain its position relative to adjacent teeth so that its occlusal level is below that of adjacent teeth. Most often seen in the primary dentition. The mechanism appears to be related to ankylosis.

submerging teeth *See* infra-occlsuion.

submucosal injection *See* injection.

submucosal vestibuloplasty (archaic) Surgical deepening of the gingival sulcus by freeing and displacing the tissue between the mucosa and the periosteum in order to allow the mucosa to become attached to the underlying bone.

submucous Beneath the mucous membrane.

subnasale Point where the lower margin columella (i.e. the terminal fleshy part of the nasal septum) meets the upper lip in the midline.

subspinale (point 'A') Deepest midline point between the anterior nasal spine and the prosthion. *See* Appendix 10.

substrate A specific substance or substances on which a particular enzyme (q.v.) acts.

substructure Metal framework, as in an implant, that is embedded beneath the tissues and in contact with the bone. Designed to support a superstructure such as an implant denture.

sucrose Cane or beet sugar. A disaccharide yielding two monosaccharides—glucose and fructose. Sucrose, together with plaque, produces lactic acid. Saliva makes a solution of such sugar which then bathes all the supragingival surfaces of teeth.

suction 1. Process of aspiration. 2. In dentistry, an inaccurate term describing the process responsible for the retention of a denture that is not retained mechanically by clasps or precision attachments. *S. apparatus.* Vacuum pump used in operating theatres and some dental surgeries to aspirate blood and debris from the field of operation.

sugar-free Term applied to foods, drinks or medicines when they do not contain fermentable sugars and so are less likely to cause a risk to dental health.

sulcus 1. Groove or furrow. 2. Space or trough, lined by mucous membrane and bounded by the cheeks on one side and the teeth and gingivae on the other. *S. deepening procedure. See* vestibuloplasty.

sulphonamide Chemical substance that prevents the growth and multiplication of a wide range of bacteria, e.g. sulfadiazine.

sulphur granules *See* actinomycosis.

super- Prefix meaning above, over, extreme or excessive.

superficial On or near the surface.

superior Above. In anatomy, refers to structures above the surface of other tissues or structures.

supernumerary In addition to the normal number. *S. teeth. See* tooth.

superstructure 1. Structure that rests on another. 2. Visible portion of an appliance. 3. Prosthesis retained and supported by an implant substructure.

supine position Position of a patient lying face upwards on the floor or a flat surface. A pad may be placed under the shoulders to extend the neck.

supplemental teeth *See* tooth.

support 1. Structure resisting masticatory forces on a prosthesis. May be classified as either tooth or mucosal. 2. Appliance that maintains a part in position.

suppuration Formation of pus as a result of inflammation.

suppurative Associated with or producing pus.

supra- Prefix denoting above or over.

suprabulge That portion of a tooth crown that converges towards the occlusal surface, i.e. is above the survey line (q.v.) of the crown and above the undercut (infrabulge) area of the tooth.

supragingival Above the gingival margin. *S. calculus. See* calculus.

supramentale (bony) (point 'B') Deepest point in the bony outline between the infradentale and the pogonion. *See* Appendix 10.

supramentale (soft tissue) Deepest point between the nose and the forehead in the midline.

supra-occlusion *See* over-eruption.

suprarenal (adrenal) gland Gland lying on each upper aspect of the kidneys, deep in the abdominal cavity. The gland has an outer cortex enclosing a medulla. The cortex secretes endocrines and is concerned with the metabolism of carbohydrates, minerals and water, and the production of sex hormones. The medulla secretes two hormones, adrenalin and noradrenalin, which under conditions of stress are released rapidly into the bloodstream to prepare the body for action.

surface Outermost or uppermost boundary of an object. *Buccal s.* Surface of molars and premolars facing the cheeks. *Distal s.* Surface of a tooth distant to the midline. *Incisal s.* Cutting surface of incisors and canines. *Labial s.* Surface of incisors and canines facing the lips. *Lingual s.* Surface of all lower teeth facing the tongue. *Mesial s.* Proximal surface of teeth facing the midline. *Palatal s.* Surface of all upper teeth facing the palate.

surface (or topical) analgesic/ anaesthetic Jelly, spray or liquid providing analgesia of the mucous membrane. Contains drugs such as benzocaine or lidocaine.

surgical spirit Methylated spirit to which is added a small amount of oil of wintergreen. Used to clean the skin before injection or surgery.

surgical template *See* template.

Surgicel® *See* oxidized cellulose.

Surgicel®

survey In dentistry, the procedure carried out by a surveyor to determine the survey line and the guiding planes of a prosthetic appliance. *S. line*. Line produced on a model by a surveyor indicating the maximum convexity of a tooth or the alveolar process in relation to the planned path of insertion and natural path of displacement of a prosthesis or the optimum position for a clasp arm.

surveyor Jointed instrument holding a lead marker or a cutting blade which is used to survey models or cut parallel surfaces.

susceptible Liable to be affected by something.

sustained release device Method of applying an antimicrobial or antibiotic to a periodontal pocket. An adjunctive treatment method for periodontal disease. Designed to provide drug delivery for up to 24 hours. Examples include: Dentomycin®, a 2% minocycline gel; Elyzol®, a 25% metronidazole gel.

suture 1. Close union between two adjoining bones of the skull. 2. Stitch used to bring together the edges of tissues or to close a wound following surgery. 3. Material used for stitching. There are two broad categories of suture: *absorbable s.*, e.g. Vicryl, and *non-absorbable s.*, e.g. silk, nylon. There are several ways to suture wounds: *Apposition s.* Used to bring together the edges of a wound. *Approximation s.* Used to bring together the deeper layers of tissues. *Continuous s.* Use of a continuous thread. *Interrupted s.* Use of several separate sutures along a wound. *Mattress s.* Suture holding together the deeper tissues, so lessening the tension on the wound edges when it approximates. *Purse string s.* Continuous suture that is drawn together when a wound has been stitched.

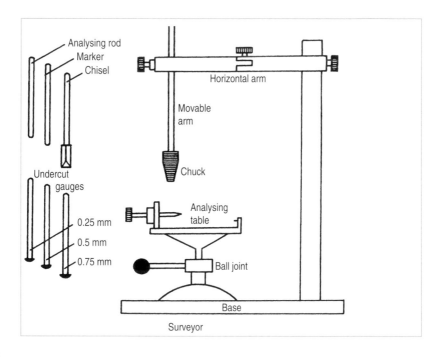

Surveyor

S. needle. Small, curved steel needle used to insert sutures. May be either cutting or round in cross-section and are now generally eyeless as the suture is attached directly to the end of the needle. Usually held in needle holder forceps.

suturing Holding together of tissues by means of a surgical stitch.

swab 1. Pledget of cotton wool or gauze wrapped around the end of a wooden stick or wire. Used to apply drugs or obtain specimens for pathological examination. 2. To clean by wiping. Sharp instrument used to cut the periodontal ligament fibres.

swage To shape metal by hammering and adapting it to a die.

swallowing *See* deglutition.

sweetener Sugars substitute, sometimes described as an alternative or artificial sweetener. Divided into 2 main types according to their properties and their purpose in the food and drinks in which they are used. *Bulk sweeteners*

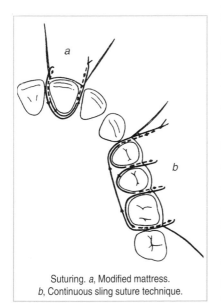

Suturing. *a*, Modified mattress.
b, Continuous sling suture technique.

(e.g. sorbitol, xylitol, maltitol, mannitol) are of low/no cariogenicity but contain calories. They are used to replace cariogenic sugars in products requiring some bulk, e.g. chocolate, baked products, and chewing gum. *Intense s.* (e.g. acesulfame K, aspartame, saccharin) contain few calories and are used in small amounts to provide an intense sweet taste in diet products which do not require any bulking agent (e.g. diet soft drinks).

swelling An enlargement of a part of the body not caused by cell proliferation. Usually associated with a disease process.

symbiosis Relationship between two organisms of different species living in close physical association in which both benefit.

sympathetic nervous system The larger part of the autonomic nervous system supplying the viscera, heart, glands, blood vessels and unstriated muscle. It responds to unusual or dangerous situations by preparing the body for action.

symphysis Junction of two bones separated by fibrocartilage. *S. menti.* Point at which the two developing bodies of the mandible join to form the chin.

symptom Abnormal condition felt by a patient, e.g. pain.

symptomatic Relating to a symptom.

syn- Prefix denoting joined or together.

synalgia *See* referred pain.

synapse Junction between two neurones that transmits nerve impulses from one to the other.

synaptic Relating to a synapse.

syncope A faint, a temporary loss of consciousness.

syndrome Combination of several signs and symptoms all occurring together, which provides a distinct clinical picture.

synergy Combined action. Co-operation of two or more muscles acting together to bring about a certain movement.

synovial fluid Fluid contained in a joint cavity acting as a lubricant. Formed from the lining membrane of the joint capsule.

synthetic Produced artificially. *S. resin.* One of a number of synthetically produced compounds on which the manufacture of a large group of plastics is based. In dentistry, the most commonly used synthetic resin is polymethyl methacrylate (q.v.).

syphilis Contagious bacterial venereal disease spread by direct contact with a person infected by *Treponema pallidum.*

syringe Hand-held device for the injection or withdrawal of fluids or pastes, or conveyance of air, water or both in the form of a spray. *Air s.* Instrument conveying cold or warmed compressed air to the mouth in order to blow away debris or to dry the field of operation. *Aspirating s.* Instrument devised to inject and withdraw fluids from tissues. A dental syringe with the facility of withdrawing the plunger of a local analgesic cartridge. It enables the clinician to see whether a blood vessel has been penetrated, so reducing the possibility of the solution passing directly into the bloodstream. *Cartridge s.* Injection syringe accommodating cartridges containing measured quantities of sterile drug solutions. Such dental syringes have a threaded end to which is screwed the hub of an injection needle. *Chip s.* Syringe with metal nozzle and soft rubber bulb, used to puff away debris and to dry tooth preparations.

Now superseded by the three-in-one (compressed air/water) s. Sometimes used to irrigate an operation site during oral surgery. *Higginson s.* A two-way rubber bulb syringe for irrigating maxillofacial wounds. *Hunt's s.* Metal syringe with spring-loaded plunger, used for irrigation. *Hypodermic s.* Syringe, usually disposable, used to inject substances below the skin. Manufactured in various sizes in plastic material and with a push-on Luer needle fitting. *Impression material s.* Syringe with detachable nozzle and plunger, used to convey mixed impression material to the site of operation. *Plastic s.* Syringe of various sizes used to convey pastes and other materials to the mouth. *Safety s.* Semi-disposable syringe that allows safe disposal without the need for removal of the needle. *Self-aspirating automatic s.* Cartridge syringe that allows aspiration without withdrawal of the syringe plunger rod. *Three-in-one s.* Combination instrument to deliver air, water or an atomized spray through a nozzle and having a variable control.

system Group of organs working together to perform a special function or functions.

systematic review Review of evidence for a particular aspect of science, approached using strict criteria for quality assessment to identify, appraise and summarize the evidence.

systemic Acting throughout the whole body.

systemic circulation That part of the cardiovascular system in which oxygenated blood is carried to all organs and tissues of the body. The blood is returned to the superior and inferior venae cavae and thence to the heart.

systole Contraction of the heart, especially of the ventricles.

TAB vaccine Combined vaccine used to provide immunization against typhoid and paratyphoid A and B.

table A horizontal flat surface serving a specific purpose. *See also* guide t.; occlusal t.

tablet In pharmacy, a measured amount of a drug compressed into a solid form.

tachy- Prefix denoting rapid or fast.

tachycardia Rapid heart beat, more than the normal 72 times per minute.

tactile Relating to or affecting the sense of touch.

tape Wide form of dental floss (q.v.).

taper To make or to become gradually more narrow. Endodontics: A. denoting the shape of root canal instruments and materials. ISO taper = 0.02 mm mm^{-1} (2%) taper. Equipment and materials may have increased tapers of 4–12%.
B. To shape or flare a root canal so that it is narrowest apically and widest coronally.

target-to-film distance *See* FFD (focus-to-film distance).

tartar Lay term for calculus (q.v.).

taste Sensitivity to chemical substances that are in solution. There are four basic tastes—sweet, sour, bitter and salt; all other tastes are combinations of these. *T. buds.* Organs of taste. Groups of cells in bundles that form papillae found on the surface of the tongue, soft palate, epiglottis and, in microscopic size, in the lingual folds. Said to be about 9000 in number and there are more in children than in adults. They are embedded within the stratified epithelium of the fungiform and circumvallate papillae of the tongue. Nerve endings in taste buds convert the chemical stimulus from a solution to a nerve impulse to be conveyed to the brain. Those in the anterior two-thirds of the tongue have nerve fibres running to the lingual nerve and those in the posterior third have nerve fibres running to the glossopharyngeal nerve.

tattoo Indelible marking on the skin or the mucosa produced by puncturing the skin and inserting a suitable pigment. *See also* amalgam tattoo.

taurodontism A variation in tooth form in which the pulp chamber is enlarged, elongated and extends into the roots.

t.d.s or t.i.d Abbreviation of Latin phrases 'ter die sumendum' and 'ter in die', three times a day. Used in prescription writing.

technician *See* dental technician.

technique Method of procedure. *T. alloy. See* student's alloy.

teeth Plural of tooth. *See* tooth.

teething Process of tooth eruption, most commonly associated with the eruption of the relatively large primary molars in 1-2 year olds. May sometimes be associated with local and systemic signs of local irritation, e.g. redness/swelling of mucosa over the erupting tooth, increased salivation and sleeplessness.

Teflon® **(polytetrafluoroethylene)** A proprietary material used in surgery as a barrier membrane. May be used in guided bone or tissue generation procedures in surgical periodontics or prior to or during implant placement.

Tegretol® *See* carbamazepine.

teicoplanin A glycopeptide antibiotic sometimes used in endocarditis prophylaxis.

telescopic crown *See* crown.

temazepam A benzodiazepine used in oral sedation.

temperature 1. Heat intensity as measured by any one of several scales. 2. Feverish condition. The normal oral temperature of a person at rest is 37°C or 98.6°F.

tempering Hardening and toughening of metals by heating and allowing them to cool.

template A pattern or mould. In prosthetics, a curved plate useful in arranging teeth along the imaginary curve of Spee (q.v.) during denture manufacture. *Surgical t.* A transparent pattern or mould used as an orientation guide for the surgical placement of asseo-integrated implants. Alternatively may aid in shaping the alveolar process prior to the insertion of immediate dentures.

temple Region of the head above and in front of each ear.

temporal Relating to the side of the head or the temporal bone. *T. bone.* Skull bone, one on each side of the head, in the region of the temple, forming part of the base of the skull and sending a process forwards to form part of the cheek. Bounded by the frontal, parietal, occipital and sphenoid bones. The external auditory meatus forms a wide passage emerging through the bone (better known as the earhole) continuous with the inner ear structures, all of which are contained within the temporal bone. Behind and below each meatus the bone forms the mastoid process containing hollow air spaces within it. *T. muscle.* Fan-shaped muscle of mastication attached to the temporal bone and the coronoid process of the mandible. Its action is to close the mouth and retrude/protrude the mandible. It

is supplied by the mandibular division of the trigeminal nerve.

temporary crown *See* crown.

temporary post crown *See* crown.

temporo- Prefix denoting the temple or the temporal lobe of the brain.

temporomandibular joint (TMJ) One of two joints lying on each side of the skull, its bony components being the condyle of the mandible and the glenoid or articular fossa of the temporal bone. The joint has two cavities divided by a flat fibrocartilage disc lying between the two bony surfaces. A loose fibrous capsule is arranged around the joint, attached to the temporal bone at the periphery of the articular fossa and eminence, and passing like a sleeve over the head of the condyle of the mandible, to be attached at its neck. It is strengthened by a stronger fibrous band laterally—the lateral ligament. The capsule, but not the disc of bony surface, is lined by a smooth shiny synovial membrane that secretes the lubricating synovial fluid filling both joint cavities. The articular disc is moulded to the rounded shape of the condylar head on its lower surface and the articular fossa and eminence of the temporal bone above it. The lateral pterygoid muscle of mastication is inserted into the articular disc, fibrous capsule and neck of the condyle. On contraction, the condylar head and disc move together to glide forwards onto the eminence. Dislocation of the joint occurs when they move beyond the height of the eminence. *TMJ dysfunction.* Uni- or bilateral disturbance of the normal function of the temporomandibular joint. Symptoms may be clicking or grating of the joint, swelling and tenderness over the joint, and areas of pain in the face, neck, and muscles of mastication. Also known as temporomandibular joint

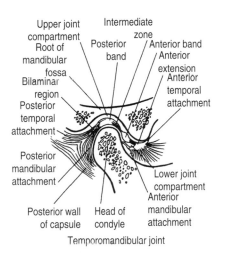

Upper joint compartment
Root of mandibular fossa
Bilaminar region
Posterior temporal attachment
Posterior mandibular attachment
Intermediate zone
Posterior band
Anterior band
Anterior extension
Anterior temporal attachment
Lower joint compartment
Anterior mandibular attachment
Posterior wall of capsule
Head of condyle

Temporomandibular joint

dysfunction syndrome (TMD) or Costen's syndrome.

tenacity State of being adhesive or holding firm.

tender 1. To offer or present. 2. Painful to pressure; sensitive, delicate.

tendon Tough whitish band of connective tissue, mainly composed of collagen fibres, that serves to attach muscle to bone.

TENS *See* transcutaneous electrical neural stimulation.

tension The act of stretching. A state of being strained or stretched.

terat- (terato-) Prefix meaning monster or abnormality.

terminal hinge axis *See* axis, transverse horizontal.

terminal hinge position record *See* record.

ternary alloy Deprecated term for high copper amalgam alloy. *See* alloy.

terra alba *See* kaolin.

test cavity Dental diagnostic test used when all other vitality tests have proved

inconclusive. The tooth is pulp-tested by cutting a small cavity in dentine (without a local analgesic) and observing the reaction.

tetanus Acute infectious disease characterized by trismus (lockjaw), general muscle spasm, arching of the back, spasm of the respiratory system and paralysis, caused by infection with *Clostridium tetani* usually by contamination of a wound with soil, dust or dirt.

tetra- Prefix denoting four.

tetracycline Broad-spectrum antibiotic drug which, if administered during the time of tooth development, may result in brown staining of the teeth.

TFD (target-to-film distance) *See* FFD (focus-to-film distance).

therapeutic Relating to medical treatment.

therapy Treatment of disease.

therm- Prefix denoting heat or temperature.

thermal Relating to heat.

thermoluminescent dosimeter (tld) Device containing a thermoluminescent material and used for detecting the amount of radiation exposure.

thermometer Graduated instrument for measuring temperature, usually by expansion of mercury or alcohol in a sealed glass tube.

thermoplastic Substance that becomes softened on warming and then hardens on cooling. *T. impression material* (or *compound*). *See* impression material.

thermostat Device intended to maintain a constant temperature.

thesis Written results of original research usually submitted by a candidate for a university degree.

thiamine (vitamin B₁) Water-soluble complex of vitamins found in egg yolks, liver and rice. Deficiency of vitamin B_1 may result in beriberi (q.v.).

Thiersch graft *See* split skin graft.

thimble In dentistry, a bridge retainer consisting of a thin, tube-like metal substructure to which a crown may be cemented. Has previously been used to overcome bridge insertion and retention problems.

thorac- (thoraco-) Prefix denoting chest or thorax.

thoracic Relating to the chest.

thorax Chest cavity bounded by the ribs, vertebrae, neck and abdomen. Contains the heart, oesophagus, trachea and lungs. Separated from the abdomen by the diaphragm.

three-in-one syringe *See* syringe.

three-quarter crown *See* crown.

threshold Point at which a defect begins to be produced. The lowest limit of stimulus that is capable of producing a response or recognition by the consciousness.

throat pack Pack made of gamgee tissue or absorbent plastic which is placed in the throat, usually during an anaesthetic, to prevent foreign bodies entering the throat or chest.

thromb- (thrombo-) Prefix meaning of a blood clot, thrombosis or blood platelets.

thrombin Enzyme converting fibrinogen to fibrin.

thrombocyte *See* platelet.

thrombocytic Relating to a thrombocyte.

thrombosis Formation of a blood clot in the interior of a blood vessel or in the heart. It causes distress, and the restoration of the blood supply takes place by another route slowly. Heart muscle has few alternative routes so that any damage may be permanent.

thrombus Blood clot.

thrush (candidiasis (q.v.) or moniliasis) Stomatitis (q.v.) caused by an infection with *Candida albicans* and characterized by white patches or a reddened inflamed surface anywhere in the mouth. Also candidiasis affecting other parts, esp. the vagina. Systemic candidiasis is rare and life-threatening.

thymol Colourless crystalline substance used as an antifungal or antibacterial medicament.

thyro- Prefix denoting the thyroid gland.

thyroid gland *See* gland.

thyrotoxicosis Condition of increased body metabolism due to excess of the hormone thyroxin. Symptoms are a high pulse rate, excessive sweating, excitability and hand tremors.

TI (treatment index) Obsolescent term based on the DMF index (q.v.)

and sometimes used to show the extent to which treatment has been successful.

tic Involuntary and repeated movement of varying complexity. Often occurs in individuals under stress, *T. douloureux*. *See* neuralgia, trigeminal.

t.i.d. Abbreviation of Latin phrase, 'ter in die', meaning three times a day. Used in prescription writing.

timer Electronic or mechanical clock used in the processing of radiographs. *X-ray t.* Electric or mechanical switch mechanism used to complete the electrical circuit during the production of X-rays.

tin White metallic element. *T. dioxide.* White insoluble compound used as a polishing agent. *Tin foil.* An extremely thin base metal foil used as a separating medium in denture construction.

tincture Alcoholic extract of an animal or vegetable drug generally prepared by a percolation or maceration process.

tine Prong, such as the point of a probe.

tinnitus A persistent noise in the ear such as ringing or buzzing.

tissue Collection of similar specialized cells formed to perform a particular function. There are four main groups of tissue in the body—connective, epithelial, muscular and nervous. Some become specialized, so producing further subdivisions. *Connective t.* Forms the means of linking up other tissues. It supports and connects the organs of the body. ADIPOSE T. Acts as a reserve store of fuel, protects underlying tissues, rounds off body prominences and produces symmetrical curves. Retains body heat and serves as a bed for the lodgement of vessels. Found subcutaneously throughout the body. AREEOLAR T. Packing agent of the body occupying the cellular intervals between other structures

and constituting the fascia of the body. BLOOD CELLS. Red and white. BONE CONNECTIVE T. Impregnated with lime salts. CARTILAGE DENSE CONNECTIVE T. Hyaline and fibrocartilage. JELLY-LIKE T. Found in the dental pulp. LYMPHOID T. Found in the lymphatic glands, tonsils and covering parts of the posterior third of the tongue. WHITE FIBROUS T. Found in all ligaments and the outer coats of arteries, the periosteum and the periodontal ligament. It will not stretch. YELLOW ELASTIC T. Found in the middle coats of arteries. *Epithelial t.* Tissue composed entirely of cells united edge to edge by cementing substances so as to form a membrane. Lines all the free surfaces of the body. When lining vessels and closed cavities it is called *endothelium*. May be simple (one layer thick), transitional, or stratified with three or more layers as in the skin. SIMPLE EPITHELIUM: There are five varieties: *pavement, columnar, ciliated, cubical* and *glandular*. Provides a smooth surface to prevent friction as in blood vessel lining. Supports tissues and permits absorption. Lines ducts of glands and the lower alimentary tract, to propel substances through the channel which it lines, e.g. the respiratory tract. Exists as a packing agent as found in the thyroid gland and bronchioles. Its function is secretion, and it lines all glands except the thyroid. STRATIFIED EPITHELIUM. Has three or more layers, is protective, forms the skin and lines the mouth. TRANSITIONAL EPITHELIUM. Has three layers and is found in the urinary tract. Prevents absorption. *Muscular t.* Most important tissue of the body forming its fleshy part. There are three kinds: STRIPED (voluntary), UNSTRIPED (involuntary) and CARDIAC (heart). Striped muscles are attached to the bony skeleton while unstriped muscles are not. *Nervous t.* Consists of nerve cells, neurones and

T

their processes, axons which are single and may be long, and dendrites which are short, numerous and branched.

tissue conditioner Type of soft liner for prostheses used for a short period and intended to improve the condition of the soft tissues lying beneath the prostheses.

tissue fluid Fluid occupying the spaces in tissue formed from the blood fluid in the capillaries and providing nutrients to the tissues at the same time as carrying products to the lymphatic system.

tissue forceps *See* forceps.

tissue surface That part of a denture that is in contact with the denture-bearing area.

titanium A metallic element used alone or as an alloy for surgical implants.

titanium oxide Pigment used to provide white colour in opaque fissure sealants.

tld *See* thermoluminescent dosimeter.

TMD Temporomandibular dysfunction.

TMJ dysfunction *See* temporomandibular joint dysfunction.

'toilet of the cavity' *See* cavity toilet.

Toller view *See* transpharyngeal projection.

-tome Suffix denoting a cutting instrument.

tomograph Radiograph produced by apparatus that allows the movement of the film and focal spot in opposite directions around a point during exposure, thus producing a distinct image of a selected tissue plane.

tomography Technique of producing a tomograph. *See* Appendix 10.

-tomy (-otomy) Suffix denoting surgical incision.

tongue Muscular organ lying in the floor of the mouth. Aids in chewing, swallowing and speech. Taste buds are located in the papillae situated on the upper surface of the tongue. *Bifid t.* Tongue that is split in the anterior region by a longitudinal fissure. *Black hairy t.* Condition characterized by elongation of the filliform papillae on the dorsum of the tongue, without desquamation, which forms a thick matted brown or black layer. Usually due to heavy smoking or to broad-spectrum antibiotic therapy. *Cleft t. See* bifid t. *Fissured, furrowed t.* Tongue with several longitudinal fissures or grooves. *Geographic t.* Tongue with several patches of papillary atrophy suggesting the appearance of a map. *Hairy t. See* black hairy t. *Magenta t.* Magenta-coloured tongue due to riboflavin deficiency. *Strawberry t.* Tongue with enlarged papillae and a whitish coat seen in scarlet fever. *T. depressor.* Flat spatula used to depress the tongue during examination of the fauces. *T. guard.* A metal device, usually attached to a saliva ejector (q.v.), designed to protect the tongue from rotating instruments during tooth preparation. *T. thrust.* Thrusting of the tongue between the teeth during the act of swallowing or speech. May cause a malocclusion. *T. tie. See* ankyloglossia.

tonsil Collection of lymphoid tissue covered by mucous membrane. *Lingual t.* Lies on the posterior third of the tongue. *Palatine t.* Lies between the pillars of the fauces on each side of the pharynx. *Pharyngeal (adenoid) t.* Lies in the nasopharynx.

tonsillectomy Surgical excision of the tonsils.

tonsillitis Inflammation of the tonsils causing pain, swelling and fever.

Streptococcal micro-organisms are the most common causal agent.

tooth (teeth) Hard calcified structures usually at the entrance of the alimentary tract and whose primary function is the comminution of food. Composed of dentine that is covered on the crown with enamel and on the root with cementum. The tooth shows a central cavity, the pulp cavity, that closely resembles the outline of the tooth. The pulp cavity consists of the pulp chamber, i.e. that portion within the crown, and the pulp or root canal lying within the confines of the root. *Accessory t. See* supernumerary t. *Acrylic (resin) t.* Tooth made of acrylic resin. *Anatomic (anatomical) t.* Artificial tooth whose crown simulates the morphology of a natural tooth. *Anchor t. See* anchorage. *Ankylosed t. See* ankylosis. *Anterior t.* One of the incisor or canine teeth. *Artificial t.* Manufactured tooth used as a substitute for a natural tooth in a prosthesis and usually made of porcelain or acrylic resin. *Avulsed t.* Tooth that has been forcibly displaced from the alveolus. *Baby t.* Colloquial name for a primary tooth. *Buck t.* Colloquialism for prominent projecting anterior maxillary teeth. *Conical (peg-shaped) t.* Malformed teeth found in ectodermal dysplasia (q.v.) and other disorders and occasionally in unaffected children. *Cracked t. See* cracked tooth syndrome. *Cuspless t.* Also known as *flat cusp teeth.* Teeth designed without cusps and used in a prosthesis where the registration of centric occlusion presents difficulties. *Dead t.* Common but erroneous term for a pulpless tooth. *Diatoric t.* Artificial tooth with holes in its base into which the denture base material flows when processed and thus attaches the tooth to the base. Also called *pinless tooth. Dilacerated t. See* dilaceration. *Double t.* Term used to describe either a geminated tooth, formed by the partial splitting of a tooth germ, or a fused tooth, formed by the fusion of two tooth germs. *Eye t. See* canine. *Embedded t.* Tooth that has not erupted because of lack of eruptive force. *Flat cusp t. See* cuspless t. *Fournier's t. See* Moon's t. *Fused t.* Teeth that have undergone partial or complete union of their tooth germs during development. *Geminated t. See* gemination. *Hereditary brown opalescent t. See* dentinogenesis imperfecta. *Hutchinson's (notched) t.* Tooth abnormality seen in congenital syphilis and affecting primarily the incisors, canines and first permanent molars. The teeth are hypoplastic and the incisors have a screwdriver or peg-shaped appearance. *Hypoplastic t. See* hypoplasia, dental. *Impacted t.* Tooth prevented from erupting normally either by overlying bone or by an adjacent tooth. *Milk t. See* primary dentition. *Missing t.* Tooth missing from the dentition because of congenital factors, exfoliation, extraction, avulsion, etc. *Molar t. See* molar. *Moon's t.* Malformed, small, domed first molars seen in patients with congenital syphilis, also known as *Fournier's teeth. Natal t.* Teeth present prior to birth. *Neonatal t.* Teeth that erupt during the first month of life. *Non-anatomic t.* Artificial tooth whose occlusal surfaces are not copies of the natural dentition, but have been given special forms designed to more nearly fulfil the requirements of mastication and tissue tolerance. *Non-functional t.* Tooth that is not in occlusion because of the absence of the opposing tooth in the other jaw. *Non-vital t.* Tooth that does not respond to normal pulp testing stimuli. Term often inaccurately used to refer to a pulpless tooth. *Notched t. See* Hutchinson's t. *Peg-shaped t. See* conical t. *Permanent t. See* permanent dentition. *Pink t.* Tooth that has undergone idiopathic internal resorption which gives it a pink coloration due to the visibility of the granulation tissue within the pulp chamber. *Pinless t. See* diatoric t. *Plastic t. See* acrylic (resin) t. *Posterior t.* Premolar and molar teeth. *Primary t. See* deciduous dentition. *Pulpless t.* Tooth from which the pulp has been extirpated. Commonly but inaccurately called a *dead* or *non-vital tooth. Secondary t. See* permanent dentition. *Steele's interchangeable t.* or *facing.* Artificial tooth manufactured with a standardized slot that fits in a matching metal backing, thus allowing its easy replacement should the facing fracture. *Supernumerary t.* Tooth of abnormal form in excess of the usual number. *Supplemental t.* Supernumerary tooth of normal appearance. *Temporary*

t. See deciduous dentition. *T. ache.* Pain in a tooth, generally due to caries or trauma producing a pulpitis. *T.-borne.* Term describing a prosthesis that relies entirely on the abutment teeth for support. *T. brush.* Manual or powered brush designed to remove plaque from teeth. *T. brush injury.* Injury to a tooth or gingiva caused by incorrect or excessive tooth brushing, or by the use of a stiff textured brush. *T. brushing. See* tooth brushing technique. *T. cleaning* or *polishing paste.* Blend of fine abrasive particles, bonding agents, flavouring and colouring matter together with medicaments and other chemicals. Used to clean and polish the surfaces of teeth and restorations. Also called *toothpaste* or *dentifrice. T. depression. See* intrusion. *See also* extrusion. *T.*

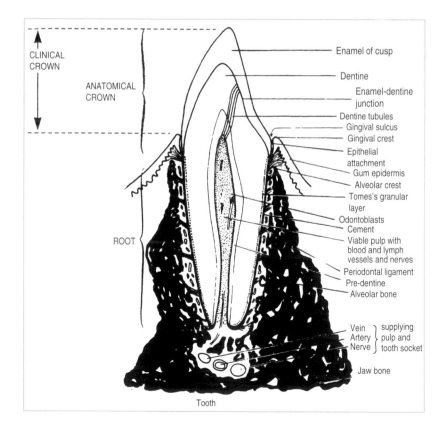

Tooth

fracture. Uncomplicated – fracture involving enamel or enamel and dentine without involving the pulp. Complicated – fracture involving enamel dentine and pulp. *T. fulcrum.* Axis about which a tooth moves when a lateral force is applied. *T. germ.* Group of embryonic cells that develop to form a complete tooth. *T. cleaning paste. See* toothpaste. *T. pick. See* wood point. *T. position.* Deprecated term for intercuspal position (q.v.). *T. preparation. See* preparation. *T. transplantation. See* transplantation. *Turner's t.* Hypoplastic permanent tooth due to injury or inflammation of the preceding primary tooth. *Tube t.* Artificial tooth constructed with a vertical circular hole in its base into which a pin or cast post can be inserted for attachment to a denture base. *Unerupted t. See* embedded t. *Wisdom t.* Lay term for a third molar.

tooth brushing technique *Bass t.b.t.* Effective method for the removal of dental plaque. The toothbrush filaments are placed at an angle of 45° to the long axis of the teeth, with the filament ends pointed towards the gingival margins. Slight pressure is then applied to remove the filaments into the sulcular regions where, once they are engaged, a vibratory motion is utilized, moving the brush back and forth with very short strokes, keeping the ends of the filaments in the sulcus. *Charter's t.b.t.* Method of cleaning utilized when the interdental papillae do not fill the embrasure spaces. The technique is contra-indicated where there are full interdental spaces. The filaments of the brush are placed at a 45° angle, directed towards the occlusal surfaces. The sides of the filaments are then placed against the marginal gingivae and the teeth, extending the filaments into the approximal spaces. A firm, rotary/vibratory movement is utilized while keeping the

filaments in position. A soft multitufted brush is recommended, particularly after periodontal surgery. *Roll t.b.t.* The toothbrush is placed buccally in the first selected quadrant with its bristles resting on the gingivae, pointing away from the teeth. The filaments are then rolled across the gingiva, up the teeth towards their occlusal surfaces, allowing the filaments to sweep into the interproximal spaces. This should be repeated about eight times before moving to another quadrant and after dealing with the lingual aspect in a similar manner.

tooth friendly *See* safe-for-teeth.

tooth surface loss Loss of surface tooth structure or toothwear due to *abrasion, attrition* or *erosion,* or a combination of these processes.

toothpaste A dentifrice. Powder or paste used on a toothbrush to clean accessible areas of teeth. Contains mild

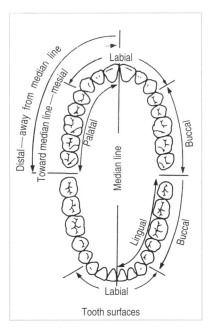

Tooth surfaces

abrasives, flavouring, colouring, often fluoride and sometimes medicaments.

topical Referring to a localized area. *T. analgesic. See* surface analgesic. *T. fluoride.* Application to the surface of the teeth of a substance containing a fluoride agent, in order to render them more resistant to caries. May be in the form of a solution, gel, foam, mouthwash, varnish or paste. *Professionally applied t. fluoride (PATF).* Topical fluoride gels, foams, solutions varnishes and prophylactic pastes applied in the dental surgery by dentists and DCPs. *Self applied t. fluoride (SATF).* Topical fluoride toothpastes and mouthrinses applied by individuals, usually at home.

topographical occlusal projection *See* oblique occlusal projection.

torus A swelling, a rounded projection. *T. mandibularis.* Developmental bony protuberance sometimes found on the lingual aspect of the mandible in the premolar region. May cause difficulty in the fitting of complete dentures. *T. palatinus.* Developmental bony eminence sometimes found in the midline of the hard palate.

total filtration In radiography, the sum of the added and inherent filtration.

Towne's projection A radiographic technique for demonstrating the occipital region of the skull. Used to demonstrate the mandibular condyles in the coronal plane. *See also* reverse Towne's projection. *See* Appendix 10.

tox- (toxi-, toxo-, toxic-) Prefix meaning poison, toxic or relating to poison or toxins.

toxaemia Condition in which toxins are present in the blood circulation giving rise to a number of systemic symptoms including malaise, fever and vomiting.

toxic Relating to toxin.

toxin Poisonous substance produced by a living organism, e.g. snake venom and a wide variety of substances produced by some fungi (mycotoxins), such as alphatoxin, and plants including many alkaloids such as hemlock. Bacterial toxins are described as either endotoxins (q.v.) or exotoxins such as botulinum toxin which causes botulism and various enterotoxins produced by pathogenic strains of *Escherichia coli* which can cause acute gut disorders.

toxoid Toxin which has been modified to reduce or eliminate its toxic properties but which is still able to elicit an immune response, e.g. tetanus *t.*

trabecula Small band of tissue passing through an organ and dividing it into chambers. Bony trabeculae occur in spongy bone.

trabeculae Plural of trabecula.

tracer 1. Diagnostic procedure in which a substance is introduced into the body in order to trace its progress and obtain information about metabolic processes. 2. In dentistry, a device to record jaw positions and movements.

trache- (tracheo-) Prefix denoting the trachea.

trachea Tube of some 10–13 cm in length, running from the larynx to the bronchus and then dividing to each lung. A rigid structure having rings of cartilage all along it to provide support and keep it patent. It is lined with ciliated mucous membrane that propels foreign bodies from the trachea to the mouth.

tracheal Relating to the trachea.

tracheostomy (tracheotomy) Operation to relieve respiratory obstruction in which an opening is made into the

246

trachea and a tube inserted to maintain the airway.

tracheotomy *See* tracheostomy.

tracing Line or pattern made on paper or a plate representing movement, such as cardiovascular activity or mandibular movement. *Arrow point t. See* gothic arch t. *Gothic arch t.* Method of illustrating, by means of a tracing, the posterior position of the mandible in determining the normal occlusion for the construction of dentures or rehabilitation cases. The horizontal tracing resembles an arrow head or gothic arch and is obtained by a series of mandibular movements using a tracing device on a horizontal recording plane. *T. stick. See* impression material, green stick.

tragacanth Gum obtained from a vegetable plant.

tragus Projection of cartilage anterior to the external opening of the ear.

tranexamic acid (Cyklokapron®) An antifibrinolytic drug that is useful in the management of patients with bleeding disorders (such as Von Willebrand's disease) who are having dental extractions or other intra-oral surgery. It can be administered orally, by injection or topically as a mouthwash.

tranquillizer Drug used to relieve anxiety, e.g. diazepam (Valium®).

trans- Prefix denoting through or across.

transbuccal or cheek wiring (archaic) Method of immobilizing fractures by wires from a halo head frame passed through the cheeks and fastened to a dental splint.

transcranial projection (of the temporomandibular joint) Radiographic technique for demonstrating the relationship of the condyle head to the glenoid fossa.

transcutaneous electrical neural stimulation (TENS) A low voltage electrical stimulation through the skin to underlying nerves said to interfere with the sensation of pain in the brain and to increase blood flow to the painful region.

transfer coping *See* coping.

transfusion Introduction of blood taken from a healthy person (the donor) into the circulation of a patient (the recipient) whose blood is deficient in quality or quantity due to accident or disease.

transient Short-lived.

transillumination Projection of light through a tissue for examination purposes. In dentistry, projection of light rays through a tooth and its associated structures in order to detect caries, calculus, debris, fractures, foreign bodies or the position of root canals.

transition Changing from one state to another.

translucent Allowing the partial passage of light without clarity of the image, e.g. ground glass, opaque light shades. *T. dentine. See* dentine.

transmaxillary projection *See* Appendix 10.

transorbital (transmaxillary) projection Radiographic technique for demonstrating the articular eminence and the head of the condyle in cross-sectional view in an oblique coronal plane.

transparent Able to see through clearly, e.g. window glass. *T. grid.* Transparent material marked with a calibrated grid and used to make accurate comparisons or measurements of drawings, radiographs, models or casts.

transpharyngeal projection (lateral transpharyngeal projection or Toller view) Radiographic technique for demonstrating the head of the condyle in lateral view.

transplantation 1. Transference of a tissue from one site to another or from a separate donor to a recipient. 2. In dentistry, the removal of a tooth from its socket and its replacement in a new position in the alveolar bone of the maxilla or mandible.

transposition 1. Movement of a tissue flap from one place to another without severing its blood supply until it is established at the new site. 2. In dentistry, the interchange of position of adjacent teeth during development and eruption.

transudate Fluid that passes through a membrane as a result of hydrostatic pressure.

transudation The passage of a fluid through a membrane.

transverse Across. *T. horizontal axis.* See axis.

trauma Any wound or injury of the tissues.

traumatic Relating to trauma. *T. exposure.* See exposure. *T. occlusion.* See occlusion.

traumatize To injure or wound.

tray Flat shallow vessel with raised edges. *See* impression tray. *T. adhesive.* Substance used to ensure adhesion of impression material to the impression tray containing it. Some adhesives are designed for use exclusively with certain materials. *T. compound.* Thermoplastic material used in making special impression trays on the preliminary models. *Special t. material* A composite resin supplied in sheet form, which cures using a visible light source. Used for the construction of special trays and temporary bases.

Treacher–Collins syndrome Mandibulofacial dysostosis. Condition characterized by hypoplasia of the facial bones, macrostomia, high palate, abnormal positioning of the teeth, atypical hair growth and possibly other skeletal deformities.

treatment The management and care of a patient in order to relieve or cure an illness or abnormality. *Conservative t.* See conservative dentistry. *Empirical t.* Treatment based on experience and observation rather than scientific knowledge. *Endodontic t.* See endodontics. *Heroic t.* Term used to describe last resort treatment of serious illness or injury, generally by unproven and unorthodox measures. *Heat t.* A method of altering the physical properties of a metal by controlled temperature changes. *Orthodontic t.* See orthodontics. *Palliative t.* Treatment aimed at the relief of acute painful symptoms rather than the curing of the disease itself. *Periodontal t.* See periodontics. *Preventive (prophylactic) t.* Treatment aimed at preventing the acquisition and development of a disease. In dentistry, the instructions given to a patient to prevent the development of dental disease particularly as related to caries and periodontal disease. *Prosthetic t.* See prosthetics. *Root canal t.* The technique of removing vital or non-vital pulp tissue from a root canal, its sterilization and preparation to receive a permanent root filling. *T. plan.* Following the examination and diagnostic procedures, the setting out of what treatment is to be undertaken for a patient, in what order and at what intervals of time.

tremor Involuntary quivering or trembling.

trench mouth Deprecated term for necrotizing ulcerative gingivitis (q.v.).

treponema Bacteria with a flexible helical structure belonging to the genus *Treponema*, (q.v. spirochaete), e.g. *T. pallidum* which is the causal organism of syphilis.

tri- Prefix denoting three.

trial denture *See* denture.

triamcinolone acetonide dental paste (Adcortyl in orabase®) A paste containing a corticosteroid anti-inflammatory drug used topically in the mouth for recurrent aphthous ulcers (q.v.).

tricuspid 1. Having three cusps. 2. Relating to the tricuspid heart valve. *T. valve.* First valve in the heart, having three cusps, and which allows blood to be pumped from the right auricle to the right ventricle but not to return.

trifurcation Anatomical area where the roots divide in a three-rooted tooth.

trigeminal Relating to the fifth cranial nerve. *See* nerve.

trigeminal neuralgia *See* neuralgia.

trigger point (area, spot) A point on the body which, when stimulated, initiates pain in another part of the body.

trimmer Machine-operated or hand instrument used to reduce the size of prostheses, models, restorations or preparations.

triple syringe *See* syringe, three-in-one.

trisaccharide A sugar which, on hydrolysis, produces three molecules of monosaccharide from each molecule.

trismus (lockjaw) Spasm of the muscles of mastication that keeps the mouth tightly closed. A symptom of tetanus or a complication of overuse of phenothiazine drugs.

trisodium orthophosphate *See* sodium phosphate.

trituration Grinding, rubbing or pounding of a mixture in order to pulverize it. In dentistry describes the process of mixing amalgam alloy particle with mercury.

troche *See* lozenge.

-trophy Suffix denoting growth or development.

-tropic Suffix denoting affinity for, turning towards or influencing.

troy System of weights used to assess quantities of precious metals.

true lateral projection Radiographic technique for demonstrating all or part of the skull by directing the central ray at right angles to the plane of the film.

true occlusal projection Radiographic technique in which the central ray is directed along the long axis of the teeth.

truncate To cut off or lop.

try in *See* denture, trial.

T-spring Removable orthodontic appliance spring, working from its palatal aspect to move a tooth or teeth buccally or labially. It is made by a double length of fine wire with a T-shaped tip.

tube Long hollow cylinder. *Endotracheal t.* Flexible tube inserted through the nose into the trachea to act as an airway during intubation. *T. head.* Protective metal head covering containing the X-ray tube, tube housing, transformers and cooling oil. The removable cone is placed at the aperture of the head.

tube side That side of an X-ray film packet or cassette which faces the source of X-rays from an X-ray machine.

tubercle 1. In anatomy, a small rounded protuberance on bone. 2. Specific lesion of tuberculosis. *T. of Carabelli.* See Carabelli's cusp.

tuberculosis Contagious disease in man caused by the bacterium *Mycobacterium tuberculosis* and in animals by related bacteria in which small nodules or tubercles develop in the body wherever the bacteria have become established, mainly in the respiratory and alimentary tracts and their associated lymphatic glands. There are various tests (e.g. Mantoux) for the disease, and immunization is by BCG (bacille Calmette–Guérin) vaccination. *Latent t.* is the condition exhibited by a symptomless person infected with *M. tuberculosis*. The disease can remain inactive for many years and become active if the infected person becomes weakened or immuno-compromised, e.g. HIV-AIDS.

tuberculous Relating to tuberculosis.

tuberculum Small rounded swelling or projection.

tuberoplasty (archaic) Surgical reshaping of the maxillary tuberosity.

tuberosity Anatomical term for a rounded eminence.

tubular Shaped like, or consisting of, a tube or tubes.

tubule Small tube. *Dentinal t.* Minute canals in the dentine running from the dental pulp to the amelodentinal junction.

tuft A cluster or bunch.

tulle gras See gauze.

tumor Swelling. One of the four classic signs of inflammation, the others being calor (heat), rubor (redness) and dolor (pain).

tumour Any swelling or abnormal growth of the body tissues. A neoplasm. Tumours may be benign or malignant.

tungsten carbide Abrasive powder used in grinding wheels and some rotary cutting instruments. Also incorporated in certain steels to produce a harder, longer-lasting cutting edge.

tunica A coat or covering. *T. media.* Middle coat of arteries and arterioles, composed of muscle and elastic tissue.

tunnel procedure See furcation t.p.

turbid Muddy and disturbed, cloudy.

turbine (turbine handpiece or air rotor) Handpiece incorporating a rotor that is driven at high speed up to 300 000 rpm by compressed air flow. The head contains a friction grip chuck and one or more water jets acting as a coolant for the burs, etc.

turgid Swollen, abnormally distended.

tussis The act of coughing.

tweed arch bending pliers See pliers.

tweezer Hand instrument with two narrow and/or pointed, straight or curved beaks used to grasp small objects. May have a locking device to maintain the beaks in a closed position until released.

twin block appliance See appliance.

twin wire arch Part of a fixed orthodontic appliance consisting of twin, fine stainless steel archwires attached to bands cemented onto the teeth or brackets bonded to the teeth. The natural effect of the wire tending to straighten itself is the force used to align such teeth.

tympan- (tympano-) Prefix denoting eardrum.

typhoid fever Acute, potentially fatal infectious disease of the digestive tract caused by the bacterium *Salmonella typhi*. Transmitted through food and water contaminated by the faeces or urine of patients or carriers.

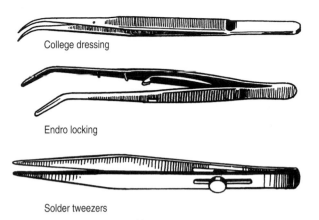

College dressing

Endro locking

Solder tweezers

Tweezers

typodont Articulated apparatus with hollowed-out upper and lower bases that can be filled with wax or acrylic to support metal or plastic teeth and on which students can practise dental techniques. Commonly used in orthodontics to practise tooth movement using appliances.

U

U-loop Orthodontic wire such as a buccal bow bent into a U-shape, to allow for adjustment by closing or opening the loop.

ulcer Open sore with loss of epithelium to its full thickness and sometimes the underlying tissues. Caused by inflammation breaking through the mucous membrane or skin. *See also* aphthous ulcer, rodent ulcer.

ulcerate To form an ulcer.

ulceration Inflammatory process causing the formation of an ulcer.

ultra- Prefix denoting beyond, excessive or extreme.

ultrasonic (ultrasound) High energy sound waves above the audible range employed in a range of diagnostic and therapeutic applications. *U. cleaning bath.* An electronic high frequency generator which agitates a cleaning solution in the bath thus loosening any debris adhering to dental instruments and appliances prior to sterilization. *U. endodontic instrumentation.* Conventional and diamond coated endodontic instruments are energized by the piezoelectric effect and used to remove pulp tissue and other debris and in enlarging and irrigating root canals. *U. instrument removal.* Use of ultrasonic energy to loosen and remove fractured instruments from root canals. *U. post removal.* Use of ultrasonic energy to loosen and remove root canal posts. *U. root-end preparation.* Cutting cavities in the root tip during endodontic surgery with ultrasonically energized instruments. *U. scaler.* Scaling instrument with interchangeable tips of several shapes. The tips vibrate at ultrasonic speeds under a water spray. Should not be used on patients with a heart pacemaker. *U. troughing.* Cutting dentine with ultrasonically energized tools to locate root canal entrances.

ultra-violet light ray Radiation having wavelength beyond that of the visible spectrum. Occurs naturally in sunlight or may be produced synthetically and used in sunlight treatment or to polymerize and harden certain fissure sealants or composite filling materials.

unconscious Insensible. State in which there is a lack of appreciation of sensory impulses reaching the cerebrum.

undercut 1. Design feature of a tooth preparation achieved by cutting away tooth substance from below, or occurring by chance or error. It prevents the displacement of a restoration when set. 2. An overhung area of a tooth beneath which a clasp or band may be placed for retention of a prosthesis as may be indicated by a survey line. *U. ridge.* Alveolar ridge in an edentulous mouth that has resorbed leaving an undercut below its crest, thus making denture construction and insertion difficult.

under-exposure Incomplete exposure time to X-rays of a radiographic film.

undulate To move up and down. To cause to vibrate.

unerupted Not yet erupted into the mouth.

uni- Prefix meaning one.

unicameral bone cyst *See* solitary bone cyst.

unilateral On one side only.

unilocular cyst *See* cyst.

union In orthopaedics, the successful healing of the fractured ends of a bone by their union with newly formed bone.

unit 1. Something that is single and complete in itself and from which more complex structures may be built up. 2. Standard by which measurements may be made. 3. Dental term for central equipment. *See* dental unit.

universal pliers *See* pliers.

universal scissors *See* scissors.

unloading reflex Reflex inhibition of the jaw closing muscles that occurs following the sudden reduction of forces between the jaws caused by the collapse of a food or other material to which a force was being applied by the muscles of mastication.

unslaked lime *See* lime.

upper respiratory tract The nasal cavity, nasopharynx, pharynx and larynx.

urea Organic compound derived from carbon compounds and which reduces caries attack.

urinary system Body system concerned with the elimination of waste products and the maintenance of a normal water balance via the tissue fluids. Consists of the kidneys, ureters, bladder and urethra.

urticaria Nettle rash. Inflammatory reaction of the skin and allergic reaction to various agents. May be localized or general and is characterized by redness and itching.

useful beam (or radiation) That part of the primary beam which is limited by a filter or collimator and which is effective in producing a radiographic image.

uveoparotid fever (Heerfordt's syndrome) Intermittent pyrexia accompanied by enlargement of the salivary glands, inflammation of the uveal tracts of the eye and cranial nerve involvement. Xerostomia (q.v.) may also occur.

uvula Flap or tag of muscle tissue suspended from the posterior border of the soft palate and which affects phonation.

The lesser palatine nerve runs from it through the lesser palatine foramen to join the maxillary branch of the trigeminal nerve.

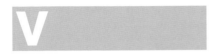
vaccinate To inoculate with a vaccine in order to produce immunity from a specific disease.

vaccination Introduction of a vaccine into the body by inoculation, to control or prevent infectious diseases by inducing an active immunity. Also known as *inoculation* or *immunization.*

vaccine Preparation which contains an antigen used to produce immunity against disease. *Component v.* is prepared using an isolated and purified component of the disease causing organism, e.g. a mixture of capsule polysaccharides from the major disease associated strains of *Streptococcus pneumoniae.* In some cases the antigen may be isolated, cloned in another organism and harvested for vaccine preparation, e.g. surface antigen from hepatitis B virus. *Conjugate v.* is prepared using, usually, a purified carbohydrate antigen attached to an unrelated protein which serves to promote an immune response, e.g. meningococcal C-conjugate vaccine. *Inactivated pathogen v.* is prepared using whole bacteria or viruses which have been killed by either heat or chemicals, usually formaldehyde, e.g. rabies, influenza and hepatitis A. *Live Attenuated v.* is prepared using live pathogen which has been weakened in some way which renders it unable to cause significant disease although it is still able to infect, e.g. BCG, MMR and oral poliomyelitis. *Toxoid v.* is prepared from toxins which have been rendered harmless by some form of chemical treatment, usually formaldehyde, but which still elicit an antigenic response in the host, e.g. tetanus. *Passive v.* is preparation of antibody produced previously in an animal which is given to a subject for immediate protection. It provides no long-term immunization, e.g. anti-tetanus antibody.

vacuole 1. Small cavity in the protoplasm of a cell. 2. Small space in tissue.

vacuum Enclosed space from which air has been removed. *V. fired porcelain. See* porcelain. *V. forming.* A method of forming flat plastic sheets into 3-dimensional shapes by the use of moulds, heat and a vacuum. *V. investing.* Investment of a waxy pattern under vacuum conditions to reduce the possibility of small air bubbles being incorporated in the investment material itself.

vagus nerve Tenth cranial nerve, having the most extensive distribution of all the cranial nerves, including the abdomen, chest, neck and head.

validity Used to describe how rigorous or sound a study, trial or experiment is and how unbiased its results are likely to be. Also used to describe how representative the results of a study are of real life, e.g. how well does the measurement being made in a laboratory represent findings in the clinical situation.

Valium® *See* diazepam.

vallate Having a rim, as in the vallate papilla of the tongue.

valve Fold in a canal or vessel that prevents the return of its contents.

valvular Relating to a valve or valves.

vancomycin A glycopeptide antibiotic sometimes used in endocarditis prophylaxis.

vaporize To change into a vapour by heating.

vaporizer Apparatus enabling a liquid to produce a vapour for inhalation.

vapour Gaseous state of a substance that is liquid or solid at ordinary temperatures but emits a vapour on heating, e.g. mercury.

varicella *See* chicken pox.

variola *See* smallpox.

varnish Solution of resin, shellac, copal, sandrac and other medicaments in a volatile solvent such as ether or alcohol. On evaporation it forms a thin protective adherent coating or film that may be a barrier against the deleterious effects of moisture, for example on glass ionomer cements. *Fluoride v.* Adherent varnish containing a high concentration (up to 23,000 ppm) of fluoride, designed for professionally applied topical use on teeth with early enamel caries to arrest and prevent caries.

vascular Pertaining to vessels or ducts containing blood or lymph. The term *vascular system* refers to all of the body blood vessels.

vasoconstriction Narrowing of the lumen of blood vessels.

vasoconstrictor Drug that causes constriction of blood vessels, especially arterioles, and is used to reduce bleeding, e.g. adrenalin 1:1000. When added in very small quantities to a local analgesic solution (e.g. adrenalin hydrochloride 1:80 000) it delays the absorption of the solution by the blood circulation and hence prolongs the effect of the analgesic.

vasodilatation Increase in the size of the lumen of a blood vessel.

vasodilator Nerve or drug that causes a blood vessel to dilate.

vegetable dye Colouring matter extracted from vegetables and used in dentistry for plaque disclosing tablets and solution, e.g. erythrocin (which is not toxic).

vegetation Abnormal deposit of fibrin and blood platelets collecting on the surface of the heart valves. Portions of this may break away and float in the bloodstream as emboli (q.v.).

vegetative 1. Concerned with growth and nutrition. 2. Resting. 3. Relating to plants.

vehicle Agent that transports drugs and may dilute or concentrate them, or increase their bulk.

vein Blood vessel with three thin coats carrying deoxygenated blood towards the heart. Larger veins may have pocket valves to prevent backflow. Lesser veins are known as *venules*. The pulmonary vein conducts oxygenated blood from the lungs to the left atrium of the heart.

veined denture base material Denture base material treated by the addition of coloured nylon threads to give an appearance of blood vessels.

vene- (veno-) Prefix denoting vein.

veneer Thin covering. In dentistry, a thin layer of tooth-shaped and tooth-coloured material, usually of composite resin or porcelain, bonded to the underlying tooth tissue to mask discoloured or malformed teeth.

venepuncture Puncturing of a vein for therapeutic purposes.

venereal disease Disease or infection communicated by sexual intercourse.

venous Describes a blood vessel carrying deoxygenated blood, e.g. a vein.

Ventolin® *See* salbutamol

ventral Relating to the abdomen.

ventricle Muscular chamber of the heart that pumps blood round the circulatory system on contraction. The right ventricle accepts blood from the right atrium via the tricuspid valve and pumps it into the pulmonary system. The left ventricle accepts blood from the left atrium via the mitral valve and pumps it into the aorta. The ventricles are composed of a specialized cardiac muscle and are lined with endocardium.

venule Small vein.

vermiform Worm-like.

vermillion border Exposed red border of the lips.

vernier Instrument used to accurately measure length.

vertebra One of a series of bones forming the vertebral column or spine. There are seven cervical (in the neck), 12 thoracic, five lumbar and five sacral vertebrae that are fused together to form the sacrum, and four coccygeal vertebrae. Each vertebra presents a body for weight bearing and a neural arch to protect the spinal cord. They are bound together by strong ligaments.

vertebral Relating to the vertebrae.

vertebral artery Artery that threads through a part of each of the first six cervical vertebrae to supply blood to the hind brain. Important to elderly persons whose carotid arteries may be considerably reduced in function. Bending the head backwards may further reduce the blood supply to the brain by compression of the vertebral arteries.

vertebrate Having a backbone or vertebral column.

vertex occlusal projection Axial true occlusal projection (q.v.) of the maxilla often used to demonstrate the buccolingual position of unerupted teeth.

vertical Perpendicular. Positioned directly above a given place or point at right angles to the horizontal plane. *V. angulation.* In radiography, the direction of the central ray in a vertical plane. *V. axis.* See axis. *V. dimension (of the face).* Measurement of the face taken by selecting two midline points above and below the mouth. A Willis facial height gauge (q.v.) may be used for this measurement. *V. overlap (v. overbite).* Overlap of the upper teeth over the lower teeth in a vertical direction when all teeth are in occlusion.

vertical subsigmoid osteotomy Osteotomy to correct mandibular prognathism by the vertical sectioning of the ramus commencing at the mandibular notch.

vertigo Dizziness or loss of balance, often accompanied by nausea.

vesicle Small blister of the skin or mucous membrane containing clear fluid.

vessel Tube or channel to carry fluid such as blood or lymph.

vestibular Relating to the space of the vestibule. *V. aspect or surface.* Surface of teeth or gingivae that face the vestibule. *V. deepening.* See vestibuloplasty. *V. surface.* See v. aspect.

vestibule Connecting passage. In dentistry, the space between the buccal and labial aspect of the teeth and gingivae, and the inner aspect of the cheeks and lips.

vestibuloplasty Surgical procedure to deepen the vestibule—often required to facilitate fitting a denture. Some techniques allow for the adjacent mucous membrane to grow together, others use skin grafts of various kinds to line the deepened area. Deepening of the vestibule may be required to facilitate the fitting of a denture.

vestige Remaining part of a structure that formerly existed in a previous stage of development.

vestigial Rudimentary.

viable Capable of living or growth.

vial *See* phial.

vibrating line Line of junction between the movable soft palate and the static tissues anterior to the soft palate.

vibrator A pulsating machine for removing air bubbles from impression and investment materials during mixing.

Vincent's angina (or disease) Deprecated term for necrotizing ulcerative gingivitis.

viral Referring to or caused by a virus.

viral hepatitis *See* hepatitis.

virology The scientific study of viruses.

virulence Degree of pathogenicity of a micro-organism.

virulent Relating to virulence. Extremely poisonous or toxic.

virus Ultramicroscopic organism with no intrinsic metabolism, comprising nucleic acid enclosed within a proteinaceous coat which has no intrinsic metabolism and which can only reproduce within a host cell. Viruses which infect bacteria are called bacteriophages. Some examples of viral diseases are the common cold, measles, poliomyelitis and parotitis (mumps).

viscid Sticky. Having a glutinous consistency.

viscous Sticky. Having a high degree of viscosity.

visible Able to be seen.

vital Necessary to life. *V. pulp*. Pulp that reacts positively to a pulp test or shown to have an intact blood supply. *V. pulpotomy*. Removal of the coronal portion of a vital tooth pulp, followed by the placement of a medicament on the remaining radicular stump, in order to retain the remaining pulp in a healthy and vital condition.

vital pulp therapy Procedures undertaken to preserve all or part of an injured dental pulp in health. See also pulp capping, pulpotomy.

vitality State of being alive and capable of responding to a stimulus.

vitality test *See* pulp test.

vitamin Naturally occurring chemical substance that is essential to health. Lack of vitamins over a period of time may cause deficiency diseases such as scurvy and rickets. The important vitamins in dentistry are *retinol (vitamin A)*, concerned with bone formation; *ergocalciferol (vitamin D)*, concerned with calcium metabolism; *ascorbic acid (vitamin C)*, concerned with healing; *thiamine (vitamin B_1)*, concerned with the breakdown of glucose, a carbohydrate; *folic acid (vitamin B_{12})*, concerned with the normal development of blood cells and the nervous system. *Vitamin K* is concerned with the clotting process of blood. Although formerly given alphabetical labels, each vitamin now has an internationally accepted name.

VMK® This abbreviation is often used to describe a porcelain fused to gold restoration. However, it is the trade mark of Vita-Zahnfabrik and stands for Vita-Metall-Keramic. The use of the abbreviation, although in common use, is deprecated.

volatile Refers to a substance that can evaporate rapidly at normal temperatures and pressures to produce vapour, e.g. ethyl chloride.

Volkmann's spoon Spoon-shaped hand instrument used as a curette, usually double ended.

Voltarol® *See* diclofenac.

volume Space occupied by matter in any state or form.

volume dose *See* integral dose.

voluntary Acting from choice, subject to the will.

vomer Bone forming part of the nasal septum.

VT Vocational training (trainee).

vulcanite Rubber to which sulphur has been added and which hardens when heated. Previously used to construct denture bases, now superseded by acrylic resins.

vulcanization Processing of rubber to form vulcanite by the application of heat under steam pressure.

vulnerable Susceptible to injury.

Ward's wax carver *See* carver.

warfarin Anticoagulant used in the treatment of thrombosis. Patients taking this drug or other anticoagulants may be liable to excessive bleeding after extractions. Trade name Marevan®.

watch spring scaler *See* scaler.

water Colourless, clear liquid, essential for life and found in all organic tissues. *Distilled w.* Purified water obtained by distillation. *W. coolant.* Water spray directed on to a tooth surface being cut by a highspeed cutting instrument, in order to reduce and prevent pulpal damage caused by friction heat.

wax Pliable substance obtained from plants and insects or synthetically produced. Has many dental applications. *Baseplate w.* A hard pink wax used in the laboratory for denture construction. *Bite w.* Bite registration material, usually in the form of thin sheets, used to register the occlusion of upper and lower teeth. *Bone w.* Wax used for filling sterile bone cavities. *Candelilla w.* Naturally occurring wax used to harden inlay casting wax obtained from the candelilla shrub. *Carnauba w.* Naturally occurring wax obtained from the Brazilian wax palm and used to harden inlay casting wax. *Carving w.* Coloured, high-melting point wax, used chiefly for instruction in tooth carving exercises. *Casting w. (inlay w.).* Mixture of waxes such as paraffin wax, beeswax, ceresin wax, carnauba wax and candelilla wax. Used for pattern making for metallic castings, such as inlays, and designed to leave no residue when burned out of investment materials. The working temperature, hardness, suppleness, expansion and contraction of casting wax are controlled by the ingredients. Blue or green in colour and obtainable in sticks, thin sheets and prefabricated shapes for clasps and bars. *Inlay wax. See* casting w. *Modelling w.* Blend of waxes, usually pink, orange or red in colour, that is pliable at room temperature. The softening temperature range varies according to its intended use. *Paraffin w.* Wax derived from crude oil and used as the major constituent in many dental waxes. *Sticky w.* Blend of waxes in the form of yellow sticks which, when heated, melt and adhere to the surface to which they are applied. Used primarily to hold components together before they are joined permanently.

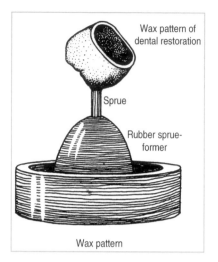

Wax pattern of dental restoration

Sprue

Rubber sprue-former

Wax pattern

Wafer w. Thin strip of wax, in which a thin metal foil is sometimes embedded, used to make interocclusal records. *W. knife.* Metal instrument used to melt, carve and convey molten wax during the construction of dentures. It has a pointed flat blade at one end and a hollowed blade at the other, separated by a wooden or plastic handle. *W. pattern.* Accurate pattern of a crown or inlay preparation made in blue or green inlay wax and used in the lost wax process during the casting of gold and other casting materials.

waxing up Use of wax by the dental technician in making trial dentures.

wear facet Characteristic polished surface of a tooth produced by moving contacts between occluding surfaces.

wedge 1. To force apart or fix firmly. 2. Wooden, plastic or metal object, thick at one end and tapered to a point, used to force apart or prevent free movement. In dentistry, a small wedge-shaped piece of wood or plastic made in various sizes and thicknesses. Used to hold a matrix band tightly against the cervical margin of a prepared cavity and also to separate teeth.

welder *See* spot welding.

welding Joining together of separate metal parts by heat and/or pressure without the use of solder. *See also* spot welding.

wetting agent Material that reduces the surface tension of a liquid thus aiding its spread over a solid surface.

Wharton's duct Submandibular salivary gland duct running from the medial aspect of the submandibular gland to open on the ridge of mucous membrane (the sublingual fold) in the floor of the mouth beneath the tip of the tongue.

wheel Disc or circular frame that revolves around a shaft or axle passing through its centre. In dentistry, an abrasive wheel mounted on a mandrel or chuck and used to reduce or polish materials.

white blood cell Leucocyte. Colourless cell that is larger than a red blood cell but fewer in number. There are numerous types, the two main ones being *granulocytes*, which have a granular cytoplasm, are formed in the bone marrow and include polymorphonuclear leucocytes, and *hyalines*, which have a clear cytoplasm and are formed in the lymphatic system. Most are capable of phagocytosis and of moving through the body tissues.

white gold casting alloy *See* semiprecious metal casting alloy.

white matter That part of the brain and spinal cord consisting of nerve fibres (axons).

white spot White area produced by acid attack from the prolonged presence of bacterial plaque which demineralizes the enamel. An early indication of dental caries.

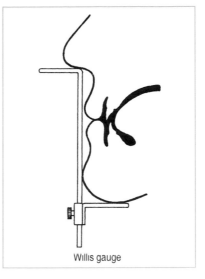

Willis gauge

Whitehead's varnish Antiseptic solution occasionally used as a dressing following some surgical procedures. It is manufactured by dissolving iodoform, green benzoin, storax and tolu balsam in ether.

whiting Finely ground white chalk used with water on a soft lathe brush to promote a high polish.

whitlow *See* paronychia.

WHO (World Health Organization) United Nations (UN) organization concerned with health on an international level.

whole (or mixed) saliva (oral fluid) Fluid present in the mouth and consisting of the combined secretions of the salivary glands, gingival fluid, cellular elements and possibly food remnants.

whooping cough (pertussis) An acute infectious disease, primarily affecting young children, caused by *Bordetella pertussis*.

William's pin Tapered plastic pin placed in prepared pin holes of an inlay or crown preparation and incorporated in a wax pattern. It burns out during the casting process.

Willis (facial height) gauge Adjustable, flat-handled metal instrument used to measure the distance between two points. May be used to decide whether the interalveolar distance is satisfactory when checking dentures, or to compare the length of incisor teeth. May also be modified to measure the length of orthodontic instruments.

window *See* exit port.

wire 1. Slender, pliable strand of metal used in surgery and dentistry. 2. To join together structures by the use of wire. *Ligature w. See* ligature. *W. brush.* Metal tube holding several strands of brass wire protruding just beyond the tube. Used to clean debris from burs and metal instruments. *W. gauge.* Metal plate perforated by holes of a known diameter through which a wire may be threaded to determine its size. *See also* archwire.

wiring Method of immobilizing bony tissues following a fracture or surgery, in order to allow them to reunite without undue disturbance. There are several types named according to their position or the technique used. *Arch w.* A bent metal bar is wired bucally to the teeth by soft stainless steel wires. *Bridle w.* A method of temporarily reducing a fracture in a dentate segment by passing a wire around teeth either side of the fracture line and twisting it clockwise. *Cheek w.* (archaic) Wires from a head halo are passed through the cheek to a splint or wires fixed to the lower teeth. *Circumferential w.* Stainless steel wires are passed from the mouth round the lower border of the body of the mandible and back into the mouth, the

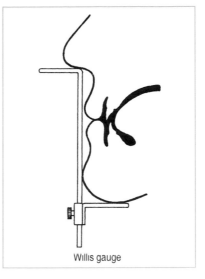

wiring

259

ends being tied over a splint or denture. *Continuous loop w.* Technique for the reduction and fixation of fractures by loop wiring the mandibular and maxillary teeth and using intermaxillary elastics. *Direct bone w.* (archaic) Used to immobilize bone fragments permanently or temporarily to allow ORIF. Holes are drilled in the bone, the fragments are repositioned and the wires passed through the holes, twisted and secured. *Inter-dental w.* The teeth are held together by passing wires round the necks of the teeth, twisting the ends together and then twisting these ends onto similar wires from the opposing teeth. *Perialveolar w.* Used in the treatment of edentulous fracture cases. A wire is passed through the maxillary alveolus, buccopalatally.

wisdom tooth *See* tooth.

Wolfe graft *See* full-thickness graft.

wood point Small, hard- or soft-wood stick, of many shapes, used to remove food debris from the inter-dental spaces and the approximal surfaces of the teeth. Some are medicated.

'wooden' jaw *See* actinomycosis.

working impression *See* final impression.

working side (ipsilateral side) Side to which a mandible moves during a lateral excursion.

working time Period of time during which a dental material can be manipulated without loss of property. Includes the mixing time (q.v.), doughing time (q.v.) for acrylics, and the manipulation time (q.v.).

wound Injury to a tissue by a cut, blow, stab or physical means.

wrought Metal that has been shaped and worked on.

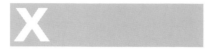

X

xantho- Prefix denoting yellow.

XCP *See* extension-cone paralleling technique.

xeno- Prefix denoting foreign, alien or different.

xenogenic graft *See* graft, xeno-.

xero- Prefix denoting dry.

xeroradiography Dry processing technique that produces paper prints of X-ray images by means of a selenium plate which records an image through the radiation-induced discharge of a positive electrostatic potential.

xerostomia Dryness of the mouth due to lack of saliva. May be due to lack of proper function of the salivary glands, blockage of the salivary ducts or the action of drugs. *See also* artificial saliva, DPF.

X-ray digitizer A computer linked to a electronic palate in order to allow the input of cephalometric orthodontic points digitally to calculate cephalometric landmarks, angles and measurements.

X-ray tracing table Illuminated table used when tracing cephalometric radiographs.

X-rays Part of the electromagnetic spectrum of radiation, having a shorter wavelength than light and more energy. When fast-moving electrons are decelerated by a solid object they produce X-rays with enough energy to produce an image on a film once they have passed through teeth, bone and soft tissue. Denser tissues stop more X-rays from passing through them than do softer tissues, hence various shades of blackness appear on the film.

Metal fillings appear white, teeth less white, and air spaces quite dark.

xylitol Bulk sweetener, with the same sweetness as sucrose. *See* sweetener.

Xylocaine® *See* lidocaine.

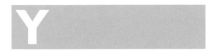

Y axis (of growth) Line joining the sella to the gnathion.

yawn Involuntary reflex action in which the mouth is opened wide and air drawn into the lungs.

yaws Contagious tropical disease caused by a spirochaete (*Treponema pertenue*), common in the West Indies, West Africa and some islands in the Pacific Ocean, which produces raspberry-like skin lesions on the face, palms of the hands and the soles of the feet.

yeast General name for fungi from various taxonomic families which are single-celled for the greater part of their lifecycle that reproduce, asexually, by budding or fission. They include *Saccharomyces cerevisiae* which is widely used commercially in the food and brewing industry and *Candida albicans* which is pathogenic.

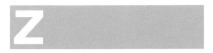

zanschonend *See* safe-for-teeth.

zero 1. Nought, nothing, nil, the figure 0. 2. Point marked zero on a graduated scale. 3. Temperature corresponding to zero.

zinc Hard bluish metal used in alloys such as brass in some dental amalgams and in galvanizing iron. Several of its salts are used in dentistry.

zinc acetate (or diacetate) Used in small quantities to accelerate the setting of zinc oxides and eugenol cements.

zinc chloride Astringent, antiseptic, styptic, caustic and obtundent. Used as an astringent with gingival retraction cord to control bleeding and temporarily displace the gingival tissues. May be used as a 40–50% solution in water and applied to desensitize a sensitive tooth area. Zinc chloride has been incorporated into toothpaste as a desensitizing agent. Has also been used diluted as a daily mouthwash. Continued use changes the composition of the saliva.

zinc free amalgam alloy *See* alloy.

zinc oxide White, amorphous, odourless and tasteless powder with mild astringent properties usually mixed with other medicaments to form creams, powders or pastes. In dentistry, widely used as a solid component in filling materials, impression materials, periodontal packs and in some polishing agents.

zinc oxide/EBA cement *See* EBA cement.

zinc oxide-eugenol cement Cement formed by mixing zinc oxide and eugenol—the principal constituent of oil of cloves. Modifiers may be added to speed up the setting reaction. Used as an obtundent, antiseptic temporary dressing in a cavity, or as a means of temporarily cementing crowns, bridges and splints into place. May also be used as a root canal filling material in combination with gutta percha.

zinc oxide–eugenol impression paste *See* impression material.

zinc phosphate cement Hard cement made of a mixture of powder containing deactivated zinc oxide and colouring matter and a solution of phosphoric acid in water. It should not be used too thin as its acidity may damage the tooth pulp. May be slaked to provide a longer working time. The synonym *zinc oxyphosphate cement* is deprecated.

zinc polycarboxylate cement (zinc polyacrylate cement) Deactivated zinc oxide powder mixed with a viscous 40% aqueous solution of polyacrylic acid to provide a non-irritant, adhesive cement. It should not be used after the cobweb stage has been reached.

zirconium oxide Finely ground powder used as a polishing agent in dentifrices.

zoster An encircling pattern as in herpes (shingles).

Zovirax® *See* aciclovir.

Z-plasty Scar incision in the form of the letter Z. The two so-formed triangles eliminate tension along the scar when sutured.

Zsigmondy charting system Charting system widely used in the United Kingdom National Health Service. Employs numerals to identify permanent teeth and alphabetical letters A–E for the deciduous teeth. *See* Appendix 3.

zygoma Malar bone. Bone forming the prominence of the cheek. The masseter muscle of mastication runs from it to be attached to the outer aspect of the ramus of the mandible.

zygomatic arch Arch of bone arising from the zygoma and passing backwards to rejoin the skull just in front of the external opening to the ear. It serves to protect the eye. The temporal muscle of mastication passes under it for attachment to the coronoid process of the mandible.

zygomatic bone One of a pair of bones forming the anterior part of the cheek bones.

Appendices

Appendix 1

Common Infectious Diseases		
	Incubation (Days)	Period of infectivity
Chicken pox	10–20	2–3 days before until 10 days after the onset of the rash
German measles	14–21	During incubation period until 2 days after resolution of symptoms
Measles	6–12	4 days before until 4 days after the rash subsides
Mumps (parotitis)	12–28	2 days before onset until symptoms are gone
Whooping cough	7–14	7 days before until 3 weeks after onset of cough

Appendix 2

Chronological Table of the Development and Eruption of the Teeth

Primary dentition

Tooth	Commences to calcify (months before birth)	Eruption (months)	Crown calcification complete (months)	Root calcification complete (months)	Resorption commences (years)
A	3–4	5–7	4	18–24	4
B	4–5	7–8	5	18–24	5
C	5	16–20	9	30–36	7
D	5	12–16	6	24–30	6
E	7–9	20–30	12	36	6

Note: 1. A=central or first incisor; B=lateral or second incisor; C=canine; D=first molar; E=second molar. 2. The lower incisors tend to erupt shortly before the upper incisors.

Permanent dentition

Tooth	Commences to calcify	Eruption (years)	Crown calcification complete (years)	Root calcification complete (years)
1	3–4 months	6–7	4–5	10
2	10–12 months	7–8	4–5	11
3	4–5 months	10–12	6–7	12–13
4	1.5–2 years	9–11	5–6	12–13
5	2–2.5 years	10–11	6–7	12–14
6	Just before birth	5–7	3	10
7	3–4 years	12–13	8	15
8	8 years	When sufficient room. Usually between 18 and 24	12–16	18–25

Note: 1. 1=central or first incisor; 2=lateral or second incisor; 3=canine; 4=first premolar; 5=second premolar; 6=first molar; 7=second molar; 8=third molar or wisdom tooth. 2. The lower incisors and canine tend to erupt 1 year earlier than the upper incisors. They also complete their calcification 1 year earlier.

Appendix 3

Tooth Notation

1. FDI two-digit system of tooth designation

Each tooth is identified by a unique two-digit combination. The first digit identifies the quadrant of the jaw, the second digit identifies the tooth within the quadrant. Quadrants are allotted the digits 1–4 for the permanent and 5–8 for the deciduous teeth in a clockwise sequence and starting at the upper right side. Teeth within the same quadrant are allotted the digits 1–8 (deciduous teeth: 1–5) from the midline backwards. The digits should be pronounced separately. Thus the permanent canines are teeth one-three, two-three, three-three, and four-three.

Permanent teeth

upper right   upper left

18	17	16	15	14	13	12	11	|	21	22	23	24	25	26	27	28
48	47	46	45	44	43	42	41	|	31	32	33	34	35	36	37	38

lower right   lower left

Primary teeth

upper right   upper left

55	54	53	52	51	|	61	62	63	64	65
85	84	83	82	81	|	71	72	73	74	75

lower right   lower left

The FDI two-digit system complies with the following basic requirements. It is—
a. simple to understand and to teach
b. easy to pronounce in conversation and dictation
c. readily communicable in print and by wire
d. easy to translate into computer 'input'
e. easily adaptable to standard charts used in general practice.

2. Zsigmondy-Palmer, 'Chevron' or set-square system

Permanent teeth

	8	7	6	5	4	3	2	1	|	1	2	3	4	5	6	7	8	
R	8	7	6	5	4	3	2	1	|	1	2	3	4	5	6	7	8	L

Deciduous teeth

	e	d	c	b	a	|	a	b	c	d	e	
R	e	d	c	b	a	|	a	b	c	d	e	L

3. European, Scandinavian or Haderup system

The mouth is viewed from the outside. The teeth in the upper jaw are identified by a + sign before or after the number, those of the lower jaw by a − sign. Deciduous teeth are identified by the figure 0 before the number, or occasionally by Roman figures.

Permanent teeth

$$R \quad \frac{8+\ 7+\ 6+\ 5+\ 4+\ 3+\ 2+\ 1+\ |\ +1\ +2\ +3\ +4\ +5\ +6\ +7\ +8}{8-\ 7-\ 6-\ 5-\ 4-\ 3-\ 2-\ 1-\ |\ -1\ -2\ -3\ -4\ -5\ -6\ -7\ -8} \quad L$$

Deciduous teeth

$$R \quad \frac{05+\ 04+\ 03+\ 02+\ 01+\ |\ +01\ +02\ +03\ +04\ +05}{05-\ 04-\ 03-\ 02-\ 01-\ |\ -01\ -02\ -03\ -04\ -05} \quad L$$

4. American system

Permanent teeth are recorded clockwise from the upper right quadrant to the lower right with figures 1–32. Capital letters are used for deciduous teeth.

Permanent teeth

$$R \quad \frac{1\quad 2\quad 3\quad 4\quad 5\quad 6\quad 7\quad 8\ |\ 9\quad 10\quad 11\quad 12\quad 13\quad 14\quad 15\quad 16}{32\quad 31\quad 30\quad 29\quad 28\quad 27\quad 26\quad 25\ |\ 24\quad 23\quad 22\quad 21\quad 20\quad 19\quad 18\quad 17} \quad L$$

Deciduous teeth

$$R \quad \frac{A\quad B\quad C\quad D\quad E\ |\ F\quad G\quad H\quad I\quad J}{T\quad S\quad R\quad Q\quad P\ |\ O\quad N\quad M\quad L\quad K} \quad L$$

Appendix 4

Average Length of Teeth (mm)							
	Central	Lateral	Canine	First premolar	Second premolar	First molar	Second molar
Upper	23	22	26.5	21	21.5	21	21
Lower	20.5	21	25	21.5	22	21	20

Appendix 5

Blood Values

BLOOD VALUES

Normal blood haemoglobin:

Males .... 15.8 g/100 ml ± 1.8 g
Females .... 13.7 g/100 ml ± 1.8 g
RBC count .... $4.5–5.5 \times 10^6/\text{mm}^3$
WBC count .... $4000–11\,000/\text{mm}^3$
Platelets .... $150\,000–400\,000/\text{mm}^3$
Bleeding time (Duke's method) .... 1–3 min
Coagulation time (Lee and White's method) .... 3–8 min

CHEMICAL BLOOD VALUES

Approximate values only:

Calcium .... 10 mg/100 ml
Cholesterol .... 200 mg/100 ml
Inorganic phosphates .... 4 mg/100 ml
Glucose .... 80 mg/100 ml

BLOOD PRESSURE

The approximate normal systolic pressure (in mmHg) is obtained by adding the patient's age to 100, e.g. patient aged 35 should have a systolic pressure of 135.

Diastolic pressure varies from about 80 mmHg in early adulthood to 90 in later years.

Appendix 6

Rules for Calculating Drug Dosage for Children

YOUNG'S RULE

$$\text{Dosage} = \frac{\text{Age} \times \text{adult dose}}{\text{Age} + 12}$$

CLARK'S RULE

$$\text{Dosage} = \frac{\text{Weight in lb} \times \text{adult dose}}{150}$$

$$\text{Dosage} = \frac{\text{Weight in kg} \times \text{adult dose}}{70}$$

Appendix 7

Length

Inches to millimetres

Inches	Millimetres	Inches	Millimetres	Inches	Millimetres
0.100	2.54	0.010	0.25	0.001	0.03
0.200	5.08	0.020	0.51	0.002	0.05
0.300	7.62	0.030	0.76	0.003	0.08
0.400	10.16	0.040	1.02	0.004	0.10
0.500	12.70	0.050	1.27	0.005	0.13
0.600	15.24	0.060	1.52	0.006	0.15
0.700	17.78	0.070	1.78	0.007	0.18
0.800	20.32	0.080	2.03	0.008	0.20
0.900	22.86	0.090	2.29	0.009	0.23

inches	$\frac{1}{64}$	$\frac{1}{32}$	$\frac{3}{64}$	$\frac{1}{16}$	$\frac{5}{64}$	$\frac{3}{32}$	$\frac{7}{64}$	$\frac{1}{8}$	$\frac{1}{4}$	$\frac{3}{8}$	$\frac{1}{2}$	$\frac{3}{4}$	1
mm	0.40	0.79	1.19	1.59	1.98	2.38	2.78	3.18	6.35	9.52	12.7	19.05	25.40

Liquid

Imperial to metric

Minim	Millilitre (ml)	Minim	Millilitre	Fluid ounce	Millilitre
½	0.03	15	1.0	1	30.0
1	0.06	20	1.2	2	60.0
2	0.12	25	1.5	4	115.0
3	0.2	30	2.0	5	140.0
4	0.25	40	2.5	6	170.0
5	0.3	45	3.0	8	230.0
6	0.4	60	4.0	10	280.0
8	0.5	90	6.0	(1 pint) 20	568.0
10	0.6	120	8.0	Gallon	Litres
12	0.8	240	15.0	1	4.546

Appendix seven

TEMPERATURE

To convert a Fahrenheit temperature to a Celsius or centigrade scale:

$$C° = \frac{F° - 32}{1.8} \quad \text{or} \quad C = (F - 32)5/9$$

To convert Celsius or centigrade to Fahrenheit:

$$F° = (C \times 1.8) + 32 \quad \text{or} \quad F = (C \times 9/5) + 32$$

Table of equivalents between Celsius (centigrade) and Fahrenheit temperature scales

Celsius	Fahrenheit	
−50	−58	
−45	−49	
−40	−40	
−35	−31	
−30	−22	
−25	−13	
−20	−4	
−15	−5	
−10	14	
−5	23	
0	32	(Freezing point of water)
1	33.8	
2	35.6	
3	37.4	
4	34.2	
5	41.0	
6	42.8	
7	44.6	
8	46.4	
9	48.2	
10	50.0	
11	51.8	
12	53.6	
13	55.4	
14	57.2	
15	59.0	
16	60.8	(Comfortable room temperature)
17	62.6	

Celsius	Fahrenheit	
18	64.4	
19	66.2	
20	68.0	
21	69.8	
22	71.6	
23	73.4	
24	75.2	
25	77.0	
26	78.8	
27	80.6	
28	82.4	
29	84.0	
30	86.0	
31	87.8	
32	89.6	
33	91.4	
34	93.2	
35	95.0	(? Human survival limit)
36	96.8	
37	98.6	(Normal body temperature)
38	100.4	
39	102.2	
40	104	
41	105.8	(Abnormal body temperature due to disease)
42	107.6	
43	109.4	
44	111.2	(Heat stroke)
45	113	
46	114.8	

Celsius	Fahrenheit	
47	116.6	
48	118.4	(Scalding hot)
49	120.2	
50	122	
60	140	
70	158	
80	176	
90	194	
100	212	

Weights: Apothecaries' To Metric

Grain	Milligram	Grain	Milligram	Grain	Gram
1/1000	0.06	1/4	15.0	20	1.0
1/200	0.3	1/3	20.0	30	2.0
1/150	0.4	1/2	30.0	45	3.0
1/100	0.6	3/4	50.0	60	4.0
1/64	1.0	1	60.0	90	6.0
1/50	1.2		Gram	120	8.0
1/40	1.5	1 1/2	0.1	150	10.0
1/32	2.0	2	0.12	180	12.0
1/25	2.5	3	0.2		
1/20	3.0	4	0.25	Ounce (avoir.)	Gram
1/16	4.0	5	0.3	1/2	15.0
1/12	5.0	6	0.4	1	30.0
1/10	6.0	8	0.5		(or nearer, 28.3)
1/8	8.0	10	0.6		
1/6	10.0	12	0.8	Pound (avoir.)	
1/5	12.0	15	1.0	1	453.59

Appendix 8

Dental Rotary Instruments

In the past the numbering of these instruments has varied according to their country of manufacture. The International Organization for Standardization (ISO), of which the British Dental Institution is a member, has agreed a universal system for designating the head size (diameter) by a figure indicating its nominal size in 10 mm. The standard specifies a range of shapes as well as of sizes.

Shapes of dental burs

	Round	Wheel	Inverted cone	Straight fissure	Straight fissure (long head)	Tapered fissure	Tapered fissure (long head)	End cutting	Pear	Pear (long head)	Domed fissure	Domed fissure (long head)
Steel	√	√	√	√	√	√	√	√				
Tungsten	√		√	√	√	√	√	√	√	√	√	√

Dimensions and ISO numbering with traditional UK, European and US number series

Diameter* mm ± 0.04	ISO numbers	UK	European	US			
				Round	Inverted cone	Fissure	Tapered fissure
0.50	005	¼	4/0	–			
0.60	006	½	3/0	½	33½		
0.70	007	–	2/0	–			
0.80	008	1	0	1	34	556	699
0.90	009	–	1	–	–	–	–
1.00	010	2	2	2	35	557	700
1.20	012	3	3	3	36	558	701
1.40	014	4	4	4	37	559	–
1.60	016	5	5	5	38	560	702
1.80	018	6	6	6	39	561	–
2.10	021	7	7	7	40	562	703
2.30	023	8	8	8	–	563	–
2.50	025	9	9	9			
2.70	027	10	10	–			
2.90	029	11	11	–			
3.10	031	12	12	11			

*This diameter refers to the maximum diameter of the head.
Note: Some shapes will not be available over the entire range of sizes.

Appendix 9

Name of gas	Symbol	Colour of cylinder body	Colour of valve end where different from body
Oxygen	O_2	Black	White
Nitrous oxide	N_2O	Blue	–
Cyclopropane	C_3H_6	Orange	–
Carbon dioxide	CO_2	Grey	–
Ethylene	C_2H_4	Violet	–
Nitrogen	N_2	Grey	Black
Oxygen and carbon dioxide mixture	$O_2 + CO_2$	Black	White and Grey
Oxygen and helium mixture	$O_2 + He$	Black	White and Brown
Oxygen and nitrous mixture	$O_2 + N_2O$	Blue	Blue and Black
Air (medical)	AIR	Grey	White and Black

Note: British Standard 1319 : 1976; Medical gas cylinders, valves and yoke connections. The colours used for gas cylinders comply with specifications in British Standards 4800 and 5252.

Appendix 10

Radiographic Technique and Anatomy

The following diagrams are reproduced, with permission, from,
BROWNE R.M., EDMONDSON H.D.
AND ROUT, P.G.J. (1983)
A Radiological Atlas of Diseases of the Teeth and Jaws,
Chichester: John Wiley

		ANGSTROM UNITS
Cosmic Rays	0.0001 Å	
Gamma Rays	0.001 Å	
X-Rays	0.1–10.0 Å	
Ultra Violet Light	100 Å	
Visible Light	5000 Å	
Infra Red	50,000 Å	
		METERS
Microwaves & Radar	0.01 M	
Television	1.0 M	
Radio	10 M–100 M	

A diagram illustrating the relative position of X-rays in the electromagnetic spectrum.

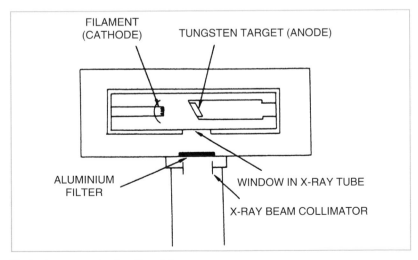

The basic components of an X-ray tube.

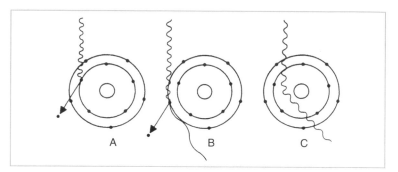

The interaction of X-rays with matter: A. Photoelectric absorption; B. Compton scatter; C. Thompson effect.

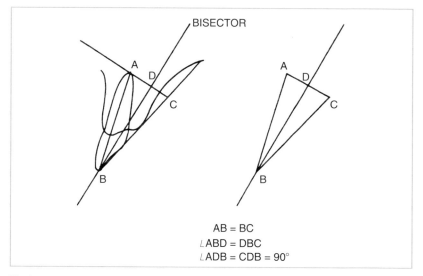

The bisecting angle technique for taking intra-oral radiographs.

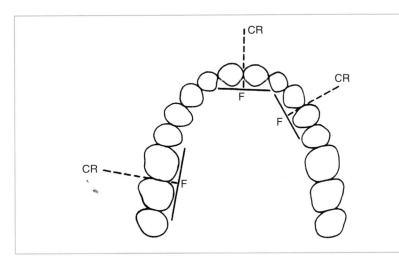

The alignment of the X-ray beam relative to the teeth in intra-oral radiographs: CR, centre ray of the X-ray beam; F, film.

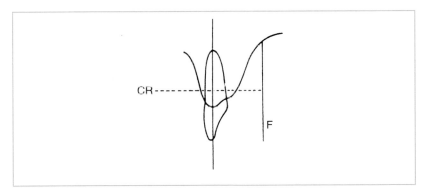

The paralleling technique for taking intra-oral radiographs: CR, centre ray of the X-ray beam; F, film.

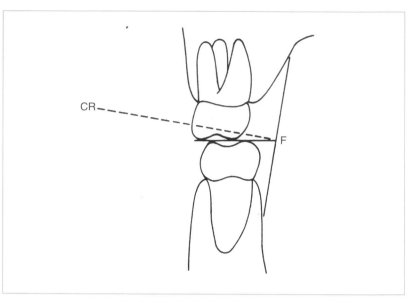

The bitewing technique in which the film (F) is held in place by occluding on a tab; CR, centre ray of the X-ray beam.

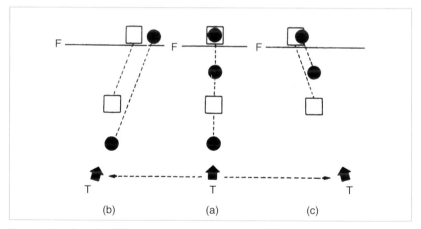

The principle of parallax. When two objects are superimposed (a) it is not possible to be certain if the reference object (open square) is nearer or further from the film (F) than the object of interest (full circle). If the object of interest is closer to the tube (T) it moves in the opposite direction (b) relative to the reference object, whereas if it is further away, it moves in the same direction (c).

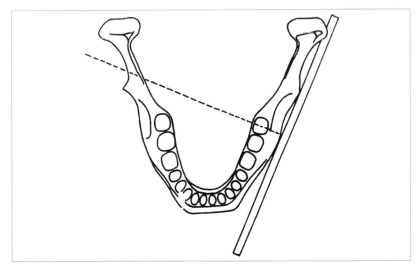

The Potter–Bucky grid. Scattered rays emerging from the object (O) are absorbed by the grid (G) and thus prevented from reaching the film (F). Only undeviated rays reach the film. CR, centre ray of X-ray beam.

Oblique lateral mandible view.

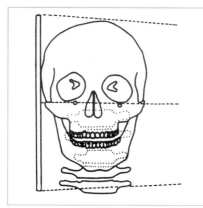

Lateral skull view.

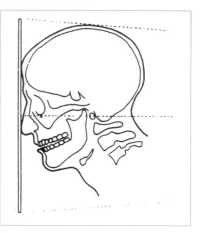

Postero-anterior view.

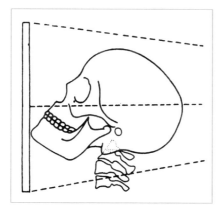

Occipito-mental view.

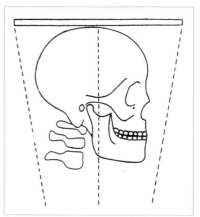

Submento-vertex (base) view.

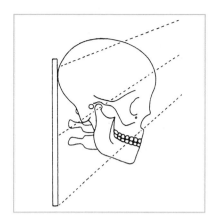

30° Fronto-occipital (Towne's) view.

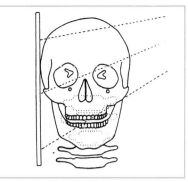

Transcranial view of the temporo-mandibular joint.

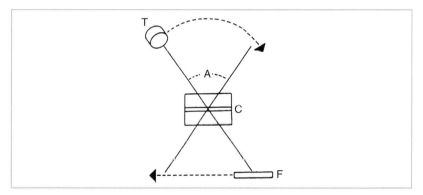

The principle of tomography. The X-ray tube (T) and film (F) rotate in opposite directions around a fixed plane (C), which remains in focus. The thickness of the plane visualized is determined by the angle of travel (A) of the tube.

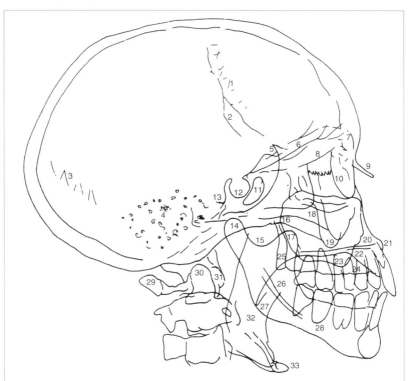

Lateral skull (L):

1 coronal suture	14 head of mandibular	24 alveolar ridge of
2 meningeal grooves	condyle	maxilla
3 lambdoid suture	15 sigmoid notch	25 pterygoid plates
4 mastoid air cells	16 posterior wall of	26 inferior alveolar
5 anterior wall of	maxillary antrum	canal
middle cranial fossa	17 coronoid process of	27 angle of mandible
6 floor of anterior	mandible	28 body of mandible
cranial fossa	18 body of zygoma	29 posterior arch of
7 frontal sinus	19 zygomatic process of	atlas vertebra
8 cribriform plate	maxilla	30 odontoid process of
9 nasal bones	20 anterior wall of	axis vertebra
10 anterior border of	maxillary antrum	31 anterior arch of atlas
lateral wall of orbit	21 anterior nasal spine	vertebra
11 sphenoidal sinus	22 hard palate	32 pharyngeal air space
12 pituitary fossa (sella	23 floor of maxillary	33 hyoid bone
turcica)	antrum	
13 clivus		

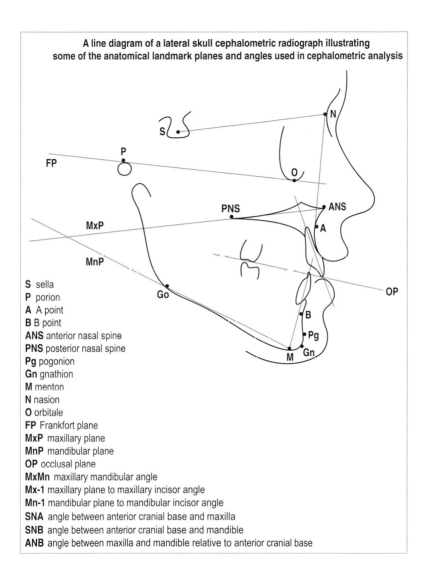

A line diagram of a lateral skull cephalometric radiograph illustrating some of the anatomical landmark planes and angles used in cephalometric analysis

S sella
P porion
A A point
B B point
ANS anterior nasal spine
PNS posterior nasal spine
Pg pogonion
Gn gnathion
M menton
N nasion
O orbitale
FP Frankfort plane
MxP maxillary plane
MnP mandibular plane
OP occlusal plane
MxMn maxillary mandibular angle
Mx-1 maxillary plane to maxillary incisor angle
Mn-1 mandibular plane to mandibular incisor angle
SNA angle between anterior cranial base and maxilla
SNB angle between anterior cranial base and mandible
ANB angle between maxilla and mandible relative to anterior cranial base

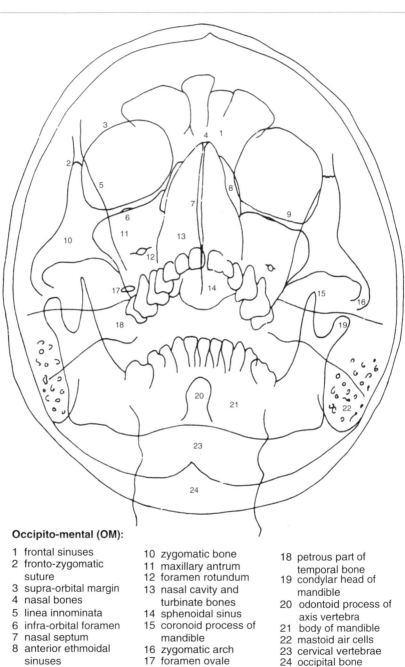

Occipito-mental (OM):

1 frontal sinuses
2 fronto-zygomatic
   suture
3 supra-orbital margin
4 nasal bones
5 linea innominata
6 infra-orbital foramen
7 nasal septum
8 anterior ethmoidal
   sinuses
9 infra-orbital margin

10 zygomatic bone
11 maxillary antrum
12 foramen rotundum
13 nasal cavity and
   turbinate bones
14 sphenoidal sinus
15 coronoid process of
   mandible
16 zygomatic arch
17 foramen ovale

18 petrous part of
   temporal bone
19 condylar head of
   mandible
20 odontoid process of
   axis vertebra
21 body of mandible
22 mastoid air cells
23 cervical vertebrae
24 occipital bone

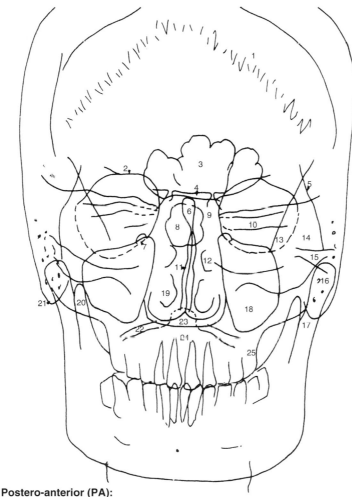

Postero-anterior (PA):

1 lambdoid suture
2 supra-orbital margin
3 frontal sinuses
4 dorsum sellae
5 zygomatic process of frontal bone
6 crista galli
7 foramen rotundum
8 sphenoidal sinus
9 ethmoidal sinuses
10 internal auditory canal
11 nasal septum

12 middle turbinate bone
13 linea innominata
14 frontal process of zygomatic bone
15 external auditory canal
16 head of mandibular condyle
17 neck of mandibular condyle
18 maxillary antrum

19 inferior turbinate bone
20 coronoid process of mandible
21 mastoid process
22 intervertebral space between atlas and axis vertebrae
23 odontoid process of axis vertebra
24 hard palate
25 alveolar process of maxilla

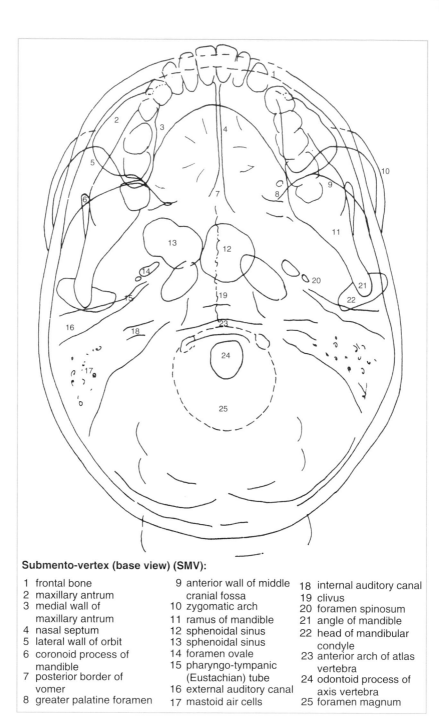

Submento-vertex (base view) (SMV):

1 frontal bone
2 maxillary antrum
3 medial wall of
  maxillary antrum
4 nasal septum
5 lateral wall of orbit
6 coronoid process of
  mandible
7 posterior border of
  vomer
8 greater palatine foramen

9 anterior wall of middle
  cranial fossa
10 zygomatic arch
11 ramus of mandible
12 sphenoidal sinus
13 sphenoidal sinus
14 foramen ovale
15 pharyngo-tympanic
  (Eustachian) tube
16 external auditory canal
17 mastoid air cells

18 internal auditory canal
19 clivus
20 foramen spinosum
21 angle of mandible
22 head of mandibular
  condyle
23 anterior arch of atlas
  vertebra
24 odontoid process of
  axis vertebra
25 foramen magnum

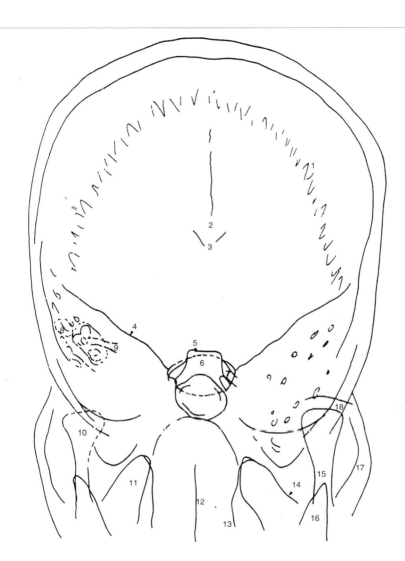

Fronto-occipital (Towne's view) (T):

1 lambdoid suture
2 internal occipital crest
3 occiput
4 petrous ridge of temporal bone
5 posterior clinoid process
6 dorsum sellae
7 foramen magnum
8 mastoid air cells
9 internal auditory canal
10 head of mandibular condyle
11 maxillary antrum
12 nasal septum
13 medial wall of maxillary antrum
14 roof and wall of maxillary antrum
15 neck of mandibular condyle
16 coronoid process of mandible
17 zygomatic arch
18 temporomandibular joint space

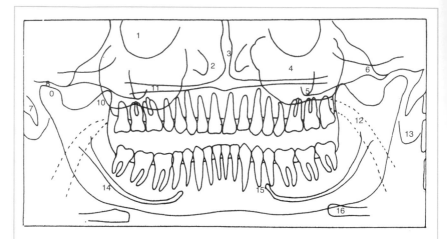

Panoramic radiograph (PR) of the jaws of an adult:

1 orbital cavity
2 nasal cavity and turbinates
3 nasal septum
4 maxillary antrum
5 root of zygoma
6 zygomatic arch
7 styloid process
8 glenoid fossa
9 head of mandibular condyle
10 coronoid process of mandible
11 hard palate
12 pharyngeal air space
13 pinna of ear
14 inferior alveolar canal
15 mental foramen
16 hyoid bone

Appendix 11

Wire Gauges

British Imperial or English Legal Standard Wire Gauge (SWG)

		Diameter	
Nearest fractional inch	Size on wire gauge	Decimal of an inch	Millimetres
$\frac{1}{2}$	7.0	0.500	12.7
$\frac{15}{32}$	6/0	0.464	11.8
$\frac{7}{16}$	5/0	0.432	11.0
$\frac{13}{32}$	4/0	0.400	10.2
$\frac{3}{8}$	3/0	0.372	9.4
$\frac{11}{32}$	2/0	0.348	8.8
	1/0	0.324	8.2
	1	0.300	7.6
	2	0.276	7.0
$\frac{1}{4}$	3	0.252	6.4
	4	0.232	5.9
	5	0.212	5.4
$\frac{3}{16}$	6	0.192	4.9
	7	0.176	4.5
	8	0.160	4.1
	9	0.144	3.7
$\frac{1}{8}$	10	0.128	3.3
	11	0.116	3.0
	12	0.104	2.6
$\frac{3}{32}$	13	0.092	2.3
	14	0.080	2.0
	15	0.072	1.8
$\frac{1}{16}$	16	0.064	1.6
	17	0.056	1.4

Nearest fractional inch	Size on wire gauge	Decimal of an inch	Millimetres
$\frac{3}{64}$	18	0.048	1.2
	19	0.040	1.0
	20	0.036	0.9
$\frac{1}{32}$	21	0.032	0.8
	22	0.028	0.7
	23	0.024	0.6
$\frac{3}{128}$	24	0.022	0.55
	25	0.020	0.5
	26	0.018	0.45
	27	0.0164	0.4
$\frac{1}{64}$	28	0.0148	0.37
	29	0.0136	0.35
	30	0.0124	0.3

Note: Hypodermic and dental needles are labelled with the SWG number, orthodontic wire with the diameter size in millimetres.